Textbook of Computer Application in Pharmaceutical Science and Management

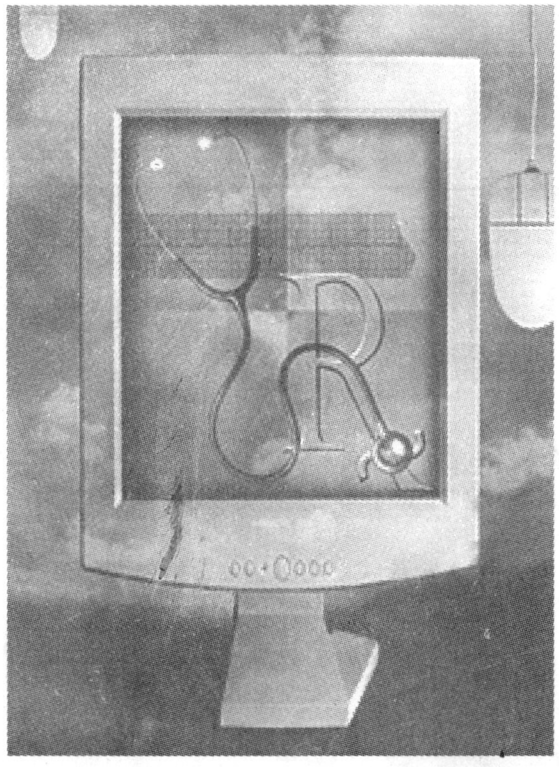

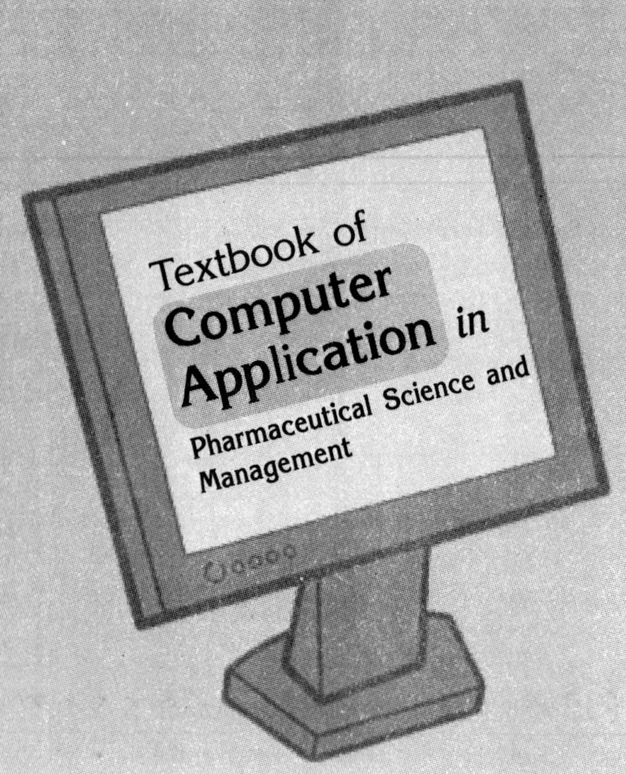
Textbook of
Computer
Application in
Pharmaceutical Science and
Management

Textbook of Computer Application in Pharmaceutical Science and Management

YS Tanwar M Pharm, PhD
Professor and Head
Department of Pharmaceutics
Bhupal Nobles' College of Pharmacy
Udaipur, Rajasthan

Nisha Tanwar MCA, MSc, M Phil
Lecturer and Head
Department of Computer Studies
Bhupal Nobles' Postgraduate College
Udaipur, Rajasthan

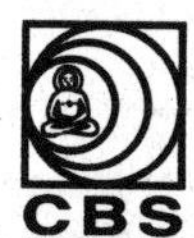

CBS Publishers & Distributors Pvt. Ltd.
New Delhi • Bengaluru • Chennai • Kochi • Kolkata • Mumbai
Hyderabad • Nagpur • Patna • Pune • Vijayawada

Textbook of Computer Application
in
Pharmaceutical Science and Management

ISBN: 978-81-239-1860-0

First Edition: 2010
Reprint: 2017, 2019

Published by **Satish Kumar Jain** and produced by **Varun Jain** for
CBS Publishers & Distributors Pvt. Ltd.,
4819/XI Prahlad Street, 24 Ansari Road, Daryaganj, New Delhi - 110002
delhi@cbspd.com, cbspubs@airtelmail.in • www.cbspd.com
Ph.: 23289259, 23266861, 23266867 • Fax: 011-23243014

Corporate Office: 204 FIE, Industrial Area, Patparganj, Delhi - 110 092
Ph: 49344934 • Fax: 011-49344935
E-mail: publishing@cbspd.com • publicity@cbspd.com

Branches:

- ***Bengaluru:*** 2975, 17th Cross, K.R. Road, Bansankari 2nd Stage, Bengaluru - 70 • Ph: +91-80-26771678/79 • Fax: +91-80-26771680 E-mail: cbsbng@gmail.com, bangalore@cbspd.com
- ***Chennai:*** No. 7, Subbaraya Street, Shenoy Nagar, Chennai - 600030 Ph: +91-44-26681266, 26680620 • Fax: +91-44-42032115 E-mail: chennai@cbspd.com
- ***Kochi:*** Ashana House, 39/1904, A.M. Thomas Road, Valanjambalam, Ernakulum, Kochi • Ph: +91-484-4059061-65 Fax: +91-484-4059065 • E-mail: cochin@cbspd.com
- ***Kolkata:*** 6-B, Ground Floor, Rameshwar Shaw Road, Kolkata - 700014 Ph: +91-33-22891126/7/8 • E-mail: kolkata@cbspd.com
- ***Mumbai:*** 83-C, Dr. E. Moses Road, Worli, Mumbai - 400018 Ph: +91-9833017933, 022-24902340/41 • E-mail: mumbai@cbspd.com

Representatives:

- Hyderabad: 0-9885175004
- Patna: 0-9334159340
- Jharkhand: 0-9811541605
- Nagpur: 0-9021734563
- Pune: 0-9623451994
- Uttarakhand: 0-9716462459

Printed at: J.S. Offset Printers, Delhi (India)

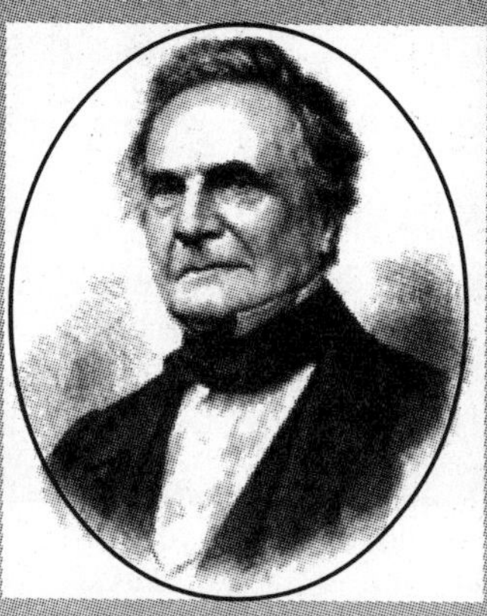

Sir Charles Babbage (1791-1871)
Father of Computers

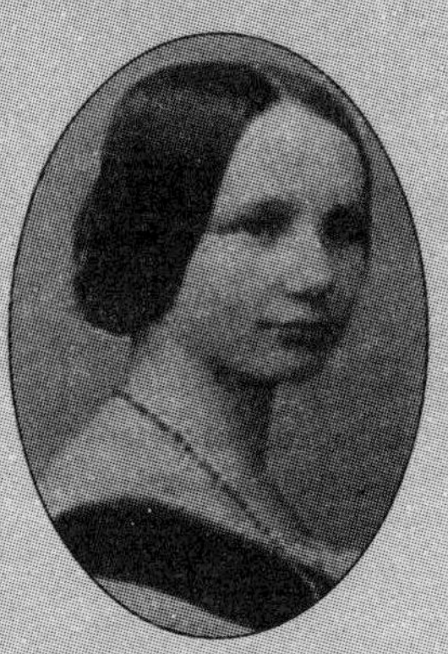

Lady Ada Lovelace (1815-1852)
First Computer Programmer

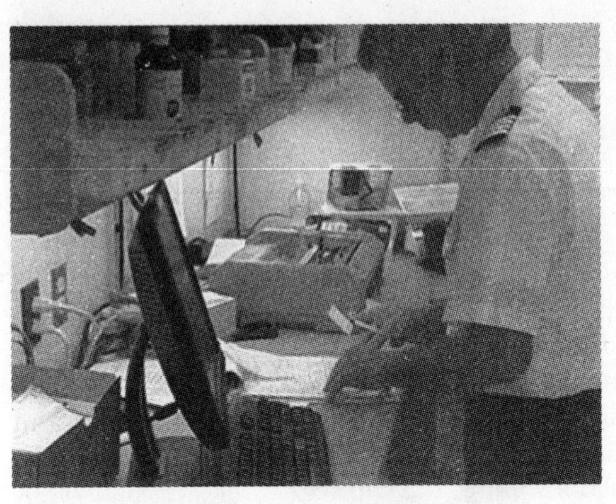

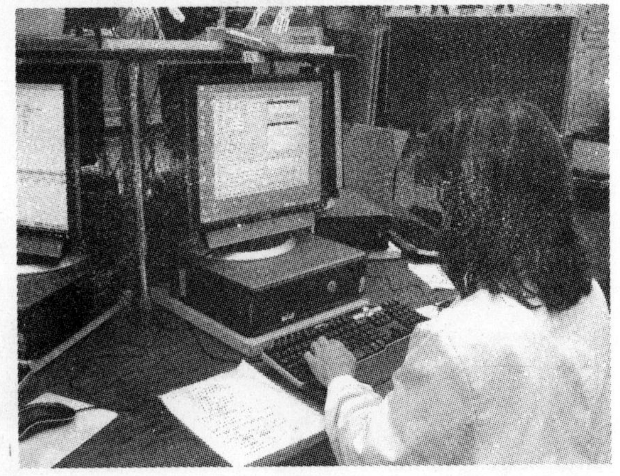

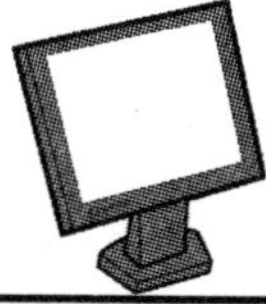

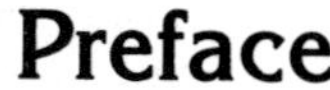

Preface

Computer application and information technology has been introduced in almost all the courses. Teachers and students felt a need for a textbook on computer application in pharmaceutical sciences and management. Teaching and research work in computer science during the last 25 years has provided enough insight in the subject.

The major objective of this edition is to serve as a textbook for graduate and postgraduate students in pharmaceutical sciences and management. All the chapters are brief, clear and concise to provide students an understandable text and recent developments in the field.

We hope the students, teachers and the professionals will like this book for their courses, and would also suggest measures to make improvements in its future editions. We will be extremely pleased if our efforts result in an improved book which could serve as a teaching and reference source in computer application.

YS Tanwar
Nisha Tanwar

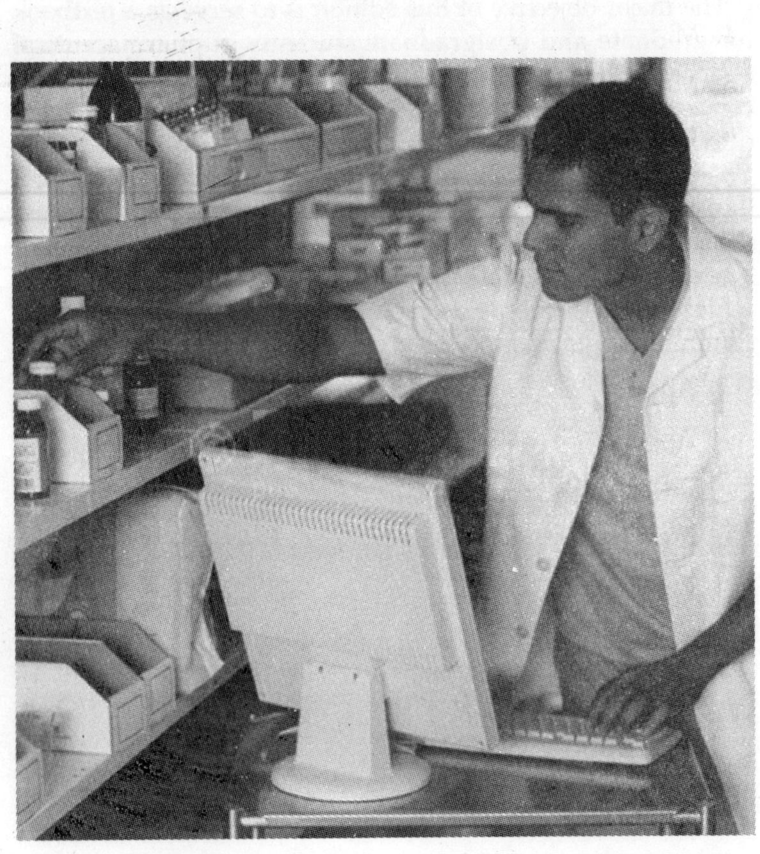

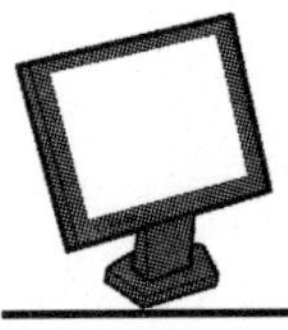

Contents

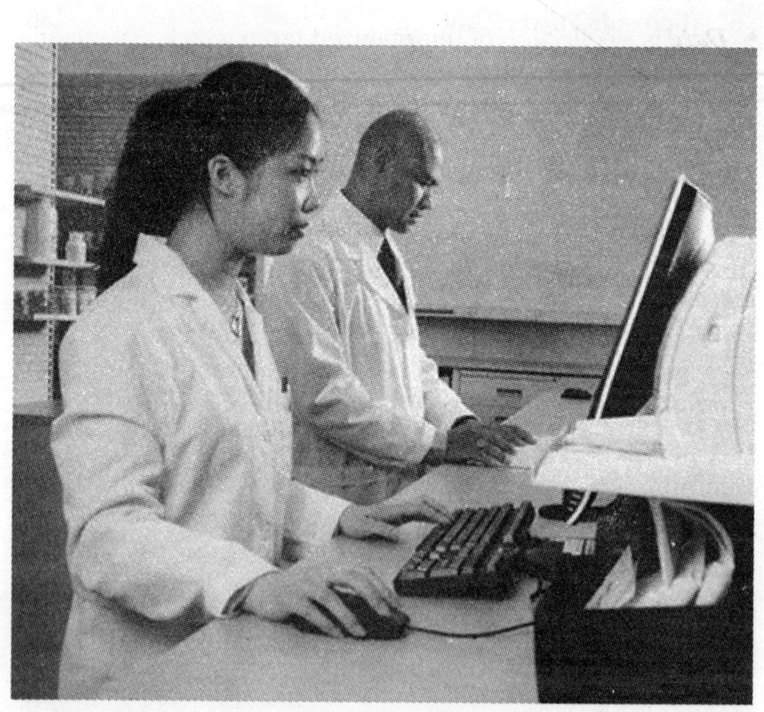

Introduction to Computers

WHAT IS A COMPUTER?

The word "computer" comes from the word "compute", which means to calculate. A computer is defined as an electronic device that can perform a variety of operations according to a set of instructions called ***program***. A computer is an electronic machine, operating under the control of instructions stored in its memory, that can accept data (input), manipulate the data according to specified rules (process), produce results (output), and store the results for future use.

- ***Data*** is a collection of unorganized facts, which can include words, numbers, images and sounds. Computers manipulate and process data to create information.
- ***Information*** is data that is organized has meaning and is useful.
- Data entered into a computer is called ***input***. The processed results are called ***output***. Thus a computer processes input to create output. A computer also can hold data and information for future use in an area called ***storage***. This cycle of input, process, output and storage is called the ***information processing cycle***.
- A person that communicates with a computer or uses the information it generates is called user.
- The electric, electronic and mechanical equipment that makes up a computer is called ***hardware***. ***Software*** is the series of instructions that tells the hardware how to perform tasks. Hardware needs the instructions provided by software to process data into information.

Characteristics of a Computer

A computer's power is derived from its capability of performing the information processing cycle with amazing speed, reliability and accuracy; its capacity to store huge amounts of data and information; and its ability to communicate with other computers.

1. ***Speed:*** Inside the system unit, operations occur through electronic circuits. When data, instructions and information flow along these circuits, they travel at close to the speed of light. This allows billions of operations to be carried out in a single second. Today, the computers are able to calculate in pico second (10^{-12} second). A powerful computer is capable of performing 3 to 4 million simple arithmetic operations per second.
2. ***Accuracy:*** The accuracy of a computer is consistently high and generates error-free results. Computers can perform all calculations and comparisons accurately, provided the hardware does not malfunction.
3. ***Reliability:*** The electronic components in modern computers are dependable as they have low failure rate. The high reliability of the components enables the computer to produce consistent results.
4. ***Storage:*** Computer has the capability to store the data on a vast scale in its memory. The capacity of memory is measured in terms of byte. For storage of data, devices like magnetic tapes, floppies, disks, etc. are used. Bubble memories can store 6,250,000 bits per square centimeter of space.
5. ***Versatility:*** Computers can perform repetitive jobs efficiently. Computers are capable of performing logical operations. They can perform the job given to them without any break for long duration. They even can work in areas where human brain can err. They can work with different types of data and information like graphics, audio, visual, characters, etc.
6. ***Communications:*** Today most computers have the capability of communicating with other computers. When two or more computers are connected together via communications media and devices, they comprise a network.

7. ***Automation:*** It is one of the most important characteristics of the computer. Once command is given to the computer, it can perform the job without the need of human intervention until the completion of the job.
8. ***Diligence:*** Unlike human beings, a computer is free from monotony, tiredness, lack of concentration, etc. and hence can work for hours together without creating any error and without grumbling.

Limitations of Computers

1. ***Lack of decision-making:*** Computers cannot decide on their own. Only the user can determine what task a computer will perform. Computers cannot make judgments on their own.
2. ***No IQ:*** Computers are dumb machines with zero IQ. They need to be told each and every step.
3. ***No heuristics:*** Heuristics refers broadly to learning from past experiences. Computer cannot learn from past experience but human beings learn from past experience very well.

THE EVOLUTION OF COMPUTERS

The earliest device that qualifies as a digital computer is the ***abacus***. The abacus was an early aid for mathematical computations. Its only value is that it aids the memory of the human performing the calculation. A skilled abacus operator can work on addition and subtraction problems at the speed of a person equipped with a hand calculator (multiplication and division are slower). The abacus is often wrongly attributed to China. In fact, the oldest surviving abacus was used in 300 B.C. by the Babylonians. The abacus is still in use today, principally in the far east. A modern abacus consists of rings that slide over rods, but the older one pictured below dates from the time when pebbles were used for counting. In 1617 Scotsman named John Napier invented *logarithms,* which are a technology that allows multiplication to be performed via addition. The magic ingredient is the logarithm of each operand, which was originally obtained from a printed table.

But Napier also invented an alternative to tables, where the logarithm values were carved on ivory sticks which are now called ***Napier's Bones***. Its upgrade versions were in use even around 1890. In 1642 Blaise Pascal, at age 19, invented the ***Pascaline*** as an aid for his father who was a tax collector. Later, in the year 1671, Baron Gottfried Wilhelm von Leibniz of Germany invented the first *calculator* for multiplication. In ***1801***, ***Joseph-Marie Jacquard*** developed a ***loom*** in which the pattern being woven was controlled by ***punched cards***. The series of cards could be changed without changing the mechanical design of the loom. This was a landmark point in programmability. Herman Hollerith invented a ***tabulating machine*** using ***punched cards*** in the 1880s. In 1833, ***Charles Babbage*** moved on from developing his ***difference engine*** to developing a more complete design, the *analytical engine*, which would draw directly on Jacquard's punched cards for its programming. In ***1835 Charles Babbage*** described his ***analytical engine***. It was the plan of a general-purpose programmable computer, employing punch cards for input and a steam engine for power. One crucial invention was to use gears for the function served by the beads of an abacus. In a real sense, computers all contain automatic abacuses (technically called the *arithmetic logic unit* or *floating-point unit*). His initial idea was to use punch-cards to control a machine that could calculate and print logarithmic tables with huge precision (a specific purpose machine). Babbage's idea soon developed into a general-purpose programmable computer, his analytical engine. While his design was sound and the plans were probably correct, or at least ***debuggable***, the project was slowed by various problems. All the parts for his machine had to be made by hand. Small errors in each item can sometimes sum up to large discrepancies in a machine with thousands of parts, which required these parts to be much better than the usual tolerances needed at the time. However, his efforts estabilished a number of principles, which have been shown to be fundamental to the design of any digital computer. Therefore *Charles Babbage* is considered to be the father of modern digital computers. The features of some of the well-known early computers are given in Table 1.1.

Table1.1: Features of some of the well-known early computers

Name of computer	*Inventor*	*Features*
The Mark I Computer (1937–44)	Howard A. Aiken of Harvard University in collaboration with IBM corporation.	• Used over 3000 electrically operated switches to control operations. • 50 feet long and 8 feet high. • Both mechanical and electronic components were used in its design. • Capable of performing 5 basic operations—addition, subtraction, multiplication, division and table reference. • A number as big as 23 decimal digits could be used. • It took about 0.3 seconds to add two numbers and 4.5 seconds for multiplication of two numbers.
The Atanasoff-Berry Computer (ABC) (1939–42)	Dr. John Atanasoff and his assistant Clifford Berry.	• Used 45 vacuum tubes for internal logic and capacitors for storage. • Solved certain mathematical equations.
The Electronic Numerical Integrator and Calculator (ENIC) (1943–46)	Prof. J. Presper and John Mauchly, Moore School of Engineering, University of Pennsylvania, USA.	• Developed as a result of military need. • It took up the wall space in a 20 x 40 sq. feet room and used 18000 vacuum tubes.

Contd..

Contd..

		• Addition of two numbers was achieved in 200 microseconds and multiplication in 2000 microseconds.
The Electronic Discrete Variable Automatic Computer (EDVAC)(1946–52)	Dr. John Von Neumann	• Designed on stored program concept. • Stored data and instructions in the binary form instead of decimal numbers.
The Electronic Delay Storage Automatic Calculator (EDSAC) (1947–49)	Group of Scientists headed by Prof. Maurice Wilkes, Cambridge University Mathematical Laboratory, U.K.	• Addition was done in 1500 microseconds and multiplication operation in 4000 microseconds. • Machine executed its first program in May 1949.
Manchester Mark (1948)	Group of Scientists headed by Prof. M.H.A. Newman	• Small experimental machine based on stored program concept. • Storage capacity of only 32 words, each of 31 binary digits.
The Universal Automatic Computer (UNIVAC) (1951)	Eckert and Mauchley	• First digital computer. • Used for business and scientific applications.

THE COMPUTER GENERATIONS

Originally the term generation was used to distinguish between varying hardware technologies. But nowadays it has been extended to include both the hardware and the software, which together make up an entire computer system.

1. ***First generation computers (1940–56):*** The first generation of computers used ***vacuum tubes*** for circuitry and *magnetic drums* for *memory*, and were often enormous, taking up entire rooms. They were very expensive to operate and in addition to using a great deal of electricity, generated a lot of heat, which was often the cause of malfunctions. First generation computers relied on *machine language* to perform operations, and they could only solve one problem at a time. Input was based on punched cards and paper tape, and output was displayed on printouts. The UNIVAC and *ENIAC* computers are examples of first generation computing devices. The UNIVAC was the first commercial computer delivered to a business client, the U.S. Census Bureau in 1951.

2. ***Second generation computers (1956–63): Transistors*** replaced vacuum tubes and ushered in the second generation of computers. The transistor was invented in 1947 but did not see widespread use in computers until the late 50s. The transistor was far superior to the vacuum tube, allowing computers to become smaller, faster, cheaper, more energy-efficient and more reliable than their first generation predecessors. Though the transistor still generated a great deal of heat that subjected the computer to damage, it was a vast improvement over the vacuum tube. Second generation computers still relied on punched cards for input and printouts for output.

Second generation computers moved from cryptic *binary* machine language to symbolic, or *assembly*, languages, which allowed programmers to specify instructions in words. *High-level programming languages* were also being developed at this time, such as early versions of ***COBOL*** and ***FORTRAN***. These were also the first computers that stored their instructions in their memory, which moved from a magnetic drum to magnetic core technology.

3. ***Third generation computers (1963–71):*** The development of the ***integrated circuit*** was the hallmark of the third generation of computers. Transistors were miniaturized and placed on ***silicon chips***, called ***semiconductors***, which drastically increased the speed and efficiency of computers. Instead of punched cards and printouts, users interacted with third generation computers through ***keyboards*** and ***monitors*** and ***interfaced*** with an ***operating system***, which allowed the device to run many different *applications* at one time with a central program that monitored the memory. Computers for the first time became accessible to a mass audience because they were smaller and cheaper than their predecessors.

4. ***Fourth generation computers (1971 onwards):*** The ***microprocessor*** brought the fourth generation of computers, as thousands of integrated circuits were built onto a single silicon chip. The Intel 4004 chip, developed in 1971, located all the components of the computer from the *central processing unit* and memory to input/output controls on a single chip. The microprocessor was a large-scale integrated circuit, which contained thousands of transistors. The transistors on this one chip were capable of performing all of the functions of a computer's central processing unit. The reduced size, reduced cost, and increased speed of the microprocessor led to the creation of the first personal computers. In 1976, Steve Jobs and Steve Wozniak built the first Apple computer in a garage in California. In 1981 IBM introduced its first computer for the home user, and in 1984 Apple introduced the Macintosh. Microprocessors also moved out of the realm of desktop computers and into many areas of life as more and more everyday products began to use microprocessors. As these small computers became more powerful, they could be linked together to form networks, which eventually led to the development of the Internet. Fourth generation computers also saw the development of *GUIs*, the *mouse* and *handheld* devices.

5. ***Fifth generation computers:*** Fifth generation computing devices, based on ***artificial intelligence***, are still in development, though there are some applications, such as *voice recognition,* that are being used today. The use of *parallel processing* and superconductors is helping to make artificial intelligence a reality. ***Quantum computation*** and molecular and *nanotechnology* will radically change the face of computers in years to come. The goal of fifth generation computing is to develop devices that respond to natural *language* input and are capable of learning and self-organization.

COMPUTER SYSTEM

A computer system is the combination of *hardware* and *software.* The simplest computer classifies as a computer system because at least two components (hardware and software) work together coherently, and these can connect into larger applications. In industry, the interconnection of ***variable-speed drives*** and ***programmable logic controllers*** (PLCs) to automate production lines and control motors is a common example of a computer system.

A typical computer system has memory, one or more processors, and a set of states that define the relationship between the system's inputs and outputs. A computer system could be varied in definition into either a chip (the *micro-controller*) or a whole system of chips, system board and peripherals, into models such as the tower, desktop, or laptop. All computer systems perform the following five basic operations:

- ***Inputting:*** The process of entering data and instructions into the computer system.
- ***Storing:*** Saving data and instructions.
- ***Processing:*** Performing arithemetic operations or logical operations on data in order to convert them into useful information.
- ***Outputting:*** The process of producing useful information or results for the user such as printed report or visual display.

- ***Controlling:*** Directing the manner and sequence in which all of the above operations are performed.

The basic organization of a computer system is shown in Fig. 1.1. The five functional units of a digital computer system correspond to the five basic operations performed by all the computer system. The details of each unit are discussed below:

1. ***Input unit:*** Input is any data or instructions entered into the memory of a computer. Four types of input are data, programs, commands and user responses. An input device converts input data and instructions into binary form for acceptance by the computer. Input devices include keyboard, pointing devices (joystick, light pen, mouse, trackballs), scanners and reading devices, digital cameras, audio and video input devices.

2. ***Output unit:*** Computer process and organize data into information, which has meaning and is useful. A computer processes input into output. Computer generates several types of output, depending on the hardware and software being used and the requirement of the user. Four common types of output are text, graphics, audio and video. Output devices such as printers, plotters, monitors and speakers are used to convey that information to the user.

3. ***Arithmetic logic unit (ALU):*** ALU of a computer system is the place where actual execution of instructions takes place during processing operation. The ALU performs arithmetic and logic operations. ALUs are designed to perform four basic operations—additions, subtraction, multiplication, division and

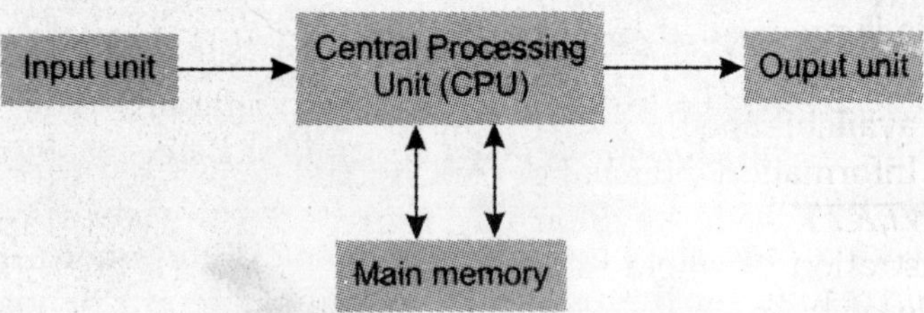

Fig. 1.1: Basic organization of a computer

logic operations or comparisons such as less than, greater than or equal to.

4. ***Control unit:*** By selecting, interpreting and seeing to the execution of the program, instructions, the control unit is execution of the program instructions; the control unit is able to maintain order and direct operation of the entire system. It manages and coordinates the entire system. It controls the entire processing. Whenever an input reaches into memory, the control unit determines what type of instruction it is. And accordingly it instructs the ALU or input/output devices. The control unit and arithmetic logic unit of a computer system are jointly known as ***central processing unit*** (CPU).

5. ***Storage unit:*** Storage refers to the media on which data, instructions and informations are kept, as well as the devices that record and retrieve these items. The functions of storage unit are to holds all data to be processed and the instructions required for processing, immediate results of processing and final results of processing. The computer makes use of two types of memory—Internal memory and External memory. The internal memory (main memory) is the built-in memory where CPU holds the programs and data being manipulated. When temporary information is to be stored permanently or semi-permanently, external memory is used.

Input Devices

1. ***Keyboard:*** It is an input device used to type letters, digits and commands. When a key is pressed a signal is sent to the computer, which is decoded there to determine which key has been pressed. For each alphabet or a symbol or a digit, etc. a code is predecided and fixed. When a key is pressed the code for that key is sent to the computer. Various types of codings are available and the most common is American Standard Code for Information Interchange (ASCII). Today most users use the ***QWERTY*** style keyboards. Figure 1.2 shows a graphic illustration of where each of the keys is on a U.S. QWERTY style keyboard. A majority of all keyboard keys produce ***letters, numbers*** or ***signs*** (characters) that are appropriate for the

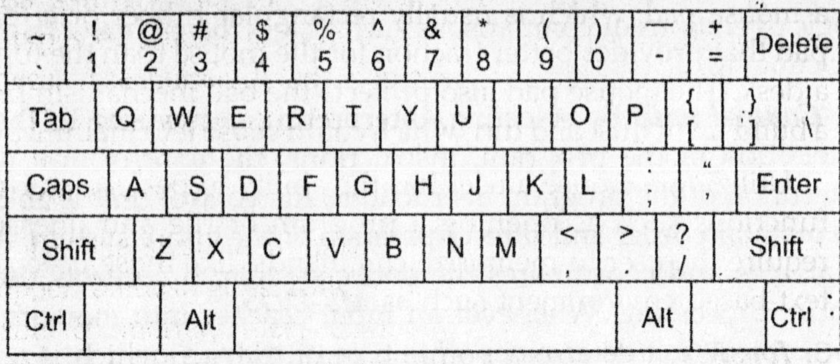

Fig. 1.2: QWERTY keyboard

operator's language. Other keys can produce actions when pressed, and other actions are available by the simultaneous pressing of more than one action key. The number of keys on a keyboard varies from the standard of 101 keys introduced in the late 1980s to the 104 key windows keyboards and all the way up to 130 keys or more, with many of the additional keys being symbol-less programmable keys that can simulate multiple functions such as starting a *web browser* or *e-mail client*. There also were "Internet keyboards", sold in the late 1990s, that replaced the function keys with pre-programmed Internet shortcuts. Pressing the *shortcut keys* would launch a browser to go to that website.

Wireless keyboards have become popular for their increased user freedom. A wireless keyboard often includes a required combination transmitter and receiver unit that attaches to the computer's keyboard port. The wireless aspect is achieved either by *radio frequency* (RF) or by *infrared* (IR) signals sent and received from both the keyboard and the unit attached to the computer. A wireless keyboard may use an industry standard RF, called *Bluetooth*.

2. ***Mouse:*** The mouse is the mostly widely used pointing device on desktop computers. The top of the mouse have one to four buttons; some also have a small wheel. The bottom of a mouse is flat and contains a multi-directional mechanism, usually either a small ball or an optical sensor, which detects movement of the mouse. Mouse devices contain a small ball often rest on

a mouse pad, which is usually rectangular rubber or a foam pad that provides better traction for the mouse than the top of a desk. The mouse pad also protects the ball mechanism from a build up of dust and dirt, which could cause it to malfunction.

Utilizing a mouse a user has the ability to perform various functions such as opening a program or file and does not require the user to memorize commands, like those used in a text-based environment such as ***MS-DOS***.

3. ***Joystick:*** It is also a pointing input device, which is used frequently in programs like video games, and on personal computers. It is an electric device used like a mouse for controlling cursor movement. It consists of four micro-switches arranged in four directions (East, West, North and South). When joystick is moved in a particular direction, the switch is activated in that direction and gives a signal to the cursor. This cursor moves in the direction in which the stick has been moved.

4. ***Light pen:*** A light pen is also a pointing device. The light pen consists of a photocell mounted in a pen shaped tube. When the pen is brought in front of a picture element of the screen, it senses light coming from a limited field of view. The light coming from the screen causes the photocell to respond by generating a pulse. This electric response is transmitted to a processor that identifies the pixel (graphic point) the light pen is pointing to. Thus to identify a specific location, the light pen is useful. The light pen is also used to draw images on the screen. With the movement of the light pen over the screen, the lines are drawn. A light pen can work with any CRT-based monitor, but not with *LCD* screens, projectors and other display devices.

5. ***Trackballs:*** This is also a pointing device. It contains a ball, which can be rotated in any direction. The user moves the ball in the desired direction to move the cursor on the screen. Speed of spin is controlled by the electronic circuit. The instructed information is sent to the processor.

6. ***Digitizer:*** A graphics tablet (or digitizing tablet, graphics pad, drawing tablet) is a computer ***input device*** that allows one to hand-draw images and graphics, similar to the way one

draws images with a pencil and paper. A graphics tablet consists of a flat surface upon which the user may "draw" an image using an attached ***stylus***, a pen-like drawing apparatus. The image generally does not appear on the tablet itself but, rather, is displayed on the computer ***monitor***.

7. ***Scanners:*** A scanner creates an electronic form of the printed image, which can later be manipulated, changed and modified according to the requirements. A scanner is commonly connected to a computer ***USB***, ***Firewire***, ***Parallel*** or ***SCSI*** port. Scanners are available in variety of sizes such as hand-held scanner, flatbed scanner and drum scanner. Hand held scanners are very small and in order to scan a single page image multiple passes are required. Flatbed scanners are large, more expensive and can scan a page in a single pass. Drum scanners are medium sized scanners with rolling drum; the drum rolls over entire sheet to be scanned.

8. ***Reading devices:*** An optical reader is a device that uses light source to read characters, marks and codes and then convert them into digital data that can be processed by a computer. Reading devices may be of different types such as optical character reader, optical mark recognition, magnetic ink character reader and bar code reader.

a. *Optical character reader (OCR):* An OCR is used to read character of special type font (or fonts) printed on conventional paper with conventional ink. The printed characters are examined by photoelectric device, which differentiates light (no ink) from inked areas and a logical system, which attempts to determine which of the possible characters is being examined. The light is absorbed by the characters and thus recognized by the OCR.

b. *Optical mark reader (OMR):* This input device read hand-drawn marks such as small circles or rectangles. It is most commonly used in evaluation of multiple choice question papers. The OMR device first reads a master document such as an answer key sheet for a test to record correct answer based on patterns of light; the remaining documents then are passed through OMR and their pattern of light are matched against the master document.

c. *Magnetic ink character reader (MICR):* A MICR is used to read characters printed on documents with magnetized ink. MICR is used by banking industry for cheque processing. Each cheque in your cheque-book has precoded MICR characters on the lower-left edge; these characters represent the bank number, your account number and cheque number. When a cheque is presented for payment, the bank uses an MICR inscriber to print the amount of the cheque in MICR characters in the lower-right corner. The cheque then is sorted or routed to the customer's bank, along with thousand of others. Each cheque is inserted into an MICR reader, which sends the check information including the amount of the cheque to a computer for processing. MICR can process 40 documents per second. A similar type of magnetic code can be seen on credit cards also.

d. *Bar code reader:* A bar code is an identification code that consists of a set of vertical lines and spaces of different widths printed on various types of products such as groceries, pharmacy, supplies, vehicles, mail and books. A bar code reader emits a beam of light (laser beam) which reflects off the bar code image. A light-sensitive detector in the bar code reader then identifies the bar code image by recognizing special bars at the both ends of the image. Once the bar code is identified, the bar pattern is converted into a numeric code that can be processed later in any manner.

9. ***Audio and video input:*** Audio input is the process of entering (recording) music, speech or sound effects. Voice recognition techniques are also used to convert voice signals into appropriate words. Video input is the process of entering a full-motion recording into a computer and storing the video on a hard disk or some other medium.

10. ***Digital camera:*** It is a type of camera that stores the pictures or video it takes in electronic format instead of to film. They record colour images as intensities of red, green and blue, which are stored as variable charges in a CCD matrix. The size of the matrix determines the resolution, but the analog-to-digital converter (ADC), which converts the charges to digital data determines the colour depth.

Output Devices

1. ***Printers:*** A printer is an output device that produces text and graphics on a physical medium such as paper or transparency film. Printers can be divided into two distinct categories—*Impact printers* and *Non-impact printers* (Fig. 1.3). In impact printers there is mechanical contact between the print head and paper whereas in non-impact printers there is no mechanical contact between the print head and paper. Two commonly used types of impact printers are dot matrix printer, line printer and daisy-wheel printer. The commonly used types of non-impact printers are ink-jet printer, laser printer and thermal printer.

a. *Dot matrix printer (DMP):* The term DOT matrix refers to the process of placing ***dots*** to form an image; the quality of the image being determined by the ***dots per inch***. Dot matrix printers were first introduced by ***Centronics*** in 1970 and is a type of printer that uses print heads to shoot ink or strike an ink ribbon to place hundreds to thousands of little dots to form text and/or images. Today, dot matrix printers are not commonly used or found because of the low quality printouts when compared to *ink-jet printers* or other later printer technologies.

b. *Line printer:* A line printer prints a complete line at a time. Printing speed varies from 150 lines to 2500 lines per minute with 90 to 100 characters on 15 inch line. There are two types of line printers—*drum printers* and *chain printers.* A drum printer

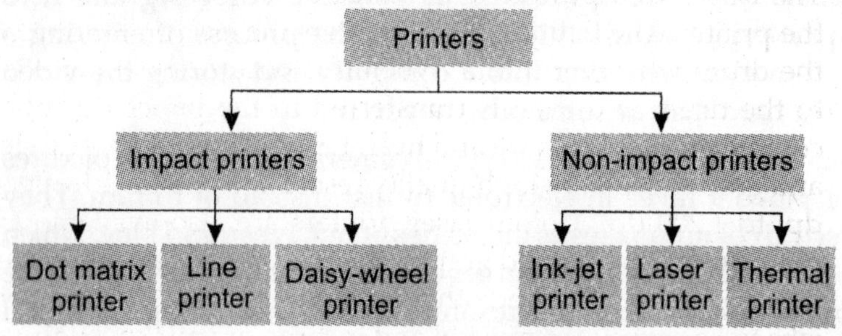

Fig. 1.3: Types of printers

consist of a cylindrical drum on which character are embossed. A chain printer consists of a steel band on which the characters are embossed.

c. *Letter quality printer:* The letter quality printer print full characters (continuous character not as the character made of dots). The most popular of such a type is ***daisy-wheel printer***. It is a solid font type character. In a daisy-wheel printer, its print head resembles a daisy flower, with its print arm appearing like the petals of the flower. It has 96 characters on its petals. While printing, the character to be printed is sent to the printer buffer. The hub is continuously rotating at high speed, and a hammer strikes the appropriate character when it is in position. The daisy-wheel printer can have speeds up to 90 characters per second.

d. *Ink-jet printer:* A popular type of printer for *home computer users* that prints by spraying streams of quick-drying ink on paper. The ink is stored in disposable ink ***cartridges***, often a separate cartridge is used for each of the major colors. These colors are usually Black, Red / Magenta, Green / Cyan, and Yellow (*CYMK*). Although ink-jet printers themselves are often relatively inexpensive, the ink cartridges used in the printers can quickly increase the overall cost of the printer.

e. *Laser printer:* First developed at *Xerox PARC* by Gary Starkweather and released in 1971, a laser printer is a type of printer that utilizes laser technology to print images on the paper. A laser printer creates images using a laser beam and powdered ink called toner, which is packaged in a cartridge. The laser beam produces an image on a special drum inside the printer. The light of the laser alters the electrical charge on the drum wherever it hits. When this occurs, the toner sticks to the drum and then is transferred to the paper through a combination of pressure and heat. Laser printers can print text and graphics in very high-quality resolutions ranging from 600 dpi to 1,200 dpi. Colour laser printers are also available and can print multicoloured graphics. Laser printers are often used in corporate, school, and other environments that require print jobs to be completed quickly and in large quantities. High-end fast laser printers are used with mainframe computers.

Depending on the amount of graphics you intend to print, a laser printer can have up to 200 MB of memory.

f. *Thermal printer:* A thermal impact printer or electro-thermal printer is a type of printer that uses heated pins to "burn" images onto heat-sensitive paper. These types of printers are commonly used in calculators and fax machines; and although they are inexpensive and print relatively fast, they produce low resolution print jobs. A thermal printer, thermal transfer printer, or thermal wax-transfer printer is a high quality printer that commonly utilizes a thermal wax ribbon that melts a colored wax onto the paper creating near photo-realistic images.

g. *Light emitting diode (LED) printer:* LED printers were developed by Casio and are capable of printing at the same or close to the same quality as most laser printers. LED printers work much like laser printers but utilize a LED panel that recreates the image on a negatively charged drum. The areas where the light hits the drum become less charged, which attracts toner. The printer then transfers the toner from the drum to the paper and applies intense heat to fuse the toner to the paper.

2. ***Plotters:*** Plotters are sophisticated output devices used to print high quality drawings such as blueprints, maps, circuit diagrams and signs. There are two types of plotters—*drum plotters* and *flat plotters.* In a drum plotter, the output paper is mounted on a rotating drum. A flat-bed plotter consist of a stationary horizontal plotting surface on which paper is fixed.

a. *Drum plotter:* The paper on which the design has to be made is placed over a drum that rotates back and forth to produce vertical motion. The mechanism also consists of one or more penholders mounted horizontally across the drum. The pen(s) clamped in the holder(s) can move to produce horizontal motion. Under the control of the computer, the drum and pen(s) move simultaneously to produce designs and graphs.

b. *Flat-bed plotter:* A flat-bed plotter plots on papers that are spread and fixed over rectangular flatbed table. The paper does not move and the pen-holding mechanism is designed to provide all the motion. This plotter uses a light pen and draws graph on the paper. Multicoloured pens are used for graphics. Pen is controlled by pen-holder. It can make graphs of small to large size depending upon the size of bed.

3. ***Monitors:*** A visual display unit (also called monitor, or screen) offers a two-dimensional visual presentation of information is a piece of *electrical equipment* which displays viewable images generated by a computer without producing a permanent record. The word "monitor" is used in other contexts; in particular in television broadcasting, where a television picture is displayed to a high standard. A computer display device is usually either a ***cathode ray tube*** (CRT) or some form of flat panel such as a TFT LCD or gas plasma monitors. The monitor comprises the display device, circuitry to generate a picture from electronic signals sent by the computer, and an enclosure or case. Within the computer, either as an integral part or a plugged-in interface, there is circuitry to convert internal ***data*** to a format compatible with a monitor. The quality of a monitor's display depends on its resolution, dot pitch and refresh rate. Resolution is expressed as two separate numbers, the number of columns of pixels and the number of rows of pixels a monitor can display. A monitor with a higher resolution displays a greater number of pixels, which provides smoother image. A screen with a 640 × 480 resolution can display 640 columns and 480 rows of pixels (or a toatal of 307,200 pixels). Most modern monitors can display 800 × 600 and 1024 × 768 pixels; some high-end monitors can display 1280 × 1024, 1600 × 1200 or even 1920 × 1440 pixels.

4. ***Speakers:*** A speaker is a *hardware device* connected to a ***computer's sound card*** that outputs sounds generated by the card. A speaker can be used for various sounds meant to alert the user, as well as music and spoken text. A sound board (or an audio card) is an *expansion card* or *integrated* circuit that provides a computer with the ability to produce sound that can be heard by the user.

Storage Devices

A storage device is a ***hardware*** device designed to store information. There are two types of storage devices used in computers; a ***primary storage*** device and a ***secondary storage*** device.

1. ***Primary storage (Internal memory):*** Presently known as memory, is the only one directly accessible to the CPU. The CPU continuously reads instructions stored there and executes them. Any data actively operated on is also stored there in uniform manner. Thus internal memory is the built-in memory where CPU holds the programs and data being manipulated. There are two types of internal memory:

a. *Random acess memory (RAM):* The internal memory that can be read from as well as written to is called RAM. RAM is read/write memory. The time taken to acess any location is the same. Read process is non-destructive, i.e. if we read data from a location, it still remains in the location. Write process is destructive, i.e. if we write data in memory location, which already has some data stored in it, the previous data disappears and is replaced by the new data. RAM is volatile, i.e. its contents are lost when power is turned off. This is the reason why we call RAM a temporary memory.

b. *Read only memory (ROM):* This memory allows only read operations and does not let us write anything on it. The information once stored remains fixed and cannot be changed. ROM can only be read. Generally ROM contains a set of start-up instructions. The contents of ROM remain stored even if power is turned off. There are various types of ROMs available nowadays, example includes—programmable read only memory (PROM), erasable programmable read only memory (EPROM) and electrically erasable PROM (EEPROM).

2. ***Secondary storage (External memory):*** Since the storage capacity of primary memory is limited and primary memory cannot store the data permanently, so we use various secondary storage devices. Most common external storage devices are—*hard drives, floppy disks, magnetic tapes, CD-ROM, video disks,* etc.

a. *Floppy disk:* A floppy disk is very small storage device which can be used as an input and output medium. It can be used both for reading and writing. This is made up of elastic plastic material and is finely coated with magnetic oxide. This disk is placed in plastic cover to avoid damage. The floppy disk is available in three standard sizes—8", 5.25" and 3.5". The storage capacity of each floppy disk is different. 5.25 inch diameter can hold 1.2 MB of data and 3.5 inch diameter floppy can hold 1.44 MB of data. The floppy is inserted into floppy drive. This rotates the floppy drive and data is stored on circular paths called tracks. The data already stored in it can be removed and new data can be fed in place of it. The storage capacity of floppy disk depends on design, density, surface and number of tracks. The formula for calculating storage capacity of floppy is:

Capacity = $N \times n \times s \times d$ where,
N = Number of tracks
n = Number of sectors
s = Number of slides
d = Data capacity.

b. *Hard disk (magnetic disk):* Hard disks consist of rigid circular platters of magnetizable material sealed in a metal box with associated read/write heads. They are usually internal to the computer. Magnetic disks are round and coated with a magnetizable recording material. Each disk has a number of concentric circles called tracks. The tracks on the disk surface are divided into sectors. Generally there are 8 sectors per track and each sector can hold upto 512 bytes. A disk pack has several disks stacked one over the other. Tracks with same number on all the disk surfaces form a cylinder. The disk is rotated by a motor at a very high speed. Data are written as tiny magnetic spots on the disk surface. The storage capacity of a disk depends upon the number of bits per track on a surface and the number of tracks per inch on the surface. Hard disks, these days are available in capacities varying from 8.1 GB to 20 GB.

c. *Magnetic tape:* One of the first storage media used with mainframe computers was magnetic tape, a magnetically coated ribbon of plastic capable of storing large amount of data and information at a low cost. This tape is similar to a tape recorder cassette and has served as efficient and reliable information storage media since the early 1950s. When we feed data in a tape, this is recorded on the tape as magnetic spots. Normally the length of the tape is 2400 feet and its standard width is ½ inch. A textbook of 400 pages with 50 lines per page and 40 letters per line can be accommodated in less than 15 feet of tape of density 6250 bpi. The storage capacity depends upon tape density, length of tape, blocking factor, inter-block gap and inter-record gap.

d. *Compact discs (CDs):* A compact disc is a flat, round, portable, metal storage medium that usually is 4.75 inches in diameter and less than one-twentieth of an inch thick. Compact discs store items such as data, instructions and information by microscopic pits (indentations) and land (flat areas) that are in the middle layer of the disc. A high-powered laser light creates the pits. A lower-powered laser light read items from the compact disc by reflecting light through the bottom of the disc, which usually is either solid gold or silver in colour. The reflected light is converted into a series of bits that the computer can process. Land causes light to reflect, which is read as binary digit 1. Pits absorb the light. This absence of light is read as binary digit 0.

- ***CD-ROMs:*** Compact disc read-only memory can contain text, graphics and video as well as sound written or recorded by the manufacturer and only can be read and used.
- ***CD-R:*** A recordable CD-ROM technology using a disc that can be written only once.
- ***CD-RW:*** A rewritable CD-ROM technology. A CD-RW disc can be rewritten. CD-RW drives can also be used to write CD-R discs and they can read CD-ROMs.

e. *Digital video disc (DVD):* A DVD resembles a CD-ROM in its appearance but the data storage technique is different. It is an extremely high-capacity compact disc capable of storing from 4.7 GB to 17 GB. DVDs are read by using a laser beam just like CD-ROM but the wavelength is smaller. This allows us to have smaller indentations and the thickness of data layer is also reduced. Thus we have the higher storage capacity in a DVD.

f. *Smart cards:* A credit card with a built-in processor and memory used for identification or financial transactions. When inserted into a reader, it transfers data to and from a central computer.

g. *Microfilm and microfiche:* Microfilm and microfiche are used to store microscopic images of documents on roll or sheet film. Microfilm uses a 100 to 215 foot roll of film. Microfiche uses a small sheet of film, usually about four inches by six inches. The images are recorded onto the film using a device called computer output microfilm (COM) recorder. The stored images are so small that they can be read only with a microfilm or microfiche reader.

TYPES OF COMPUTERS

The types of computers range from the hybrid to the analog types. The computers we come across in the daily course of your day range from laptops, palmtops and towers, to desktop computers, to name a few. Different categories of computes have been devised in keeping with our varied needs (Fig. 1.4).

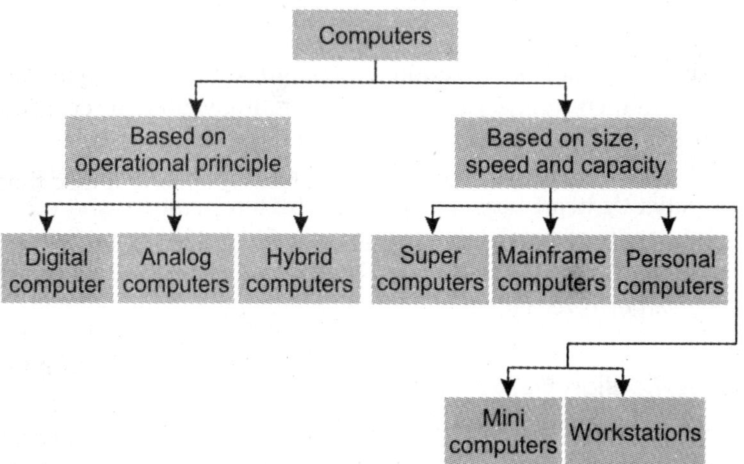

Fig. 1.4: Types of computers

Classification Based on Operational Principle

a. ***Digital computers:*** The digital computers work upon discontinuous data. They convert the data into digits (binary digits 0 and 1) and all operations are carried out on these digits at extremely fast rates. Digital computers are much faster than analog computers and far more accurate. Digital computers are classified as special-purpose computers and general-purpose computers. Microcomputers are examples of digital computers.

b. ***Analog computers:*** The analog computer is almost an extinct type of computer these days. It is different from a digital computer in respect that it can perform numerous mathematical operations simultaneously. It is also unique in terms of operation as it utilizes continuous variables for the purpose of mathematical computation. It utilizes mechanical, hydraulic, or electrical energy for operation. Computations are carried out with physical quantities such as voltage, current, temperature, etc. Their accuracy is poor as compared to digital computers.

c. ***Hybrid computers:*** These types of computers are, as the name suggests, a combination of both analog and digital computers. The digital computers which work on the principle of binary digit system of "0" and "1" can give very precise results. But the problem is that they are too slow and incapable of large-scale mathematical operation. In the hybrid types of computers the digital counterparts convert the analog signals to perform robotics and process control. Hybrid computers are best used in hospital where analog part is responsible for measurement of patient's heart beat, blood pressure, temperature and other vital signs and then the operation is carried out in digital fashion to monitor patient's vital signs. Hybrid computers are also used in weather forecasting.

Classification Based on Size, Capacity, Speed Reliability and Use

a. ***Supercomputers:*** A supercomputer contains a number of CPUs, which operate in parallel to make it faster. Although some supercomputers are single computer systems, most are comprised of multiple high performance computers working in parallel as a single system. A supercomputer is capable of processing more than 64 billion instructions in one second. Supercomputers are used for applications requiring complex, sophisticated mathematical calculations. The speed of a supercomputer is generally measured in ***FLOPS***. The distinction between supercomputers and mainframes can be difficult to define at times. Supercomputers tend to be custom built and focus on processing power to do one task. Mainframes, while providing a lot of processing power, focus more on data throughput and generally perform many datahandling operations involving minor computations. They are used for weather forecasting, nuclear energy research, rocketing, aerodynamics, seismology, petroleum exploration and plasma physics. Examples of supercomputers are—PARAM, CRAY 3, HITAC S-300, etc. IBM's Blue Gene/L is the fastest supercomputer in the world.

b. ***Mainframe computers:*** The term mainframe computer was created to distinguish the traditional, large, institutional computer intended to service multiple users from the smaller, single user machines. Mainframe computers have more memory, speed and capabilities than workstations and are usually shared by multiple users through a series of interconnected computers. A mainframe speed is so fast that it is measured in millions of tasks per milliseconds (MTM). These are computers used by large organizations like meteorological surveys and statistical institutes for performing bulk mathematical computations. They are core computers, which are used for desktop functions of over one hundred people simultaneously. Examples of mainframe computers are—IBM 4300 series, IBM 3090 series, HP 9000 model 870S/400, HP 9000 model 870S/300, etc.

c. ***Personal computers:*** A personal computer (PC) is a computer that can perform all of its input, processing, output and storage activities by itself, i.e. it contain at least one input device, one output device, one storage device and a processor. The processor is a central processing unit (CPU) on a single chip and is the basic building block of a PC. PCs were first known as *microcomputers* because they were a complete computer but built on a smaller scale than the huge systems in use by most businesses. Two major sub-categories of personal computers are desktop computers and portable computers (laptops and palmtops).

- *Desktop computers:* A desktop computer is designed in such a way that the system unit, input devices, output devices and any other devices fit entirely on or under a desk or table. They have large amounts of internal memory to store hundreds of programs and documents.
- *Laptop computers:* Laptop computers are so called as they can sit on a Lap. Laptop computers (also called notebooks) can be carried out in brief cases. Laptop computers usually have similar hardware and software as PCs but they are more compact and have flat, lightweight LCDs instead of video display monitors. Laptops are portable computers that integrate the display, keyboard, a pointing device or trackball, processor, memory and hard drive all in a battery-operated package slightly larger than an average hardcover book. Most laptop computers can run either on batteries or using a standard power supply.
- *Palmtops:* More commonly known as ***Personal Digital Assistants*** (PDAs), palmtops are tightly integrated computers that often use flash memory instead of a hard drive for storage. These computers usually do not have keyboards but rely on touchscreen technology for user input. Palmtops are typically smaller than a paperback novel, very lightweight with a reasonable battery life. A slightly larger and heavier version of the palmtop is the hand-held computer.

d. ***Workstations:*** Workstations are computers that are intended to serve one user and may contain special hardware enhancements not found on a *personal computer*. Workstations are similar to PCs but they have greater memory and more extensive mathematical abilities and they are connected to other workstations or personal computers to exchange data. They run operating systems that are normally associated with mainframe computers, usually one of the variants of the UNIX operating system. It is a desktop computer that has a more powerful processor, additional memory and enhanced capabilities for performing a special group of task, such as 3D Graphics or game development. User in fields such as engineering, desktop publishing and graphic art use work-station.

e. ***Minicomputers:*** Minicomputers fall in between micro-computers (PCs) and mainframes (enterprise servers). Minicomputers are normally referred to as mid-range servers now. Mini computers were much smaller, less powerful, and much less expensive than *Mainframe Computers.* The first mini computers generally only performed one task at a time, while bigger computers ran multi-tasking operating systems, and served multiple users. Mini computers were typified by small word sizes such as 8 or 16 bits whereas larger machines had larger word sizes. Mini computers like the mainframe computers are used by business organization. The difference being that it can support the simultaneous working of up to 100 users and is usually maintained in business organizations for the maintenance of accounts and finances. A minicomputer is more powerful and larger than workstation.

f. ***Servers:*** Server usually refers to a computer that is dedicated to the task of storing and retrieving large amounts of data. For example, a large computer dedicated to a database may be called a "database server". "File servers" manage a large collection of computer files. "Web servers" process web pages and web applications. This tends to distinguish them from "mainframes", which were generally intended to handle a variety of tasks. In some instances, a computer that was once considered a mainframe is given the role of *server.* This is because the actual data processing is taken over by individual personal computers. Many smaller servers are actually personal computers that have been dedicated to the task of storing data for other personal computers. In other instances, many small computers (essentially specialised personal computers) are designed to work in concert as a single server.

g. ***Embedded computer systems:*** Embedded computers are general purpose *CPUs* that are a part of a machine or device. This computer runs a program that is stored in read only memory (ROM) and is only intended to operate a specific machine or device. They are intended to operate this single machine or a single function of that machine. Embedded systems are typically required to operate continuously without being reset or rebooted, and once employed in their task the software usually cannot be modified. An automobile may contain a number of *embedded systems*; however, a washing machine and a DVD player would contain only one. The CPUs used are slower and less expensive than those found in a personal computer, but they generally only have to conduct a single function.

BASIC APPLICATIONS OF A COMPUTER

Every day, numerous users rely on different types of computers for a variety of applications. Some major applications of computers are listed below:

1. ***Computers at home:*** Computer can be used for different purposes by members of family including entertainment, research and education, personal financial management, home business management, personal and business communication, web acess, shopping, etc. Softwares also provide hours of education as well as entertainment.

2. ***Education:*** Computers are effectively used in classrooms, museums and libraries. In classroom computers are used to develop projects, prepare reports, gather information and as an interactive learning tool. Nowadays online learning and training is possible through networks.

3. ***Science, research and engineering:*** Scientists and Engineers use the computer as a tool to experiment, design and develop their ideas/projects. For example, impact of earthquakes on buildings can be predicted using computers. Various three-dimensional objects can be designed, rotated, viewed in detail, examined internally or externally through Computer Aided Designing (CAD). Computer Aided Engineering (CAE) allows

designers to specify the type of material to be used for each part, calculate whether the part could withstand necessary stresses and temperatures.

4. ***Communications:*** Computers can be used for communicating to different parts of world. This could be done through e-mail, chat or video confrencing. Events occurring at a place can be viewed instantly all across the world through computer networks.

5. ***Manufacturing:*** Computers play an important role in manufacturing. For example, in power plants that generate steam for electricity, computer can monitor pressures and temperatures at hundred of critical points. If pressure or temperature in a tank or pipe exceeds a specified level, computer can regulate the process by instructing valves to turn and burners to adjust.

6. ***Computers at railway stations and airports:*** Reservation of tickets is done with the help of computers. The schedule of flights and trains is maintained with the help of computers. Railway and flight enquiry is done by the use of computer technology.

7. ***Computers at banks:*** All details of computer accounts are fed into the computer. If you deposit or withdraw money from your account, balance will be updated automatically in the computer. Money can be withdrawn at any time from ATM of your bank.

8. ***Computers at hospital:*** Computers are helpful in maintaining the details of patients and their diseases. With the application of computer technology, doctors monitor patient's blood pressure, heart beat and other functions of the body.

9. ***Computers in entertainment:*** Computers are used as a creative tool for music, movies, animation cartoons and games. Film and television use computers to incorporate special effects. Movies may now contain many visual tricks with the aid of computers. Animation is created by displaying a series of still images in rapid sequence is also done on computers.

10. ***Desktop pubilishing:*** Newsletters, brochures, advertisements, postcards, greeting cards, letterheads, calendars, logos,

magzines, newspapers, books, etc. are produced using computers.

APPLICATIONS OF COMPUTER TECHNOLOGY IN PHARMACEUTICAL AND MEDICAL SCIENCES

1. ***Drug information-storage and retrieval system:*** The drug information about pharmacological actions, adverse effects, toxicity, drug interactions, etc. is necessary for pharmacist and this search has been simplified by the use of computers. For retrieval of medical information international data banks are available, example includes:

- *Excerpta medica:* It is an information system that provides abstracts of more than 2,500,000 items, covers 400 biomedical journals. The system was computerized in 1968.
- *MEDLARS:* Medical Literature Analysis and Retrieval System is one of the best known and most widely used service by National Library of Medicine. There are within several subdivisions such as Toxline, Cancerline, Chemline. This information base contains 2,500,000 articles, books and scientific articles. In 1971 afast working system was developed which is Medline.
- *Bitnet:* It is a worldwide network of universities and research institutions for exchanging files that contain data, reports, drafts of papers, messages and memoranda.
- *Biosis:* It is a database containing biological abstracts produced by Bioscience Information.
- *Ama/net:* It is a disease information base that contains descriptions and diagnostic symptoms for more than 3,500 diseases.

2. ***Teaching and training:*** The use of technology in teaching has been increasing over the past few years with the expectation that technology can lead to better student learning. The use of the World Wide Web in teaching becomes very beneficial when the capabilities of this new technology are utilized to create new teaching-learning experiences that can improve student learning. In this basic pharmacokinetic class, the World Wide

Web provided a medium for instructor-student-content interactions. The interactive modules enables the delivery of the course content in an appealing format and the pharmacokinetic simulation exercises provided the students with learning experiences that cannot be duplicated by textbooks.

Computer simulations in clinical pharmacy education help expose students to clinical patient management earlier and enable training of large numbers of students outside conventional clinical practice sites. The development of multimedia computer simulations in clinical pharmacy has two important advantages:

i. It enables students to be exposed to clinical patient management earlier in the educational process.

ii. It allows for the clinical training of large numbers of students outside of conventional clinical practice sites. Multimedia simulations are used as a means of exposing students to clinical simulations earlier in the educational process and of supplementing clinical experiences, allowing them to be better prepared for actual clinical experiences. With today's user friendly software, the availability of extensive multimedia files on the Internet, and the affordability of the necessary computer hardware, we would like to encourage all clinical pharmacy educators (though this is certainly applicable to other disciplines) to consider developing multimedia simulations.

Multimedia computer simulations provide numerous advantages in teaching clinical pharmacy. They allow large numbers of student's early exposure to clinical practice via computer simulation without increased demands on clinical faculty. They enable students living outside of commuting distance to schools of pharmacy to continue to participate in the education process and allow certain flexibility in clinical teaching. Since multimedia programs can incorporate pictures, sounds and even full-motion video, realistic simulations of patient care are possible. In addition, multimedia computer simulations provide certain inherent advantages over traditional teaching methods. Students have the opportunity to move at their own pace, choose their own direction through material and repeat material as often as desired. Medical videos are available on the Internet in various file formats or (Table 1.2), alternatively, digitized video files can pictures be created by connecting a VCR to a video capture card.

3. ***Hospital and clinical pharmacy:*** Computer technology is becoming more universally accepted in hospital pharmacy, and this acceptance will continue to increase. Maintenance of patient census lists and patient billing are the most frequent uses of computers. Computers are used in hospitals to maintain patient record database which is continually updated to reflect the current status of all patients. The information stored

Table 1.2: Medical images websites

Title (Description)	*Address*
Cardiax (cardiology study cases with sounds, videos)	http://www.med.umich.edu/lrc/cardiax/cardiax.html
The human visible project	http:/www.nlm.nih.gov/research/visible/human.html
Jonathan Tward's multimedia medical reference library	http://www.med-library.com
Pulmonology images/cases	http://indy.radiology.uiowa.edu/Providers/ProviderOrgSys/OSPulmonary.html
Dermatology images	http://www.uni-erlangen.de/docs/FAU/fakultaet/med/kli/derma/bilddb/db.html
Neurology images/cases	http://count51.med.harvard.edu/AANLIB/home.html
Pediatric cases	http://www.rad.washington.edu/PedERCaseList.html
Human anatomy images	http://www.cc.emory.edu/ANATOMY/Radiology/Home.Page.MENU.HTML
Medical image teaching files on WWW (list of links to medical images sites)	http://www.si.umich.edu/impact/Fali95/Papers-projects/ Papers/Scherer/#list

include—name, age, sex, weight, height, allergies, physician, present diagnosis, other diseases, drugs prescribed and special notes. The primary use also includes preparation of letters and labels. For drug store maintenance, purchase and inventory control in hospital pharmacy computers are very useful.

The clinical pharmacist may use computer for therapeutic drug monitoring, which is required in cases of drugs which have narrow therapeutic range. Computer programs are used to calculate drug dosage schedules to suit the individual patient. The adaptive programs use feedback from drug concentration measurements to predict future dosage needs of the patients. Apart from this drug interactions may be screened using programs like MEDIPHOR (Monitoring and Evaluation of Drug Interactions by Pharmacy Oriented Reporting) and PADIS (Pharmacy Automated Drug Interaction Screening).

4. ***Drug information center:*** All countries should provide drug information services either independently or as part of a regional network. The service should include collecting, reviewing, evaluating, indexing and distributing information on drugs to health workers. Drug and poisons information centers are best established within major teaching hospitals. This allows access to clinical experience, libraries, research facilities and educational activities. Drug and poisons information centers should be supported by government authorities. They require clinically trained staff with access to specialist support. In some cases drug information services can be provided in conjunction with toxicology services and pharmacovigilance programs. WHO recognizes independent drug information centers as a core component of national programs to promote the rational use of drugs. Pharmacists and other health care workers routinely provide drug information to the community. Basic equipment required for a centre includes:

- Furniture—desks, chairs, shelving;
- Communications—telephones, facsimile;
- Internet access;

- Computers—including external data backup;
- Printer;
- Software—for word processing, spreadsheets, databases and presentations;
- Photocopier;
- Textbooks and electronic information resources.

Recognizing the need to provide organized drug information to health care professionals as well as consumers, the WHO India Country Office in collaboration with the Karnataka State Pharmacy Council (KSPC) is supporting the establishment of five drug information centers. These centers have been established in Haryana (Sirsa), Chhattisgarh (Raipur), Rajasthan (Jaipur), Assam (Dibrugarh), and Goa (Panaji). These centers seek to provide authenticate, unbiased drug information to health care professionals; provide tailor-made counseling and drug information to patients / consumers as well as monitor and document adverse drug reactions within the hospital.

Drug information centers should be organized on a cooperative model involving a multidisciplinary team. Where possible, existing resources such as a libraries, computers and databases should be used. Cooperation between drug information centers can help to optimize limited resources and enhance overall service levels. Networking can involve two or more centers, and includes regional, national and international links.

5. ***Computer-assisted drug design:*** The search for new, effective and safe drugs has become increasing, sophisticated and costly. The process of drug discovery and development is a long, tedious and difficult one. Occasionally new drugs are found by accident. More frequently they are developed as a part of an organized effort to discover new ways to treat human disease but also to improve the quality of life. In general the computer aided drug design technique has the ability to accomplish both these goals and to improve the efficiency of the process as well.

- *Computer-assisted drug design (CADD):* It involves all computer-assisted techniques used to discover, design, and optimize biologically active compounds with effective use as drugs.
- *Computer-assisted molecular design (CAMD):* It involves all computer-assisted techniques used to discover, design, and optimize compounds with desired structure and properties.
- *Computer-assisted molecular modeling (CAMM):* It involves the investigation of molecular structures and properties using computational chemistry and graphical visualization techniques.

Computer graphics has many uses in drug design and related fields—crystallography, receptor mapping, molecular mechanics and dynamics, NMR, molecular docking, quantum mechanics, Structure Activity Relationship (SAR), QSAR, etc. The most extensive use of molecular graphics to date has been in the field of structure activity relationship. Some recent examples of CADD are:

- Design of thymidylate synthetase inhibitor as anticancer agents.
- Design of HIV protease inhibitors as antiviral agents.
- Design of CAI as antiglaucoma agents.
- Design of neutrophil elastase.
- Discovery of novel sweeteners using a sweet taste receptor model.

Computerized molecular modeling can provide scientists with few major types of information that are important for mechanistic design of drugs—three-dimensional structure of molecules; chemical and physical characteristics of molecule; comparison of the structure of one molecule with other different molecules; visualization of complex formed between different molecules and prediction about how related molecules might look.

The predominant systems for molecular modeling calculations are work stations with UNIX operating system, e.g. three-dimensional graphics work station from Silicon Graphics, Sg. Inc and Evans and Sutherland multipicture systems. The entire range of computer hardware being used are Desktop, Macintosh, MS-Dos PC, Computer servers, Super-Computer as Cray super computers. The software used by molecular modelers ranges from simple programs that perform just a single task to highly complex packages that integrate many different methods. Molecular modeling programs like AMBER, CHARMM and GROMACS are widely used to carry out molecular dynamic simulations. Carrying out large realistic simulations on biomolecules necessitate the use of high performance computing machines. Codes like AMBER, CHARMM and GROMACS have been ported and optimized on PARAM Padma, a supercomputer. Using such codes on the PARAM system, it is possible to carry out large simulations of biomolecules for structural studies.

Some examples of softwares are described below:

- ***Alchemy:*** Molecular mechanics and display program powerful display options with real-time rotation. Functionalities similar to those of SYBYL, runs on MS-Dos PC, with math coprocessor is recommended.
- ***Amber:*** Molecular mechanics and molecular dynamics program.
- ***ChemOffice:*** Molecular mechanics, conformational searching, molecular dynamics. Runs on windows.
- ***CS Chem Finder:*** Electronic features and SAR, docking studies.
- ***ASP:*** Predicts binding affinity of a potential drug were structure of binding site is unknown.

6. ***Applied biopharmaceutics:*** Pharmacokinetics is the study of the time course of drug and metabolite levels in different fluids, tissues, and excreta of the body. The availability of computers and improvements in bioanalytical chemistry has greatly accelerated the development of pharmacokinetics. Computer software programs now allow for the rapid solution of complicated pharmacokinetic equations and rapid modeling of pharmacokinetic processes. Computers simplify tedious calculations and allow more time for the development of new

approaches to data analysis and pharmacokinetics modeling. In addition, computer software is used for the development of experimental study designs, statistical data treatment, data manipulation, graphical representation of data, pharmacokinetic model simulation, and projection or prediction of drug action.

Computer-aided pharmacokinetic, pharmacodynamic, and pharmacokinetic/pharmacodynamic methods are commonly applied to quantify the disposition and the pharmacological effects of the drug, to explore exposure-response relationships, and to predict safety and efficacy outcomes. Use of modeling and simulation throughout the drug development continuum can support more efficient preclinical and clinical study design and interpretation. Mechanism-based approaches where sound biological understanding exists provide meaningful quantitative comparisons between candidates and are sought to support science-based decisions. Simulations from these models allow for scientists to investigate a variety of trial designs where assumptions are clearly stated.

A good pharmacokinetic program should:

- Provide fail-safes, such as checks on age and weight, lab values, etc.
- Check against standard kinetics values and warn of +/– 2 standard deviations from the norm.
- Have storage capability to view what you did the day before or when the patient was in the ICU versus stabilized.
- Allow appropriate equation flexibility for all ages.
- Offer compatibility with numerous printers.
- Be easy to learn and use.
- Be capable of doing steady-state as well as non-steady-state.
- Perform Bayesian analysis.
- Change parameters according to renal or liver function.
- Feel right, in your clinical judgement.

In 1969 Metzler introduced the first package NONLIN, which fit the non-linear data to a predetermined pharmacokinetic model using least square regression analysis. Examples of commonly used pharmacokinetic software's are listed in Table 1.3.

Table 1.3: Examples of pharmacokinetic softwares

Software	*Salient features*
PharMod	Powerful but very friendly pharmacokinetic modeling program. Models 2 different pharmacokinetic situations including linear and non-linear elimination.
MacDope	Computer simulation of pharmacokinetics which enables patient factors and drug factors to be changed. Changes are reflected in drug concentrations in biological fluids.
ADAPT II	Models are specified using FORTRAN statements. Requires a FORTRAN compiler as each model is recompiled before use. Simulation can be error free of with noise or based on population values. Uses the LSODA method for numerical integration (which is suitable for non-stiff and stiff problems). The program will perform simplex optimization, maximum likelihood and Bayesian fitting or will develop optimal sampling designs.
NONMEM	Computer program for fitting non-linear mixed effects (statistical regression-type) models. These techniques are particularly useful where the data are population pharmacokinetic data and when there are few measurements from each subject and/or the variation between subjects is considerable.
SAAM30 and CONSAM	Computer programs for performing non-linear regression analysis. Models are specified by means of various parameters or free-form equations. SAAM30 is operated in batch mode while CONSAM is more interactive. Numerical integration routines are available non-stiff and stiff systems.
Boomer and MultiForte	Weighted non-linear regression, simulations, Bayesian analysis, and Iteratively Reweighed Least Squares analyses are possible. In MultiForte models are specified by modifying model definition subroutines in FORTRAN. In Boomer the model is defined by the selection of parameters such as dose, first-order rate

Contd..

Contd..

	constant, volume, etc. Integrated and differential equation type models are possible. Fitting algorithms include Gauss-Newton, Marquardt, and simplex. Numerical integration routines include Runge-Kutta, Runge-Kutta-Fehlberg, and Gears.
Kinetics	Multiple creatinine clearance methods: Cockcroft and Gault, Jelliffe, MDRD, Salazar and Corcoran. *Population analysis tool*, *Bayesian analysis*, *Drug model database*, *Patient database management*, *Serum level plots* for 1 and 2-compartment models, Non-steady-state analysis of 1-compartment models.
PK Solutions	It offers a fast and easy way to compute, graph, and analyze the most commonly used pharmacokinetic parameters associated with blood (plasma, serum) concentration-time data following extravascular (such as oral) and intravenous dosing. In the data manager, Pk-fit includes the non-compartmental analysis module, the compartmental analysis module, the non-linear kinetic process module, the drug absorption module, the pharmacodynamic data modeling module, the simultaneous fitting module, and the user-defined library module. Approximately 75 pharmacokinetic parameters are computed for each data set, including tables and graphs projecting multiple dose results based on single dose values.

7. ***Pharmaceutical analysis:*** The applications of computers include data handling, processing, storing, file search or display. The results in analysis of drugs, pesticides, herbal extracts, etc. are generated in graphical form as a spectrum containing number of peaks. The computer compares the spectrum of given sample with spectrum of pure compound with the use of library systems available in the software of the analytical instruments (HPLC, HPTLC, GLC, MS, IR, etc.). These library may contain few thousand spectra to more than 1,50,000 spectra. For example, when gas-liquid chromatography (GLC) with mass spectrometry (MS) is used for separation and identification of complex mixtures. GLC separates the individual component and MS identifies it. Commercial software packages are available for Infrared (IR)

spectra such as Sadtler Standard Infrared Collection and Sadtler Commercial Infrared Collection.

8. ***Pharmaceutical manufacturing industry:*** The successful manufacturing requires integration of many previously compartmentalized activities, plus new knowledge and greater understanding of manufacturing processes, product design methods, and manufacturing system design methods.

There are many computer aids available for manufacturing bulk drugs and pharmaceutical products. Computer Aided Manufacturing (CAM) softwares are usually product oriented. Process synthesis and flow-sheet programs are commonly used. It involves generating a flow sheet for a process to produce a particular product from a specific raw material. Spread sheet software has been found useful for material and energy balancing, cost estimation, and economic analysis. The commercial flow sheet programs include COPE by Exxon, COPES by Du Pont, IPES by Union Carbide, etc.

9. ***Bioinformatics:*** Bioinformatics is the combination of biology and information technology. The discipline encompasses any computational tools and methods used to manage, analyze and manipulate large sets of biological data. Bioinformatics is the comprehensive application of mathematics, statistics, biochemistry, biophysics and computer algorithms to analyze biological data. Essentially, bioinformatics has three components:

- The creation of databases allowing the storage and management of large biological data sets.
- The development of algorithms and statistics to determine relationships among members of large data sets.
- The use of these tools for the analysis and interpretation of various types of biological data, including DNA, RNA and protein sequences, protein structures, gene expression profiles, and biochemical pathways.

Everyday bioinformatics is done with sequence search programs like ***Blast***, sequence analysis programs, like the EMBOSS and Staden packages, structure prediction programs like ***Threader*** or ***PHD*** or molecular imaging/modeling programs like ***RasMol*** and ***What If***.

Bioinformatics is the application of computer technology to the management of biological information. Computers are used to gather, store, analyze and integrate biological and genetic information which can then be applied to gene-based drug discovery and development. The need for bioinformatics capabilities has been precipitated by the explosion of publicly available genomic information resulting from the Human Genome Project for determination of the sequence of the entire human genome (approximately three billion base pairs). The science of bioinformatics, which is the melding of molecular biology with computer science, is essential to the use of genomic information in understanding human diseases and in the identification of new molecular targets for drug discovery. In recognition of this, many universities, government institutions and pharmaceutical firms have formed bioinformatics groups, consisting of computational biologists and bioinformatics computer scientists. Such groups will be key to unraveling the mass of information generated by large scale sequencing efforts underway in laboratories around the world.

10. ***Data mining:*** Data mining also called Knowledge-Discovery in Databases (KDD) or Knowledge-Discovery and Data Mining, is the process of automatically searching large volumes of data for patterns using tools such as classification, association rule mining, *clustering*, etc. It is non-trivial retrieval of implicit previously unknown and potentially useful information from various sources of data. The ever fast developing "Biopharmaceutical Industry" in the world is profusely using enormous quantum of databases that are virtually flooded with a plethora of vital information, retrieved from a variety of data mining methodologies such as:

- Annotated databases of disease profiles.
- Molecular pathways involved in dreadful human diseases.
- Quantitative structure activity relationship (QSAR).
- Precise chemical structures of combinatorial libraries of compound.
- Results of clinical trials of new molecules.

11. ***Neural networks in medicine:*** Artificial neural networks (ANN) is currently a 'hot' research area in medicine and it is believed that they will receive extensive application to biomedical systems in the next few years. At the moment, the research is mostly on modeling parts of the human body and recognizing diseases from various scans (e.g. cardiograms, CAT scans, ultrasonic scans, etc.). Neural networks are used experimentally to model the human cardiovascular system. Diagnosis can be achieved by building a model of the cardiovascular system of an individual and comparing it with the real time physiological measurements taken from the patient.

12. ***eHealth:*** The use of electronic technologies for exchanges of communication, interaction and decision-support regarding health is known as eHealth. This includes activities between providers, payers, regulators, communities, individual consumers and suppliers. eHealth is a wide and fast-growing field with many implications on how health care will be delivered in the future. Now, medical knowledge is an eagerly sought public commodity on the Internet. It seeks to explore ways to use emerging technologies to improve the health and well being of all people, including the underserved. eHealth is the use of emerging technologies, especially the Internet, to improve or enable health and health care.

eHealth, by making use of computers and telephone technologies, now makes it possible for an increasing range of medical services to be available locally. An example of a current telemedicine service is NHS Direct, has been extended to provide advice services to the whole country. In some parts of the country traditional hospital based outpatient clinics are being replaced with nurse-run clinics in GP practices. The nurses talk to the patient, collect all the information required on a computer and send this "electronic patient record" over the phone lines to a specialist. The specialist could be located anywhere. The specialist views the record (which could include photographs, X-rays, ECGs or other details as well as text) and uses his computer to send a report back to the patient's GP.

Minor injury units are now being linked to trauma centre. If you attend such a unit, the nurse can send X-rays over the phone line, for a radiologist to view and report back. She can also videoconference with a consultant in the trauma centre in order to discuss how to manage an injury. These sorts of approaches enable care and advice to be made available much more locally and often more quickly than the traditional approaches.The range of eHealth service is increasing rapidly and will become a core feature of the NHS. Access to expertise regardless of where you live should help to ensure fair provision of services for all. Access to good quality health information over the Internet, digital TV and via multimedia kiosks will give us all an opportunity to maintain better health.

NUMBER SYSTEM

Many number systems are used in digital technology. The most common are the decimal, binary, octal, and hexadecimal systems. The decimal system is clearly the most familiar to us because it is a tool that we use every day.

1. ***Decimal:*** Decimal has 10 digits which are 0, 1, 2, 3, 4, 5, 6, 7, 8, 9. Decimal is also called base 10 because it has 10 digits. The reason why people started counting in decimal is because it has 10 digits and we have 10 fingers and people used to use their fingers for counting.

A ***digit*** is a symbol given to an element of a number system. The *radix,* or base of a counting system is defined as the number of unique digits in a given number system.

2. ***Binary:*** Binary uses only 2 digits which are 0 and 1 and is also called base 2. Binary is what computers use for counting because inside a computer you get things that are like little switches that can be either off or on (0 or 1). A subscripted 2 is placed after a binary number so that it can be recognized as being a binary number like in the following example-$\mathbf{1001_2}$.

We already know that when we count we add 1 to the current number each time to get the next number. If we start at 0 and then add 1 we get 1. Now we have to add 1 to 1 but we have run out of digits because there are only 2 digits in binary. When we get to 9 in decimal and add 1 we first change the number to a 0 and then add 1 to the imaginary 0 to the left of it which gives us 10. If we apply this to binary then we change the 1 to 0 and then increase the imaginary 0 to the left of it which gives us 10 but this 10 is actually 2. The following sequence shows you how to count to 5 in binary-**0 1 10 11 100 101**.

3. ***Hexadecimal:*** The word hexadecimal is made up of 2 parts which are hex (6) and decimal (10). If you add 6 and 10 together you get 16 and that is how many digits there are in hexadecimal. Hexadecimal is sometimes called hex or base 16. To get 16 digits we have to use letters of the alphabet and those 16 digits are 0, 1, 2, 3, 4, 5, 6, 7, 8, 9, A, B, C, D, E, F. Hexadecimal is often used instead of binary numbers because just 2 hexadecimal digits can make the same numbers as 8 binary digits which in turn make up a byte. A subscripted 16 is used to show that a number is hexadecimal-$\mathbf{7F_{16}}$.

4. ***Octal:*** Octal uses 8 digits which are 0, 1, 2, 3, 4, 5, 6, 7 and is also called base 8. We use a subscripted 8 to show that a number is octal-$\mathbf{275_8}$.

Converting Binary to Decimal

The following steps are used to convert binary to decimal:

1. Get the last digit of the hex number; call this digit the ***current digit***.
2. Make a variable, let's call it ***power***. Set the value to 0.
3. Multiply the *current digit* with (2^*power*), store the result.
4. Increment *power* by 1.
5. Set the *current digit* to the previous digit of the hex number.
6. Repeat step 3 until all digits have been multiplied.
7. Sum the result of step 3 to get the answer number.

Example: Convert Binary **11101** to Decimal

Steps	Multiplication	Result
Start from the last digit, which is 1 multiply that digit with 2^0, note that the power	1 × (2^0)	1

Contd..

Contd..

of 0 of any number is always 1 1110**1** (current digit is in bold)		
Process the previous digit, which is 0, multiply that digit with the increasing power of 2 111**0**1 (current digit is in bold)	0 × (2^1)	0
Process the previous digit, which is 1, note that 2^2 means 2 × 2 11**1**01 (current digit is in bold)	1 × (2^2)	4
Process the previous digit, which is 1, note that 2^3 means 2 × 2 × 2 1**1**101 (current digit is in bold)	1 × (2^3)	8
Process the previous digit, which is 1, note that 2^4 means 2 × 2 × 2 × 2 **1**1101 (current digit is in bold)	1 × (2^4)	16
Here, we stop because there is no more digit to process		
This number comes from the **sum** of the results	**Answer**	**29**

Basically, this is the same as saying:

$$1 \times (2^4) + 1 \times (2^3) + 1 \times (2^2) + 0 \times (2^1) + 1 \times (2^0) \text{ or}$$

$$1*(16) + 1*(8) + 1*(4) + 0*(2) + 1*(1) = 29$$

Converting Decimal to Binary

To convert from decimal to binary, you can repeatedly divide the decimal by two until the result of the division is zero. Starting from the rightmost bit, write 1 if the division has a remainder, zero if it does not.

Example: Convert the 74_{10} into binary number system.

74 / 2 = 37 remainder 0;	0
37 / 2 = 18 remainder 1;	10
18 / 2 = 9 remainder 0;	010
9 / 2 = 4 remainder 1;	1010
4 / 2 = 1 remainder 0;	01010

2 / 2 = 1 remainder 0; 001010

1 / 2 = 0 remainder 1; 1001010

$$1001010_2 = 1 \times 2^6 + 1 \times 2^3 + 1 \times 2^1 = 64 + 8 + 2 = 74$$

Converting Decimal to Hexadecimal

The following steps are used to convert decimal to hexadecimal:

1. Divide the decimal number by 16. Treat the division as an integer division.
2. Write down the remainder (in hexadecimal).
3. Divide the result again by 16. Treat the division as an integer division.
4. Repeat step 2 and 3 until result is 0.
5. The hex value is the digit sequence of the remainders from the last to first.

Hexadecimal

0 1 2 3 4 5 6 7 8 9 A B C D E F

Decimal

0 1 2 3 4 5 6 7 8 9 10 11 12 13 14 15

Example: Convert the number **1128** decimal to hexadecimal.

Steps	*Division*	*Result*	*Remainder (in hexadecimal)*
Start by dividing the number by 16. In this case, 1128 divided by 16 is 70.5. So the integer division result is 70 (throw out anything after the decimal point). The remainder is (70.5–70) multiplied with 16; or (0.5 times 16), which is 8.	1128/16	70	**8**
Then, divide the result again by 16 (the number 70 on the division column comes from the previous result).	70 / 16	4	**6**

Contd..

Contd..

In this case, 70/16 = 4.375. So the integer division result is 4 (throw out anything after the decimal point). The remainder is (0.375 multiplied with 16, which is 6.			
Repeat. Note here that 4/16 = 0.25. So the integer division result is 0. The remainder is (0.25–0) multiplied with 16, which is 4.	4 / 16	0	4
Stop because the result is already 0 (0 divided by 16 will always be 0)			
Well, here is the answer. These numbers come from the Remainder column values **(read from bottom to top)**		**Answer**	**468**

Converting Hexadecimal to Binary

Convert the hexadecimal number to its equivalent decimal and then again convert the decimal number to its equivalent binary form. But we will use the shortcut method, where we directly write the equivalent binary of each, hexadecimal digit in 4 bits form. Before solving the example we give the binary representation of the decimal integers from 0 to 15 in 4 bits form and also the binary representation.

Decimal	*Binary*		*Hexadecimal*
0	0000	0	0
1	0001	1	1
2	0010	0	2
3	0011	1	3
4	0100	0	4
5	0101	1	5
6	0110	0	6

7	0111	1	7
8	1000	0	8
9	1001	1	9
10	1010	0	A
11	1011	1	B
12	1100	0	C
13	1101	1	D
14	1110	0	E
15	1111	1	F

Example: Convert 7F.2C to its equivalent binary form.

We write the equivalent binary of each hexadecimal digit in 4 bits form.

7	F	.	2	C
0111	1111	.	0010	1100

Equivalent binary is **01111111.00101100**

Converting Hexadecimal to Decimal

The following steps are used to convert hexadecimal to decimal:

1. Get the last digit of the hex number; call this digit the *current digit.*
2. Make a variable, let's call it *power*. Set the value to 0.
3. Multiply the *current digit* with (16^*power*), store the result.
4. Increment *power* by 1.
5. Set the *current digit* to the previous digit of the hex number.
6. Repeat from step 3 until all digits have been multiplied.
7. Sum the result of step 3 to get the answer number.

Example: Convert the number 1128 hexadecimal to decimal.

Steps	Multiplication	Result
Start from the last digit of the number. In this case, the number is 112**8**.	8 × (16^0)	8

Contd..

Contd..

The last digit of that number is **8**. Note that the power of 0 of any number is always 1.		
Process the previous, which is **2**. Multiply that number with an increasing power of 16.	2 × (16^1)	32
Process the previous digit, which is **1**, note that 16^2 means 16 × 16.	1 × (16^2)	256
Process the previous digit, which is **1**, note that 16^3 means 16 × 16 × 16.	1 × (16^3)	4096
Here, we stop because there is no more digit to process.		
This number comes from the **sum** of the results.	8 + 32 + 256 + 4096	**4392**

Once discerned, notice that the above process is essentially performing this calculation:

$$1 \times (16^3) + 1 \times (16^2) + 2 \times (16^1) + 8 \times (16^0) = 4392$$

Converting Binary to Hexadecimal

We convert the binary number to its equivalent decimal and then again convert the decimal number to its equivalent hexadecimal form.

In short-cut method we group the binary digit into 4 bits form beginning from right to the left, writing extras zeros on left side, if needed to make number of bits into a multiple of 4. Then we can directly write the equivalent decimal number for each group to get the equivalent octal number.

Example: Convert 1011011100.01001110_2 to its equivalent hexadecimal form.

We group the binary digits into 4 bits form beginning from right to the left, writing two extras zeros on the left side to make the number of bits a multiple of 4.

0010	1101	1100	.	0100	1110
2	D	C	.	4	E

Therefore, $1011011100.01001110_2 = 2DC4E_{16}$

Converting Binary to Octal

Each octal digit is represented by exactly three bits. This becomes obvious when you consider that the highest octal digit is seven, which can be represented in binary by 111_2.

To convert a binary number to octal, group the bits in groups of three starting from the rightmost bit and convert each triplet to its octal equivalent. For example,

$$100010011101_2 = (100\ 010\ 011\ 101)_2 = (4\ 2\ 3\ 5)_8 = 4235_8$$

Converting Octal to Binary

To convert an octal number to binary, simply write the equivalent bits for each octal number.

Example: Convert 752_8 to its equivalent decimal form.

$$752_8 = (111\ 101\ 010)_2 = 111101010_2$$

Converting Octal to Decimal

Any octal number can be converted to its equivalent decimal forms, exactly by the similar method we have used in case of binary to decimal conversion. But in this case the base or radix of the system is 8.

Example: Convert 223.12_8 to decimal form.

8^2	8^1	8^0	.	8^{-1}	8^{-2}
2	2	3		1	2

Therefore,

$$223.12_8 = (2 \times 8^2 + 2 \times 8^1 + 3 \times 8^0 + 1 \times 8^{-1} + 2 \times 8^{-2})_{10}$$
$$= (128 + 16 + 3 + 0.125 + 0.03125)_{10}$$
$$= 147.15625_{10}$$

BIT, BYTE, NIBBLE AND WORD

- ***Bit:*** Digital computers use the binary number system, which has two digits '0' and '1'. A binary digit is called a bit.
- ***Byte:*** A set of 8 bits is called a byte.
- ***Nibble:*** A set of 4 bits is called a nibble.
- ***Word:*** A group of bits which is used to represent a number in binary form or a computer instruction or one or more characters is known as word.

ALGORITHM AND FLOW CHART

Algorithm

An algorithm is a sequence of steps used to complete a task. An algorithm is a general solution of a problem which can be written as a verbal description of a precise, logical sequence of actions. It is the most fundamental concept in computer science. Algorithms may be presented:

- In words
- As a flow chart
- In structured code.

A computer program is an algorithm written for a computer in a special programming language. Structural diagrams and flow charts are tools that make the job of writing the algorithm easier, especially in complex programs. The final refined algorithm should use the same type of constructs as most programming languages. Once an algorithm is developed, the job of writing a program in a computer language is relatively easy; a simple translation of the algorithm steps into the proper statements for the language. Programs that follow the algorithmic logic will then be easy to implement. Languages that include the above types of include languages such as C, Pascal, and Fortran.

Flow Chart

A flow chart is a drawing that shows the steps in an algorithm. Flow charts describe algorithms and programs by means of a set of graphical symbols (Alternate Process, Process, Sub-process, Data, Decision, etc.) interconnected by arrows. The flow charts follow some strict rules for their visual appearance:

- A flow chart starts with a start symbol and ends with a stop symbol.
- The variables and constants must be initialized before use.
- Processes / Sub-processes has only one input and one output. Decisions have only one input and two outputs, correspondingly.
- The flows of symbol sequences are oriented vertically on the page. The main flow is directed from the upper side to the lower side of the column. Secondary backward flows are directed in the opposite direction. Horizontal expansions of flow charts are due to the secondary forward and backward flows.
- A flow chart should be placed on a single column and should not continue to another column.

Flow charts most often use five basic symbols. At times other symbols, usually computer symbols, are also used. Symbols are connected with arrows pointing in the direction of flow. The convention is for flow to move from left-to-right, or top-to-bottom if space necessitates.

1. ***Terminal:*** The oval is used to indicate the beginning and end points of a flow chart.
2. ***Input and output:*** The parallelogram is used to represent both input and output.
3. ***Assignment:*** A rectangle is used for assignment statements, or calculations.
4. ***Decision:*** The diamond is used for decisions. A Boolean condition (an expression that will evaluate to either true or false) is shown inside the diamond. There will always be 2 lines out of the diamond: one marked T (true) and one marked F (false). Evaluate the Boolean expression to determine which line to follow.
5. ***Procedures and functions:*** A procedure is a group of statements that can be grouped together logically to perform

a task such as printing a heading, calculating a bonus, or printing a check. A procedure is represented by a rectangle with a bar on each side. Each procedure within a program will have its own flow chart.

6. ***Connector:*** Used to connect to other pages in the flow chart or to other flow charts.
7. ***Flow lines:*** The directions of flow in a flow chart is indicated by arrows (→↑←↓) known as flow lines.

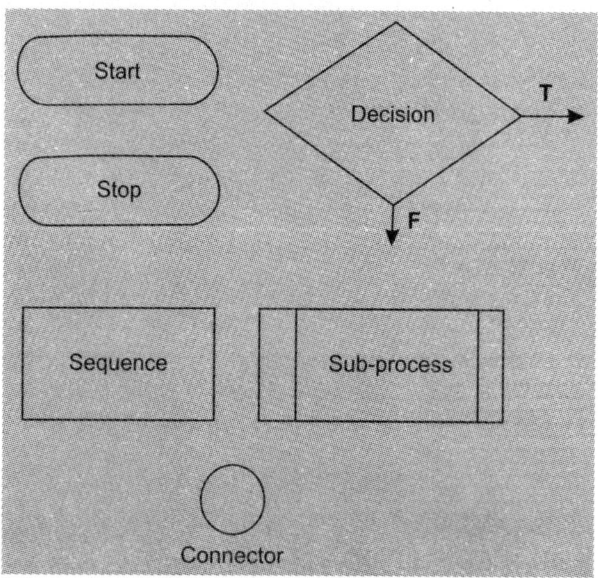

Examples

1. Develop an algorithm and draw a flow chart to find the largest of three distinct numbers X, Y, Z.

Algorithm:

- *Step 1:* Read X, Y, Z.
- *Step 2:* Initialize A = X.
- *Step 3:* If A > Y, then the value of A remains unaltered otherwise the previous value of A is replaced by Y.

- *Step 4:* If A > Z, then the value of A remain unaltered otherwise the previous of A is replaced by Z.
- *Step 5:* Print A, the largest of the three numbers and the algorithm is terminated.

Flow Chart: 1.1

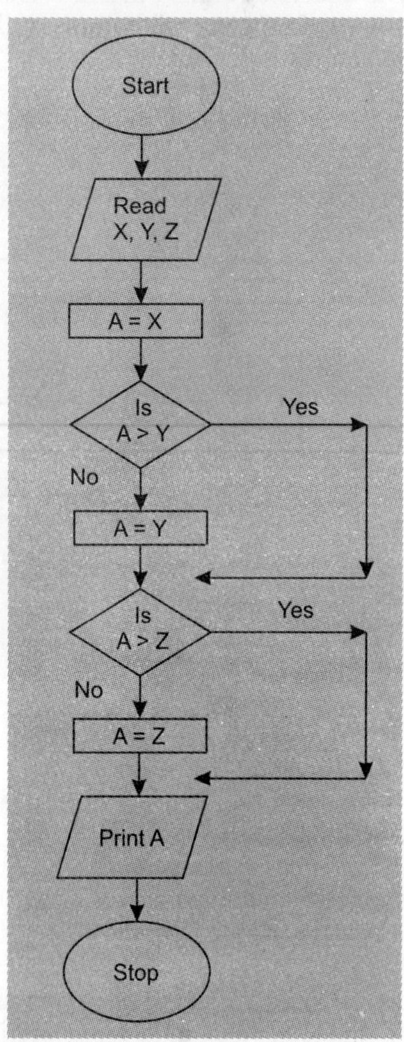

2. Develop an algorithm and draw a flow chart for computing surface area and volume of a sphere with a given radius.

Algorithm:

- *Step 1:* Read 'r', the radius of the sphere.
- *Step 2:* Compute the surface area and volume by using the formula: $S = 4 \pi r^2$, $V = (4/3) \pi r^3$.
- *Step 3:* Print the surface area and volume of the sphere and terminate the algorithm.

Flow Chart: 1.2

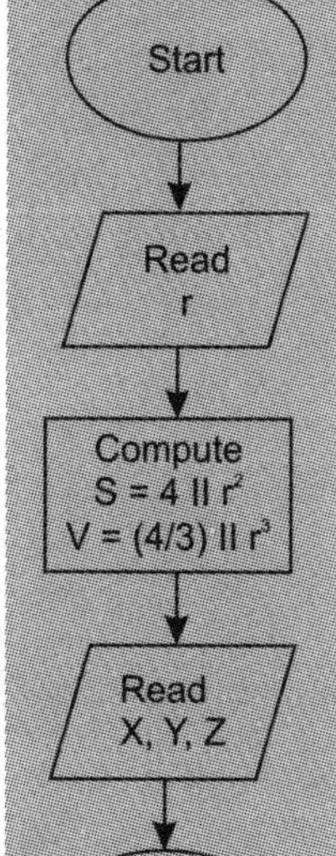

3. Design an algorithm and draw a flow chart to compute the factorial of a positive integer *n*.

Algorithm:

- *Step 1:* Read the positive integer *n* whose factorial is to be computed.

- *Step 2:* Initialize the product p = 1 and i = 1.
- *Step 3:* Compute p = p . i.
- *Step 4:* If i = n, print factorial of the number and terminate the algorithm, otherwise replaced i by i +1 and go to step 3.

Flow Chart: 1.3

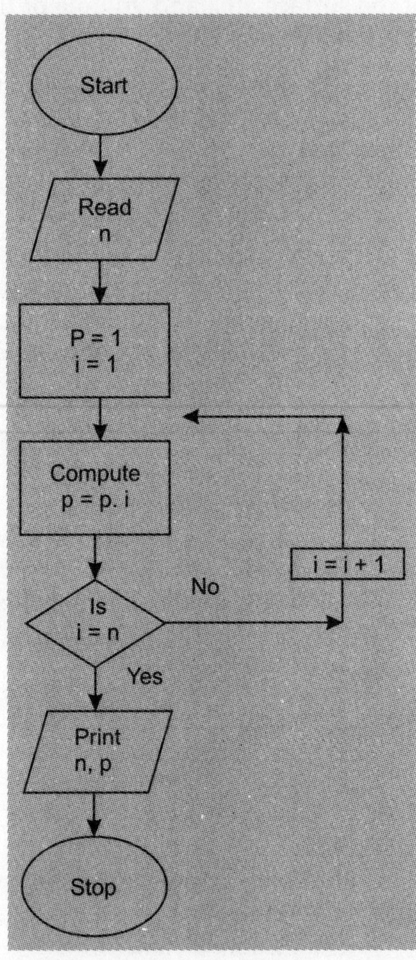

2 Computer Software

WHAT IS SOFTWARE?

A computer cannot do anything without instructions from the user. In order to do any specific job the user has to give a sequence of instructions to the computer. This set of instructions is called a computer program. Software refers to the set of computer programs, procedures that describe the programs, how they are to be used. We can say that it is the collection of programs, which increase the capabilities of the hardware. Software guides the computer at every step where to start and stop during a particular job. The process of software development is called programming. Software and hardware are complementary to each other. Both have to work together to produce meaningful result.

Types of Software

Computer software is normally classified into two broad categories—Application software and System software. Figure 2.1 shows the relation between hardware, software and user of computer system.

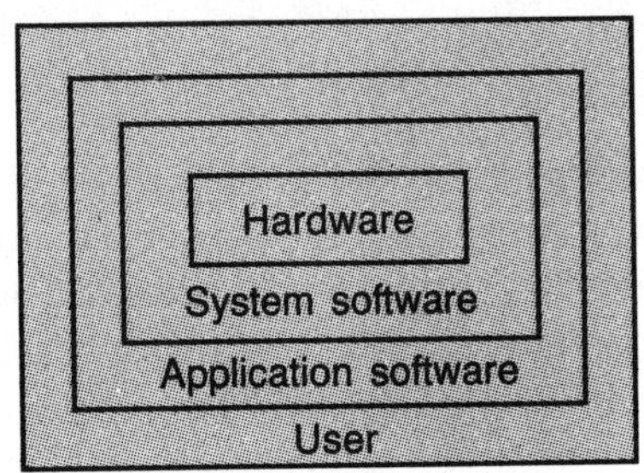

Fig. 2.1: Relation between hardware, software and user

1. ***Application software:*** Application software is a set of programs to carry out operations for a specific application. For example, payroll is an application software for an organization to produce pay slips as an output. Application software is useful for word processing, billing system, accounting, producing statistical report, analysis of numerous data in research, weather forecasting, etc. MS Word, Lotus 1-2-3 and dBASE III Plus are examples of application software's. Applications are software programs that perform specific tasks for us and following are some common ones:

- Activity management programs like calendars and address books.
- Word processing applications for creating documents that are attractively formatted.
- Spreadsheet applications for creating documents to manage and organize numerical data.
- Presentation applications for making slide shows.
- Graphics applications for creating pictures.
- Database applications for developing databases that can organize and retrieve large amounts of information.
- Communications programs like e-mail and faxing software for sending and receiving messages.
- Multimedia applications for creating video and music.
- Utilities for performing a variety of tasks that maintain or enhance the computer's operating system. Utility programs are generally fairly small. Each type has a specific job to do. Utility software has long been integrated into most major operating systems. Table 2.1 shows the descriptions of some utilities.

2. ***System software:*** An instruction is a set of programs that has to be fed to the computer for operation of computer system as a whole. When the computer is switched on the programs written in ROM is executed which activates different units of your computer and makes it ready for you to work on it. This set of program can be called system software. Therefore, system software may be defined as a set of one or more programs

Table 2.1: Examples of some utilities

Utility program	*Description*
Anti-virus applications	Protect computer from the damage that can be caused by viruses and similar programs.
Compression utilities	Make files smaller for storage (or sending over the Internet) and then return them to normal size.
Data recovery utilities	Attempt to restore data and files that have been damaged or accidentally deleted.
Disk defragmenters	Reorganize the data stored on disks so that it is more efficiently arranged.
Firewalls	Prevent outsiders from accessing your computer over a network such as the Internet.

designed to control the operation of computer system. The two types of system software are operating systems and language processors.

System software contrasts with application software, which are programs that enable the end-user to perform specific, productive tasks, such as word processing or image manipulation. System software are general programs designed for performing tasks such as controlling all operations required to move data into and out of the computer. It communicates with printers, card reader, disk, tapes, etc. monitor the use of various hardware like memory, CPU, etc. Also system software is essential for the development of applications software. System software allows application packages to be run on the computer with less time and effort. It is not possible to run application software without system software. So without system software it is impossible to operate the computer. Therefore, system software is any computer software which manages and controls computer hardware so that application software can perform a task.

Development of system software is a complex task and it requires extensive knowledge of computer technology. Computer manufactures build and supply this system software with the computer system. DOS, UNIX and WINDOWS are some of the widely used system software. Out of these UNIX is a multi-user operating system whereas DOS and WINDOWS are PC-based.

OPERATING SYSTEMS

An operating system (OS) is the software that manages the sharing of the resources of a computer and provides programmers with an interface used to access those resources. An operating system processes system data and user input, and responds by allocating and managing tasks and internal system resources as a service to users and programs of the system. At the foundation of all system software, an operating system performs basic tasks such as controlling and allocating memory, prioritizing system requests, controlling input and output devices, facilitating networking and managing file systems. Most operating systems come with an application that provides a user interface for managing the operating system, such as a command line interpreter or graphical user interface. The operating system forms a platform for other system software and for application software. There are different types of OS available, which require different types of hardware to run upon. The OPs are classified as single program OS, multiprogram OS, time sharing OS, real-time OS and multiprocessing OS (Table 2.2). The most commonly-used contemporary desktop and laptop (notebook) OS is Microsoft Windows. More powerful servers often employ Linux, FreeBSD, and other Unix-like systems. The Macintosh OS is commonly used on machines built by Apple Computer, Inc. There are only a few operating systems that are commonly used on microcomputers.

There are four main jobs an operating system is responsible for:

i. It provides a user interface (Fig. 2.2). The user interface lets you give commands to the OS.
ii. It gives instructions to the computer hardware, such as the printer and monitor.
iii. It manages the way in which the computer stores data and applications.

iv. It keeps track of different jobs. For example, if you are using both a spreadsheet and a word processing application at the same time, the OS will run both of these applications and let you switch back and forth between them.

Table 2.2: Types of operating systems

Type	*Characteristics*	*Example*
Single program operating system	Single user OS, only one program can be supported and executed by it at any point of time.	MS-DOS
Multiprogramming operating system XP	Supports multiprogramming, more than one user can be supported and executed by it at the same time.	UNIX, Windows 95, 98, 2000, LINUX
Time sharing operating system	The OS uses time sharing technique. Each active user program is given a fair share of CPU time, if time elapses or an I/O operation is reques-ted, CPU shifts over to the next job waiting and the previous program is put to wait or handed over to I/O manager. The active programs are scheduled for execution using certain job scheduling techniques.	---
Real time operating system	The jobs have fixed deadlines and the jobs have to be comple-ted within their deadlines	LINUX
Multiprocessing operating system	Capable of handling more than one processor, as the jobs have to be executed on more than one processor.	---
Network operating system	Developed to control networks. Supports communication between the users and system.	Novell Netware, Windows NT

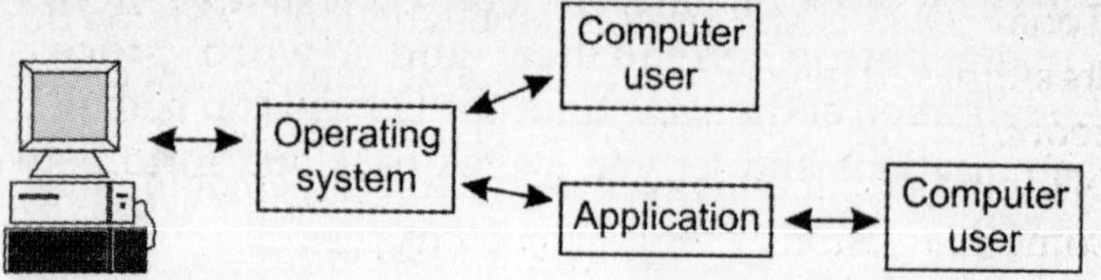

Fig. 2.2: Operating system act as an interface between computer hardware and user

Operating systems, such as Microsoft Windows, Mac OS X or Linux are prominent examples of system software.

Microsoft Disk Operating System (MS-DOS)

MS-DOS is an operating system commercialised by Microsoft. It was the most commonly used member of the DOS family of operating systems and was the dominant operating system for the PC compatible platform during the 1980s. It has gradually been replaced on consumer desktop computers by various generations of the Windows operating system. MS-DOS was originally released in 1981 and had eight major versions released before Microsoft stopped development in 2000. It was the key product in Microsoft's growth from a programming languages company to a diverse software development firm. It also provided the platform on which early versions of Windows ran.

- MS-DOS employs a command line interface and a batch scripting facility via its command interpreter, COMMAND.COM. MS-DOS was designed so users could easily substitute a different command line interpreter, for example 4DOS.
- MS-DOS was not designed to be a multi-user or multitasking operating system, but many attempts were made to add these capabilities.
- There were computers that used MS-DOS but could not run all the software that an IBM-Compatible machine could. An example is the Morrow Pivot, which used MS-DOS but was not IBM-Compatible.

- Today, DOS is still used in embedded x86 systems due to its simple architecture, and minimal memory and processor requirements. The command line interpreter of Windows NT, cmd.exe, maintains most of the same commands and some compatibility with DOS batch files.

Microsoft Windows

Microsoft Windows is the name of several families of software operating systems by Microsoft (Table 2.3). Microsoft first introduced an operating environment named Windows in November 1985 as an add-on to MS-DOS in response to the growing interest in graphical user interfaces (GUIs). Microsoft Windows eventually came to dominate the world's personal computer market, overtaking Mac OS, which had been introduced previously. Windows has about 91.80% of the client operating system market. The current client version of Windows is Windows Vista. The current server version of Windows is Windows Server 2003. The successor to Windows Server 2003, Windows Server 2008, is currently being beta tested.

a. *16-bit windows versions:* The early versions of Windows were often thought of as just graphical user interfaces, mostly because they ran on top of MS-DOS and used it for file system services. Unlike MS-DOS, Windows allowed users to execute multiple graphical applications at the same time, through cooperative multitasking. Finally, Windows implemented an elaborate, segment-based, software virtual memory scheme, which allowed it to run applications larger than available memory: Code segments and resources were swapped in and thrown away when memory became scarce, and data segments moved in memory when a given application had relinquished processor control, typically waiting for user input. 16-bit Windows versions include Windows 1.0 (1985), Windows 2.0 (1987).

b. *Hybrid 16/32-bit windows versions:* Windows 3.0 (1990) and Windows 3.1 (1992) improved the design, mostly because of virtual memory and loadable virtual device drivers (VxDs)

Table 2.3: Timeline of various versions of windows

Product name	*Year of release*
Windows 1.01	November 1985
Windows 2.03	November 1987
Windows 2.11	March 1989
Windows 3.0	May 1990
Windows 3.1	March 1992
Windows for Workgroups 3.1	October 1992
Windows NT 3.1	July 1993
Windows for Workgroups 3.11	December 1993
Windows 3.2 (released in simplified Chinese only)	January 1994
Windows NT 3.5	September 1994
Windows NT 3.51	May 1995
Windows 95	August 1995
Windows NT 4.0	July 1996
Windows 98	June 1998
Windows 98 SE	May 1999
Windows 2000	February 2000
Windows Me	September 2000
Windows XP	October 2001
Windows XP 64-bit Edition 2003	March 2003
Windows Server 2003	April 2003
Windows XP Professional x64 Edition	April 2005
Windows Fundamentals for Legacy PCs	July 2006
Windows Vista	November 2006 (volume licensing)/January 2007 (retail)
Windows Home Server	July 2007
Windows Server 2008	February 2008 (planned)
Windows 7 (code-named Blackcomb, then Vienna)	2010 or later (planned)

which allowed them to share arbitrary devices between multitasked DOS windows. For Windows 3.0, Microsoft also rewrote critical operations from C into assembly, making this release faster Windows 95 introduced Long File Names, reducing the 8.3 file name DOS environment to the role of a boot loader. MS-DOS was now bundled with Windows; this notably made it (partially) aware of long file names when its utilities were run from within Windows. The most important novelty was the possibility of running 32-bit multi-threaded preemptively multitasked graphical programs. Microsoft's next OS was Windows 98; there were two versions of this (the first in 1998 and the second, named "Windows 98 Second Edition", in 1999). In 2000, Microsoft released Windows Me (Me standing for Millennium Edition), which used the same core as Windows 98 but adopted the visual appearance of Windows 2000, as well as a new feature called System Restore, allowing the user to set the computer's settings back to an earlier date.

c. *32-bit windows versions:* The first release was Windows NT 3.1, which was followed by NT 3.5 (1994), NT 3.51 (1995), and NT 4.0 (1996); NT 4.0 was the first in this line to implement the "Windows 95" user interface. Microsoft then moved to combine their consumer and business operating systems. Their first attempt, Neptune was cancelled and replaced with a new project, Whistler, which later became Windows XP, which came in both home and professional versions and improved backwards compatibility. Then, Windows Server 2003 brought Windows Server up to date with Windows XP. Since then, a new version, Windows Vista was released and Windows Server 2008 will bring Windows Server up to date with Windows Vista. Windows CE, Microsoft's offering in the mobile and embedded markets, is also a true 32-bit operating system that offers various services for all sub-operating workstations.

d. *64-bit windows versions:* Versions of NT from 3.1 to 4.0 were 64-bit processors, although the operating system treated them as 32-bit processors. Itanium versions of Windows XP and Windows Server 2003 were then released. Windows Vista is the first end-user version of Windows that Microsoft has released simultaneously in 32-bit and x64 editions. The modern

64-bit Windows family comprises AMD64/Intel64 versions of Windows Vista, and Windows Server 2003, in both Itanium and x64 editions.

Unix

Unix operating systems are widely used in both servers and workstations. The Unix environment and the client-server program model were essential elements in the development of the Internet and the reshaping of computing as centered in networks rather than in individual computers. Both Unix and the C programming language were developed by ATandT and distributed to government and academic institutions, causing both to be ported to a wider variety of machine families than any other operating system. As a result, Unix became synonymous with "open systems". As of 2007, the owner of the trademark UNIX is The Open Group, an industry standards consortium.

Unix was designed to be portable, multi-tasking and multi-user in a time-sharing configuration. Unix systems are characterized by various concepts: The use of plain text for storing data; a hierarchical file system; treating devices and certain types of inter-process communication (IPC) as files; and the use of a large number of small programs that can be strung together through a command line interpreter using pipes, as opposed to using a single monolithic program that includes all of the same functionality.

Under Unix, the "operating system" consists of many of these utilities along with the master control program, the kernel. The kernel provides services to start and stop programs, handle the file system and other common "low level" tasks that most programs share, and, perhaps most importantly, schedules access to hardware to avoid conflicts if two programs try to access the same resource or device simultaneously.

Linux

Linux is a Unix-like computer operating system. Linux is a widely ported operating system. The name "Linux" comes from the Linux kernel, started in 1991 by Linus Torvalds. The system's utilities and libraries come from the GNU operating system, started in 1983 by Richard Stallman. Linux is one of the most prominent examples of free software and open source development; typically all underlying source code can be freely modified, used, and redistributed by anyone. Predominantly known for its use in servers, Linux is supported by corporations such as Dell, Hewlett-Packard, IBM, Novell, Oracle Corporation, Red Hat, and Sun Microsystems. It is used as an operating system for a wide variety of computer hardware, including desktop computers, supercomputers, video game systems, such as the PlayStation 2 and PlayStation 3, several arcade games, and embedded devices such as mobile phones and routers. Linux is a modular Unix-like operating system. Linux uses a monolithic kernel, the Linux kernel, which handles process control, networking, and peripheral and file system access. Device drivers are integrated directly with the kernel. The GNU (General Public Licence) userland is an important part of most Linux systems, providing the shell and Unix tools which carry out many basic operating system tasks. On top these tools form a Linux system with a graphical user interface that can be used, usually running in the X Window System. Linux can be controlled by one or more of a text-based command line interface (CLI), graphical user interface (GUI) (usually the default for desktop), through controls on the device itself (common on embedded machines). As well as those designed for general purpose use on desktops and servers, distributions may be specialized for different purposes including: Computer architecture support, embedded systems, stability, security, localization to a specific region or language, targeting of specific user groups, support for real-time applications, or commitment to a given desktop environment.

Mac OS X

Mac OS X is a line of graphical operating systems developed, marketed, and sold by Apple Inc., the latest of which is pre-loaded on all currently shipping Macintosh computers. Mac OS X is the successor to the original Mac OS, which had been

Apple's primary operating system since 1984. Unlike its predecessors, Mac OS X is a Unix-based operating system built on technology that had been developed at NeXT through the second half of the 1980s until Apple purchased the company in early 1997.

The first version released was Mac OS X Server 1.0 in 1999, and a desktop-oriented version, Mac OS X v10.0 followed in March 2001. Since then, five more distinct "end-user" and "server" versions have been released, most recently Mac OS X v10.5 in October 2007. Releases of Mac OS X are named after big cats, for example, Mac OS X v10.5 is usually referred to by Apple and users as "Leopard".

LANGUAGE PROCESSORS/TRANSLATORS

A program written by user in language other than low-level language is called source code or source program. When source program is translated into machine language it is called object code or object program. Computer has a translator, which translates our language into computer's language and after processing vice versa. There are three types of translators:

1. ***Assembler:*** This language processor converts the program written in assembly language into machine language. Assemblers are generally simpler to write than compilers for high-level languages. Most assemblers also include macro-facilities for performing textual substitution, e.g. to generate common short sequences of instructions to run inline, instead of in a subroutine.

2. ***Compiler:*** A compiler is also used to translate HLL program into machine language but the conversion manner is different than interpreter. It is called compiler because it compiles machine language instructions for every program instructions of higher-level language. It converts the entire HLL program in one go, and reports all the errors of the program along with line numbers. After all the errors are removed, the program is recompiled, and after that the compiler is not needed in memory as the object program is available. Compilers are faster than interpreters and are more popular. A compiler can

translate only those source programs, which have been written, in that language for which the compiler is meant for. For example, FORTRAN compiler will not compile source code written in COBOL language. Object program generated by compiler is machine dependent. It means programs compiled for one type of machine will not run in another type. Therefore, every type of machine must have its personal compiler for a particular language.

3. ***Interpreter:*** It converts the entire high-level language (HLL) program into machine language by converting and executing it line by line. If there is any error in any line, it reports it at the same time and program execution cannot resume until error is rectified. It must always be present in computer memory every time the program is executed; as everytime the program is run, it is first interpreted and then executed. It differs from compiler, which translate the entire source program into machine code and does involve in its execution. The advantage of interpreter compared to compiler is its fast response to changes in source program (Table 2.4). It eliminates the need for a separate compilation after changes to each program. Interpreters are easy to write and do not require large memory in computer.

Table 2.4: Comparison between interpreter and compiler

Interpreter	*Compiler*
It converts source code into object code online at a time.	It converts the whole source code into object code in one go.
Errors for one line are displayed only when errors for previous lines are fully removed or corrected.	Errors for the whole source code are displayed together.
Object code cannot be stored and executed at a later stage.	Object code once generated, can be saved and reused.
Throughout the program execution, the interpreter is required to be loaded in the main memory.	Once the object code has been formed, we no longer require the software for compiler to execute the program.
It is more time consuming, e.g. BASICA for BASIC language.	It is less time consuming, e.g. TURBOC for C++.

The disadvantage of interpreter is that it is time-consuming method because each time a statement in a program is executed then it is first translated.

PROGRAMMING LANGUAGES

A computer program is a set of instructions that directs a computer to perform the tasks necessary to process data into information. A program written for a computer is known as software. A computer programmer write these instructions using a programming language, which are set of words, symbols and codes used to create instructions a computer can process and execute. The program is stored in RAM. The CPU takes one instruction of the program at a time from RAM and executes it. The instructions are executed one by one in sequence and finally produce the desired result. A programming language is an artificial language that can be used to control the behavior of a machine, particularly a computer. Programming language contains the series of commands that create software. A particular language is suitable for a particular program. There are two major types of programming languages—Low Level Languages (LLL) and High Level Languages (HLL). Low level languages are further divided in to Machine language and Assembly language.

Machine Language

The only language that the computer directly understands is machine language, also called first generation language. No conversion is to be done as the computer can directly apprehend the code. Machine language use a series of binary digits (0s and 1s) that correspond to the on and off electrical states of a computer. 0 was used to represent OFF state and 1 for ON state. An instruction written in binary form has at least two parts:

- *Op-code:* It specifies the operation or function to be performed.
- *Operand:* It tells the computer the data or address of the data/instruction that is to be processed.

For example, a program instruction may look like this:

1011000111101

It is not an easy language for you to learn because of its difficult to understand. It is efficient for the computer but very inefficient for programmers. It is considered to the first generation language. It is also difficult to debug the program written in this language.

Advantage

The only advantage is that program of machine language run very fast because no translation program is required for the CPU.

Disadvantages

- It is very difficult to program in machine language. The programmer has to know details of hardware to write program.
- The programmer has to remember a lot of codes to write a program, which results in program errors.
- It is difficult to debug the program.

Assembly Language

Assembly languages were first developed in the 1950s, when they were referred to as second generation programming languages. They eliminated much of the error-prone and time-consuming first generation programming needed with the earliest computers, freeing the programmer from tedium such as remembering numeric codes and calculating addresses. They were once widely used for all sorts of programming. With an assembly language instructions are written using abbreviations and codes. It implements a symbolic representation of the numeric machine codes and other constants needed to program a particular CPU architecture. This representation is usually defined by the hardware manufacturer, and is based on abbreviations (called mnemonics) that help the programmer remember individual instructions, registers, etc. An assembly language is thus specific to a certain physical or virtual computer architecture. The programmer can refer to storage locations with symbolic addresses.

Examples of mnemonics:

- ADD is mnemonic for addition.
- SUB is mnemonic for substraction.
- MUL is mnemonic for multiplication.

A set of assembly language commands would somewhat look like:

Command	*Action*
INP A	Inputs a number in memory location alloted to A.
INP B	Inputs another number in memory location alloted to B.
LDA A	Loads the contents of A is an accumulator which is a special memory used to temporarily store intermediate results.
ADD B	Add the contents of B to accumulator.
STA C	Stores the contents of accumulator in memory location alloted to C.
OUT C	Print the contents of C.

Advantages

- The symbolic programming of Assembly Language is easier to understand and saves a lot of time and effort of the programmer.
- It is easier to correct errors and modify program instructions.
- Assembly Language has the same efficiency of execution as the machine level language. Because this is one-to-one translator between assembly language program and its corresponding machine language program.

Disadvantage

One of the major disadvantage is that assembly language is machine dependent. A program written for one computer might not run in other computers with different hardware configuration.

High-Level Language

The term "high-level language" does not imply that the language is always superior to low-level programming languages—in fact, in terms of the depth of knowledge of how computers work required to productively program in a given language, the inverse may be true. Rather, "high-level language" refers to the higher level of abstraction from machine language. Rather than dealing with registers, memory addresses and call stacks, high-level languages deal with variables, arrays and complex arithmetic or boolean expressions. In addition, they have no opcodes that can directly compile the language into machine code, unlike low-level languages like assembly language. Other features such as string handling routines, object-oriented language features and file input/output may also be present.

Higher-level languages are problem-oriented languages because the instructions are suitable for solving a particular problem. For example, COBOL (Common Business Oriented Language) is mostly suitable for business oriented language where there is very little processing and huge output. There are mathematical oriented languages like FORTRAN (Formula Translation) and BASIC (Beginner's All Purpose Symbolic Instruction Code) where very large processing is required. Thus a problem-oriented language designed in such a way that its instruction may be written more like the language of the problem. For example, businessmen use business term and scientists use scientific terms in their respective languages (Table 2.5).

Advantages

1. Higher-level languages (HLLs) are simple languages that use English and mathematical symbols like +, –, %, /, etc. for its program construction.
2. HLLs are easy to learn and use.
3. Programs are portable.
4. Writing of program in HLL is easier and faster than assembly languages.
5. It has easier documentation.
6. Allocation of memory locations for instructions and data is done by computer.

7. Modification in program could be done easily.
8. Programs in HLL are independent of the structure of computer.
9. HLL are problem-oriented rather than machine-oriented.
10. Number of instructions given to computer are reduced in HLL compared with machine or assembly language.

Disadvantages

1. Speed of operating HLL is slow.
2. Extensive hardware support is required.
3. Computation time is more with machine language.
4. One has to learn specific rules for writing programs in a particular language.
5. A program in HLL occupies large memory.
6. A compilier is to be provided for converting HLL into machine language.

Table 2.5: HLLs used for various purposes

Scientific languages	*Commercial languages*	*Special purpose languages*	*Multipurpose languages*
ALGOL	PL/I	IQL	PASCAL
BASIC	COBOL	APL 360	PL/I
PASCAL		CORAL-66	BASIC
COMAL		LOGO	
FORTRAN		PILOT	
ADA		SNOBOL	

General Description of Some High-Level Languages

1. ***Basic:*** This language was developed by John Kemeny and Thomas Kurtz at Dormouth college in the year 1960. This is a very simple language and taught to begineers in computer programming. It was standardized by ANSI in the year 1978. Mostly this is used for scientific or mathematical operations. Most microcomputers have a BASIC interpreter which translates each line of BASIC into machine code instruction.

IBM-PC, uses latest interpreter of BASIC called GWBASIC. This advanced interpreter of BASIC has a lot of other facilities like graphic designing. Presently advanced versions of this language are available and used in variety of fields such as Buisness, Science and Engineering.

2. ***FORTRAN:*** This language was developed by IBM in 1954, it was the first major scientific programming language. This has been modified since then many times and these versions were given names like FORTRAN II, FORTRAN III, FORTRAN IV. Its syntax is very rigid. Main use of FORTRAN is in engineering and scientific calculations as there are almost all symbols used in aforesaid applications (Table 2.6).

3. ***COBOL:*** This language was developed by CODASYL in the year 1960. COBOL is file oriented language and similar to English language. It is a useful language to solve buisness problems. COBOL is a powerful language for various institutions like banks, insurance, manufacturing industries, public utilities, etc. Many enhanced versions (MF COBOL, RM COBOL, MS COBOL, CICS COBOL) have been released to optimize the performance of specific machines.

4. ***PASCAL:*** This language was developed by Niklaus Wirth at University of Zurich and has been named after Blaize Pascal, the great French mathematician. This language was developed as a simple language for the purpose of teaching and constructing compilers and interpreters. It was derived from ALGOL-60. PASCAL is block structured language. It supports structured programming in a simple manner.

5. ***C-language:*** This language was developed in 1972 by Bell Laboratories in USA. Widely used to develop commercial applications. UNIX operating system is written in C. C++ is an extension to C-language. BORLAND C++ and TURBO C++ are its new transformation.

6. ***C++:*** This language was developed by Bjarne Stroustrup in early 1980s. It is the superset of C that supports object-oriented features. This language is used effectively in developing system software as well as application software.

7. ***LOGO:*** This is a very simple language and has been developed for school going kids. This is basically a graphic-based language and the kids can do the work of graphics in it.

8. ***Java:*** Originally it was called Oak. This general-purpose language was developed by Sun Microsyatems of USA in 1991. Java was designed for the development of software for consumer electronic devices. Java came out to be simple reliable, portable and a powerful language. Like C++ Java is an object-oriented language.The capabilities and functionalities of Java has brought this language to the forefront of the programming world. Java's rapidly growing popularity is due to the web. Sun's Java is used to create client/server applications on intranets and the web.

Table 2.6: Applications of some high-level languages

Language	*Full name*	*Use*
FORTRAN	Formula Translation	Used for scientific and mathematical calculations.
BASIC	Beginner's All Purpose Symbolic Instruction Code	Used by begineers.
PASCAL	Named after the French Physicist Blaise Pascal	A general purpose language and best suited for small computers.
COBOL	Common Business Oriented Language	Commonly used for large data handling purposes in commercial and business application.
LOGO	Logic Oriented Graphic Oriented	Used for graphics.
C	--	Used for system programming.
C++	Superset of C language, which supports Object Oriented Programming Structure (OOPS)	Used in developing system software as well as application software.
Java	Originally called Oak	Development of softwares.

Microsoft Windows

INTRODUCTION

Microsoft Windows is a GUI based operating system that adheres to the features of a good GUI. The Windows operating system uses both mouse and keyboard as input devices. Microsoft Windows is the application that runs all of your programs. Windows stores files in items called folders on different drives.

1. ***Drives:*** Drives are devices used to store data. Most computers have at least two drives: A hard drive C:\ (which is the main means of storage) and a floppy drive (which stores smaller volumes of data (1.44 Mb) on 3.5" disks—floppy disks). The hard drive is typically designated the C:\ drive and the floppy drive is typically designated the A:\ drive. If you have an additional floppy drive, it is typically designated the B:\ drive. You will also have network drives on your computer, depending on authorization and rights of each user. This drives will typically be labeled F:\ or H:\ or G:\

2. ***Folders:*** Folders are used to organize the data stored on your drives. Think of your drives as filing cabinets. You want to sort your filing cabinets with folders that store different files. The files that make up a program are stored together in their own set of folders. You will want to organize the files you create in folders. You will probably want to store files of a similar kind in a single folder.

3. ***Directory:*** A Directory is the path given to a folder on a drive. For example, a text file called Phone Numbers is located in the My Documents directory on the C:\ drive. It would, therefore, read "C:\My Documents\PhoneNumbers.txt"

4. ***File extensions:*** File Extensions are the ending letters associated with a file and an application that it can be manipulated in. This way Windows 98 knows to tell which program to open the file you want to manipulate. For example, a text file has an extension of .txt, so a text file created in Notepad called Phone Numbers would look like this PhoneNumbers.txt ... You do not have to assign a file extension to a file that you create. The program you use will automatically do this for you. All you need to do is give it a filename. Some other common extensions are as follows:

.doc	=	Microsoft word document
.xls	=	Microsoft excel document
.ppt	=	Microsoft powerpoint presentation
.mdb	=	Microsoft access database
.bmp	=	Windows bitmap picture
.wav	=	Sound file
.html or .htm	=	Internet document

5. ***Icon:*** An icon is a graphic image. Icons help you execute commands quickly. Commands tell the computer what you want the computer to do. To execute a command by using an icon, double-click on the icon.

FEATURES OF WINDOWS XP

Windows XP provides the tools you need to work and play in today's high-speed communications environment. Your toolbox includes system tools that help you set and adjust system resources, users and user groups, and scheduled system tasks. Accessories help you get the job done, no matter what the job is. You can create documents and images, calculate figures, schedule your time, and have online meetings with co-workers. When it's time to enjoy some music, browse the Internet, or play a few games. Your communications and entertainment tools will help you relax.

Among the new features available in Windows XP, there are new security tools that you can use to help keep your computer more secure, and new technologies that run in the background, making your computer run more efficiently and reliably.

Windows XP has improved upon security, including the new security center, which allows you to check the status of the important security elements on your computer—Windows firewall, automatic updates, and virus protection software, making it easier for you to understand how to keep your computer better protected against viruses and other security threats. Performance is at an all-time high. You can now use more programs at the same time and they will run faster than ever. Windows XP is dependable and stable, so you can always rely on the performance and effectiveness of your computer.

Improvements have also been made on many features that make using your computer more effective and useful. For example, you can use Remote Desktop to access your work computer and its resources from home, and to view files and documents on your computer's desktop from a co-worker's computer. With NetMeeting you can have virtual meetings with anyone, anywhere, and you can participate in discussions using audio, video, or chat. Getting help has never been easier. With Remote Assistance, you just send an invitation (either in e-mail or Instant Messenger) to your favorite computer expert or support professional, and they can help you fix a problem from their location. Windows XP provides extensive online help for all operating system features, as well as a digital tour to help you discover the possibilities awaiting you.

WINDOWS DESKTOP

When starting your computer, the desktop is the first thing you. The desktop is the area you work in. Windows XP combines a bright, fresh new look with a simple-to-use design. The desktop and taskbar are less cluttered. The Start menu provides easier access to your programs. And there are more options for customizing your desktop environment.

The on-screen work area on which windows, icons, menus, and dialog boxes appear. You can add shortcuts to your Desktop for frequently used programs, files, and folders. To add a shortcut to your Desktop, right-click a blank area on your Desktop, point to **New**, and then click **Shortcut**.

Name	*Picture*	*Description*
Taskbar	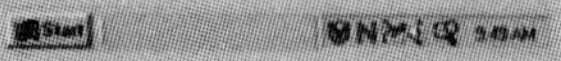	The taskbar is usually located on the bottom of the desktop. The start button, active program buttons, and the system tray are located on the Taskbar.
System Tray	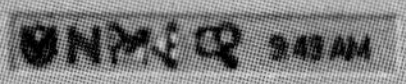	You will typically find the system tray in the lower right hand corner of the Windows Desktop. The system tray contains a display of the current computer time, and the icons representing the programs activated when Windows first starts up.
My Computer	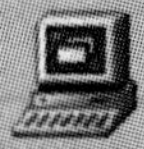	My Computer icon provides access to the different parts on your computer. You can access the different drives (Hard Drive, Floppy Drive, Network Drives) inside My Computer. My Computer shows you the contents of your floppy disk, hard disk, CD-ROM drive, and network drives. You can also search for and open files and folders, and gain access to options in Control Panel.
Recycle Bin	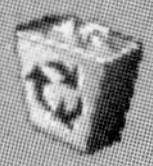	When you delete an object, Windows 98 sends it to the Recycle Bin. You can restore objects that are located in the Recycle Bin or you can permanently delete them by right clicking on the Recycle Bin and select Empty Recycle Bin.

My Documents	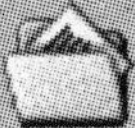	The My Documents folder is nothing more than a regular folder that resides on your Windows Desktop. However, it offers an easy-to-reach location where you can store and retrieve important data, and the icon is always available in Explorer Windows and on the desktop.
Internet Explorer	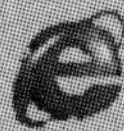	The Internet Explorer icon launches the Internet Explorer browser. The Internet Explorer browser is what you will use to access the Internet and the World Wide Web.
Shortcut Icons	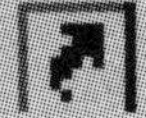	Icons with an arrow in the lower left corner (picture on left) are shortcut icons. If you double click on them they will open up the program that the icon displays on it.

1. ***Themes:*** You have no doubt already noticed the new look of the taskbar, Start button, dialog boxes, and other desktop elements. This new look is part of a theme, which is intended to both unify and clear up your desktop. You can switch themes, customize a theme, or revert to the Windows Classic look.

2. ***Start menu:*** The new Start menu is smarter and provides you with more customization options. It shows you who is logged on. It automatically adds the most frequently used programs to the top-level menu. It enables you to move any programs you want to the Start menu. Items such as the My Pictures and My Documents folders and Control Panel are also now available from the top level.

3. ***Taskbar:*** When many document and program windows are open, taskbar grouping creates more available space on the taskbar. For example, if you have 10 windows open and three of them are Wordpad documents, the three Wordpad

document taskbar buttons will group together into one button named "Wordpad". Click this button and then click one of the documents to view it. To reduce taskbar clutter, icons in the notification area (next to the clock) are hidden from view when they have not been used in a while. If an icon becomes hidden, click the arrow (‹) to temporarily display the hidden icons. If you click one of these icons, it is displayed again.

4. ***Control panel:*** Control Panel includes a new view- Category view that groups together similar items. Classic view continues to display all of the items individually. Choose the view-Category view or Classic view that works best for you.

5. ***Keep your desktop clean:*** Use the Desktop Cleanup Wizard to remove shortcuts that you do not use from your desktop. The wizard automatically runs every 60 days, or you can start it yourself whenever you want.

START MENU

The new Start menu is smarter and provides you with more customization options. It shows you who is logged on. It automatically adds the most frequently used programs to the top-level menu. It enables you to move any programs you want to the Start menu. Items such as the My Pictures and My Documents folders and Control Panel are also now available from the top level.

Clicking Start displays a menu that lets you easily access the most useful items on your computer. You can click Help and Support to learn how to use Windows, obtain troubleshooting information, receive support, and more. Clicking All Programs opens a list of programs currently installed on your computer.

The list of programs on the Start menu is divided into two parts: The programs displayed above the separator line (also known as the pinned items list) and the programs displayed below the separator line (also known as the most frequently used programs list). The programs on the pinned items list remain there and are always available for you to click to start them. You can add programs to the pinned items list.

Programs are added to the most frequently used programs list when you use them. Windows has a default number of programs that are displayed on the most frequently used programs list. When that number of programs is reached, the programs you have not opened recently are replaced by the programs you used last. You can change the default number of programs displayed on the most frequently used programs list. You can customize the Start menu by adding a folder called My Recent Documents that contains the files you opened most recently.

MY COMPUTER

My Computer shows you the contents of your floppy disk, hard disk, CD-ROM drive, and network drives. You can also search for and open files and folders, and gain access to options in Control Panel to modify your computer's settings. To open My Computer, click Start, and then click My Computer.

You can use My Computer Information to view detailed information about your computer's hardware and software, examine diagnostic information, or view computer information on another computer.

To see what is on your computer:

1. Open My Computer.

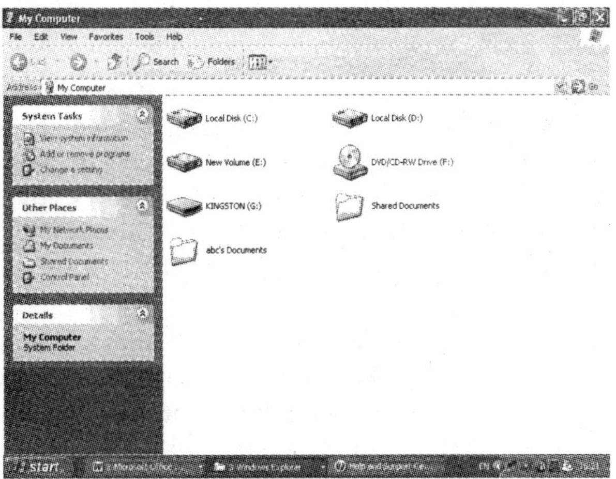

2. To see what is on your hard drive, under Hard Disk Drives, double-click the drive you want to see. or

   To find a file or folder on a floppy disk, CD-ROM, or other media, under Devices with Removable Storage, double-click the item you want to see. or

   To find a file in a folder, under Files Stored on This Computer, double-click a folder.

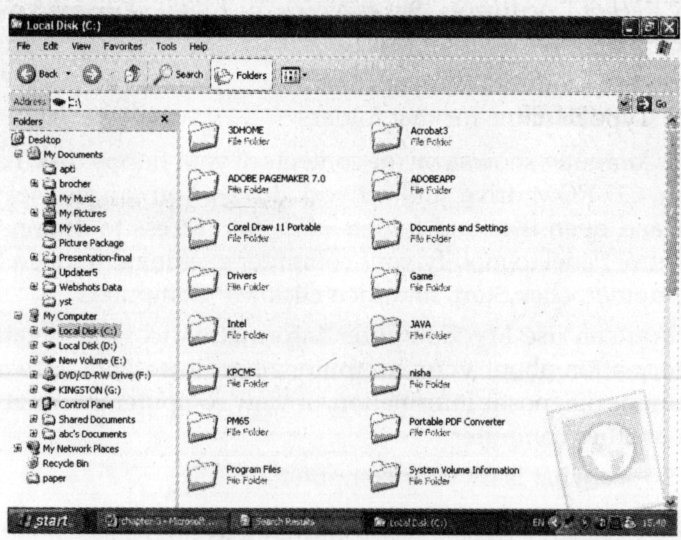

WINDOWS EXPLORER

Windows Explorer displays the hierarchical structure of files, folders, and drives on your computer. It also shows any network drives that have been mapped to drive letters on your computer. Using Windows Explorer, you can copy, move, rename, and search for files and folders. For example, you can open a folder that contains a file you want to copy or move, and then drag the file to another folder or drive.

Windows Explorer is a program which allows you to view all of your folders, and the files that belong in those folders. It is divided into 2 panes. On the left side the drives and folders. The right pane shows the files and subfolders of the folder or drive you have chosen from the left pane.

1. Click on the start at bottom left corner of screen.
2. Click on programs.
3. Select windows explorer.

Creating a Folder

1. Select the drive or folder you want to create your folder in.
2. Right click in the right pane in the white area.
3. Select new.
4. Select folder.
5. Type in name for that folder.

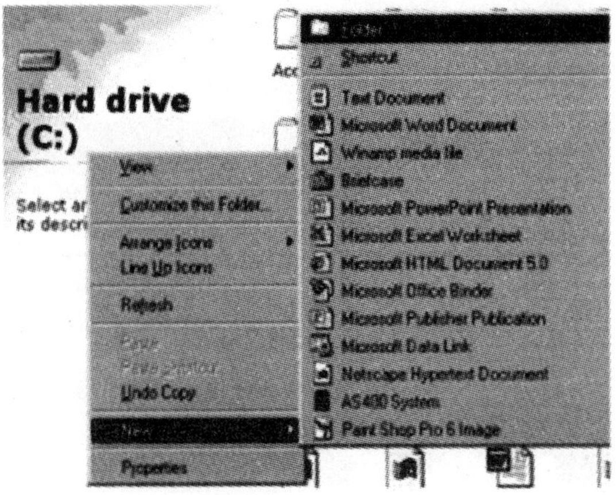

Deleting a File or Folder

1. Select the file/folder you want to delete.
2. Hit the delete key on the keyboard.
3. Confirm deletion.

Moving/Copying Files to Different Folders

1. Select the folder you want to move or copy.
2. To Move File—Simply drag it to the destination you want it to go to.

3. To Copy File—Click on Edit ' Copy from the top of the screen. Then go to the destination folder and click Edit ' Paste.

Copying a File/Folder to a Floppy Disk

1. Select the folder you want to move or copy.
2. Right click on the file or folder in the right pane.
3. Select Send To.
4. Select 3.5 Floppy (A).
5. You can also drag the file to 3.5" Floppy (A:\) in the left pane.

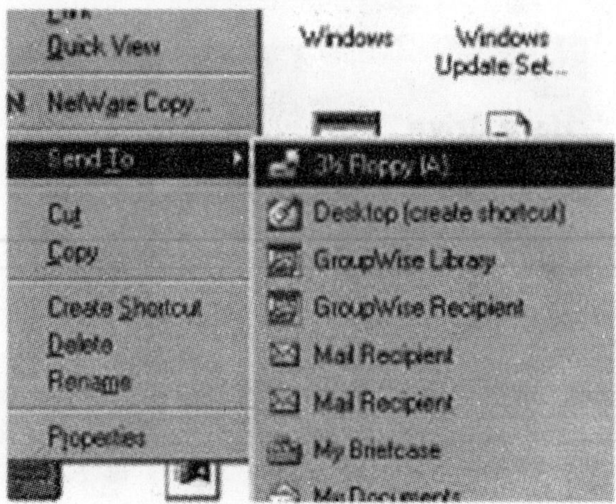

Copying a File/Folder from a Floppy Disk to Other Drive

1. Select 3.5 floppy (A: in the left pane).
2. Select the file/folder you want to copy from in the floppy drive.
3. Drag it to your destination.

Renaming a File or Folder

1. Select the file or folder you want to rename.
2. Right click on it.

3. Select rename.
4. Rename file.

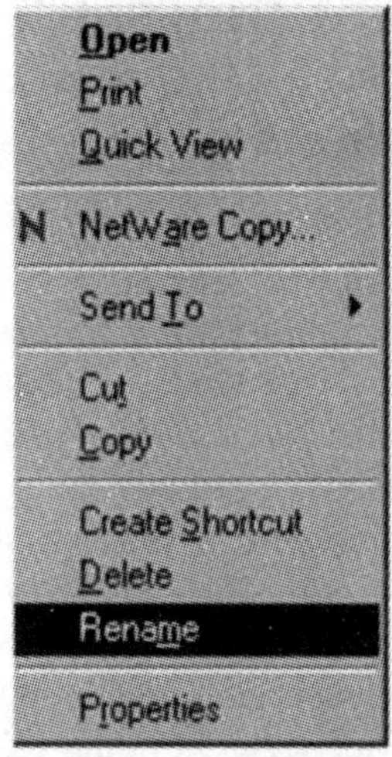

RECYCLE BIN

The Recycle Bin provides a safety net when deleting files or folders. When you delete any of these items from your hard disk, Windows places it in the Recycle Bin and the Recycle Bin icon changes from empty to full. Items deleted from a floppy disk or a network drive are permanently deleted and are not sent to the Recycle Bin.

Items in the Recycle Bin remain there until you decide to permanently delete them from your computer. These items still take up hard disk space and can be undeleted or restored back to their original location. When it fills up, Windows automatically cleans out enough space in the Recycle Bin to accommodate the most recently deleted files and folders.

If you are running low on hard disk space, always remember to empty the Recycle Bin. You can also restrict the size of the Recycle Bin to limit the amount of hard disk space it takes up.

Windows allocates one Recycle Bin for each partition or hard disk. If your hard disk is partitioned, or if you have more than one hard disk in your computer, you can specify a different size for each Recycle Bin. To empty the Recycle Bin:

1. On the desktop, double-click Recycle Bin.
2. On the file menu, click Empty Recycle Bin.

WINDOWS COMPONENTS

Accessories

1. ***Calculator:*** You can use calculator in standard view to do simple calculations, or in scientific view to do advanced scientific and statistical calculations. You can use calculator to perform any of the standard operations for which you would normally use a handheld calculator. Calculator performs basic arithmetic, such as addition and subtraction, as well as functions found on a scientific calculator, such as logarithms and factorials. To open calculator, click Start, point to All Programs, point to Accessories, and then click Calculator. You can also use your numeric keypad to type numbers and operators by pressing NUM LOCK.

2. ***Character map:*** You can use Character Map to copy and paste special characters into your documents, such as the trademark symbol, special mathematical characters, or a character from the character set of another language. To open Character Map, click Start, point to All Programs, point to Accessories, point to System Tools, and then click Character Map.

3. ***Notepad:*** Notepad is a basic text editor you can use for simple documents or for creating Web pages. You can use WordPad to create or edit text files that contain formatting or graphics. Use Notepad for basic text editing or for creating Web pages. To create or edit files that requires formatting, use WordPad. To open Notepad, click Start, point to All Programs, point to Accessories, and then click Notepad. Notepad is a basic text editor that you can use to create simple documents. The most common use for Notepad is to view or edit text (.txt) files, but many users find Notepad a simple tool for creating Web pages.

Because Notepad supports only very basic formatting, you cannot accidentally save special formatting in documents that need to remain pure text. This is especially useful when creating HTML documents for a Web page because special characters or other formatting may not appear in your published Web page or may even cause errors. You can save your Notepad files as Unicode, ANSI, UTF-8, or big-endian Unicode. These formats provide you greater flexibility when working with documents that use different character sets.

4. ***Wordpad:*** You can use WordPad to create or edit text files that contain formatting or graphics. Use Notepad for basic text editing or for creating Web pages. To open WordPad, click Start, point to All Programs, point to Accessories, and then click WordPad. With WordPad, you can create and edit simple text documents or documents with complex formatting and graphics. You can link or embed information from other documents into a WordPad document. You can save your WordPad file as a text file, rich text file, text file for MS-DOS, or Unicode. These formats provide greater flexibility when working with other programs. Documents that use multiple languages should be saved as rich text files.

5. ***Outlook express:*** Outlook Express is an e-mail program that lets you exchange mail with friends and colleagues, and join newsgroups to trade ideas and information. You can manage multiple mail and news accounts, keep your mail on a server so you can view it from more than one computer, and add stationery or a personal signature to your messages. To open Outlook Express, click Start, point to All Programs, and then click Outlook Express.

If you have several e-mail or newsgroup accounts, you can work with all of them within one window. You can also create multiple users, or identities, for the same computer. Each identity has unique e-mail folders and an individual Address Book. Multiple identities make it easy for you to keep work e-mail separate from personal e-mail, and also to keep individual users' e-mail separated. Using the message list and preview pane, you can view a list of messages and read individual messages at the same time. The folders list contains e-mail folders, news servers, and newsgroups, and you can easily switch among them.

You can also create new folders to organize and sort messages, and then set up message rules so that incoming e-mail that meets your criteria automatically goes to a specific folder. You can also create your own views to customize the way you look at your e-mail.

If your Internet service provider (ISP) uses an Internet message access protocol (IMAP) e-mail server for incoming e-mail, you can read, store, and organize your messages in folders on the server without downloading the messages to your computer. That way, you can view messages from any computer that can connect to that server. You can save names and addresses in the Address Book automatically by simply replying to a message.

You can also import names and addresses from other programs, type them into the Address Book, add them from e-mail messages you receive, or add them from a search of popular Internet directory services (white pages). The Address Book supports Lightweight Directory Access Protocol (LDAP) for viewing Internet directory services. You can insert essential information into outgoing messages as part of your personal signature, and you can create multiple signatures to use for different purposes.

You can also include a business card with more detailed information. To make your messages look more attractive, you can add stationery patterns and backgrounds, and you can change the color and style of the text. You can digitally sign and encrypt messages by using digital IDs. Digitally signing your message assures recipients that the message is really from you. Encryption ensures that only intended recipients can read the message. To use your online time efficiently, you can download messages, so you do not have to be connected to your ISP to read messages.

You can also download message headers only for offline viewing and then mark the headers of the messages you want to read; then the next time you are connected, Outlook Express downloads the message text. You can also compose messages offline and send them the next time you reconnect.

6. ***Paint:*** Paint is a drawing tool you can use to create black-and-white or color drawings that you can save as bitmap (.bmp) files. You can also use Paint to send your drawing in e-mail, set the image as a desktop background, and save image files using different file formats. To open Paint, click Start, point to All Programs, point to Accessories, and then click Paint.

Paint is a drawing tool you can use to create simple or elaborate drawings. These drawings can be either black-and-white or color, and can be saved as bitmap files. You can print your drawing, use it for your desktop background, or paste it into another document. You can even use Paint to view and edit scanned photos. You can also use Paint to work with pictures, such as .jpg, .gif, or .bmp files. You can paste a Paint picture into another document you have created, or use it as your desktop background.

7. ***Control panel:*** Control Panel is full of specialized tools that are used to change the way Windows looks and behaves. Some of these tools help you adjust settings that make your computer more fun to use. For example, use Mouse to replace standard mouse pointers with animated icons that move on your screen, or use Sounds and Audio Devices to replace standard system sounds with sounds you choose. Other tools help you set up Windows so that your computer is easier to use. For example, if you are left-handed, you can use Mouse to switch the mouse buttons so that the button on the right performs the primary functions of selecting and dragging.

To open Control Panel, click Start and then click Control Panel. If your computer is set up in Classic view using the more familiar Start menu, click Start, point to Settings, and then click Control Panel.

The control panel includes:

- Appearance and themes.
- Network and Internet connection.
- Add or remove programs.

- Sound, speech and audio devices.
- Performance and maintenance.
- Printers and other hardware.
- User account and password.
- Date, time, language and regional options.
- Accessibility options.
- Security center.

System Tools

1. ***Backup:*** The Backup utility helps you create a copy of the information on your hard disk. In the event that the original data on your hard disk is accidentally erased or overwritten, or becomes inaccessible because of a hard disk malfunction, you can use the copy to restore your lost or damaged data. To start Backup, click Start, point to All Programs, point to Accessories, point to System Tools, and then click Backup.

2. ***System properties:*** System properties is a Windows Management Instrumentation (WMI) tool that lets you view and change system properties on a remote computer or local computer. Using System Properties, you can restart a remote computer to apply settings changes or to detect new hardware, view the computer name and domain information for other computers on your network, and change the settings for the virtual memory paging file on a computer that might run programs requiring a lot of memory. Open Computer Management (Local). In the console tree, right-click Computer Management (Local), and then click Properties.

3. ***System information:*** System information collects and displays your system configuration information. Support technicians require specific information about your computer so they can resolve your system problem. You can use System Information to quickly find the data they need. To open System Information, click Start, and then click Run. In the Open box, type msinfo32.exe.

4. ***Local users and groups:*** Local users and groups manages users and groups of users for your computer. You can create

new users and groups, add users to groups, remove users from groups, disable user and group accounts, and reset passwords. Open Computer Management (Local). In the console tree, click Local Users and Groups.

5. ***Removable storage:*** Removable storage makes it easy for you to track your removable storage media (such as tapes and optical discs) and to manage the libraries that contain them (such as changers and jukeboxes). To open Computer Management, click Start, and then click Control Panel. Click Performance and Maintenance, click Administrative Tools, and then double-click Computer Management. In the console tree, click Removable Storage.

6. ***Computer management:*** Computer management helps you manage local or remote computers using a single, consolidated desktop tool. It combines several Windows administration utilities into a single console tree, providing easy access to a specific computer's administrative properties and tools. To open Computer Management, click Start, and then click Control Panel. Click Performance and Maintenance, click Administrative Tools, and then double-click Computer Management.

7. ***Disk cleanup:*** Disk Cleanup helps free up space on your hard drive. Disk Cleanup searches your drive, and then shows you temporary files, Internet cache files, and unnecessary program files that you can safely delete. You can direct Disk Cleanup to delete some or all of those files. To open Disk Cleanup, click Start, point to All Programs, point to Accessories, point to System Tools, and then click Disk Cleanup.

8. ***Disk defragmenter:*** Disk Defragmenter consolidates fragmented files and folders on your computer's hard disk, so that each occupies a single, contiguous space on the volume. As a result, your system can gain access to your files and folders and save new ones more efficiently. By consolidating your files and folders, Disk Defragmenter also consolidates the volume's free space, making it less likely that new files will be fragmented. To open Disk Defragmenter, click Start, point to All Programs, point to Accessories, point to System Tools, and then click Disk Defragmenter.

9. ***Device manager:*** Device Manager provides you with information about how the hardware on your computer is installed and configured, and how the hardware interacts with your computer's programs. With Device Manager, you can update the device drivers for hardware installed on your computer, modify hardware settings, and troubleshoot problems. To open Device Manager, click Start, and then click Control Panel. Click Performance and Maintenance, and then click System. On the Hardware tab, click Device Manager.

10. ***Event viewer:*** Event viewer maintains logs about program, security, and system events on your computer. You can use Event Viewer to view and manage the event logs, gather information about hardware and software problems, and monitor Windows security events. To open Event Viewer, click Start, click Control Panel, click Performance and Maintenance, click Administrative Tools, and then double-click Event Viewer.

11. ***Windows task manager:*** Windows Task Manager provides information about computer performance and displays details about programs and processes running on your computer. If you are connected to a network, you can also view network status and see at a glance how your network is functioning. Depending on your work environment and whether you share your computer with other users, you can view additional information about those users. Using Windows Task Manager, you can also end programs or processes, start programs, and view a dynamic display of your computer's performance. To open Windows Task Manager, right-click an empty space on the taskbar, and then click Task Manager.

Communications and Entertainment

1. ***Volume control:*** You can use Volume Control to adjust the volume, balance, bass, and treble settings for sounds played on your computer or by multimedia applications. You can also use Volume Control to adjust the level of system sounds, microphones, CD audio, line-in, synthesizer, and wave output. To open Volume Control, click Start, point to All Programs, point to Accessories, point to Entertainment, and then click Volume Control.

2. ***Sound recorder:*** You can use Sound Recorder to record, mix, play, and edit sounds. You can also link sounds to or insert sounds into a document. To open Sound Recorder, click Start, point to All Programs, point to Accessories, point to Entertainment, and then click Sound Recorder.

3. ***Windows media player:*** With Windows Media Player, you can play CDs and DVDs, create your own CDs, listen to radio stations, search for and organize digital media files, and copy files to a portable device. You can play many types of audio and video files by using Windows Media Player. You can also play and make copies of your CDs, play DVDs (if you have DVD hardware), listen to Internet radio stations, play clips from a movie, or view a music video on a Web site. You can also use Windows Media Player to make your own music CDs. To open Windows Media Player, click Start, point to All Programs, point to Accessories, point to Entertainment, and then click Windows Media Player.

4. ***Windows games:*** Windows provides several games on the Start menu. You can add others using Add or Remove Programs in Control Panel. To open a game, click Start, point to All Programs, point to Games, and then click the game you want to open.

- Freecell.
- Hearts.
- Minesweeper.
- Solitaire.
- Spider solitaire.
- Space cadet 3D pinball.

5. ***Windows messenger:*** Windows Messenger is an instant messaging program that enables you to:

- See who is online.
- Send an instant message.
- Call a contact's computer.
- Send someone a file.
- Have an instant message conversation with a group of friends.

You can open it by clicking Start, pointing to All Programs, and then clicking Windows Messenger.

6. ***Windows movie maker:*** With Windows Movie Maker, you can transfer recorded video and audio from a source, such as an analog camcorder or digital video camera, to your computer. In addition to using your own recorded content, you can also import existing audio and video files to use in the movies you create. After you create a movie, you can share it with family and friends directly through Windows Movie Maker by sending your movie in an e-mail message or by posting it to a Website. To open Windows Movie Maker, click Start, point to All Programs, point to Accessories, and then click Windows Movie Maker.

7. ***Outlook express:*** Outlook Express is an e-mail program that lets you exchange mail with friends and colleagues, and join newsgroups to trade ideas and information. You can manage multiple mail and news accounts, keep your mail on a server so you can view it from more than one computer, and add stationery or a personal signature to your messages.

Advanced Tools

1. ***Indexing services:*** Indexing Service creates indexes of the contents and properties of documents on your local hard drive and on shared network drives. You can also control the information included in the indexes. Indexing Service is designed to run continuously and requires little, if any, maintenance.

2. ***Network service:*** Network services provide features such as file and printer sharing. For example, the File and Printer Sharing for Microsoft Networks service allows other computers to access resources on your computer using a Microsoft network. The procedure below describes how to add a network service to your computer. To add a network service to your computer:

- Open Network Connections.
- Under LAN or High-Speed Internet, click Local Area Connection.

- On the File menu, click Properties.
- In the Local Area Connection Properties dialog box, click Install.
- In the Select Network Component Type dialog box, click Service, and then click Add.
- In the Select Network Service dialog box, click the service you want to install, and then click OK.

3. ***Computer management:*** Computer Management helps you manage local or remote computers using a single, consolidated desktop tool. It combines several Windows administration utilities into a single console tree, providing easy access to a specific computer's administrative properties and tools.

4. ***IP security policy management:*** Internet Protocol security (IPSec) is a key line of defense against internal, private network, and external security attacks. IPSec uses cryptographic security services to provide data integrity, data authentication, data confidentiality, and replay protection for TCP/IP traffic. IPSec behavior is controlled using an IPSec policy that you configure and assign using the IP Security Policy Management snap-in. To install an IP Security Policy Management snap-in:

- Click Start, and then click Run.
- In the Open box, type mmc, and then click OK.
- On the File menu, click Add/Remove Snap-in.
- Click Add, and then double-click IP Security Policy Management.
- Follow the instructions on your screen.

5. ***WMI control:*** The WMI (Windows Management Instrumentation) Control is a tool that lets you configure WMI settings on a remote computer or local computer. Use the WMI Control to set permissions for authorized users and groups, turn error logging on or off, back up the WMI repository, or perform other configuration tasks. To open the WMI Control console, click Start, and then click Run. In the Open box, type wmimgmt.msc, and then click OK.

WINDOWS SECURITY CENTER

Windows Security Center checks the status of your computer for the three security essentials—Firewall, Virus protection software and Automatic updates. If a problem is detected with any of the three essentials (for example, if your antivirus program is out of date), the Security Center sends you an alert and provides recommendations for how to better protect your computer. To open the Security Center, click Start, click Control Panel, and then click Security Center.

Firewall

A firewall helps protect your computer by preventing unauthorized users from gaining access to it through a network or the Internet. Windows Firewall is built into Windows XP and is turned on automatically, helping to protect your computer against viruses and other security threats. Windows checks to see if your computer is protected by a software firewall. To open Windows Firewall, click Start, click Control Panel, click Network and Internet Connections, and then click Windows Firewall.

A firewall is different from antivirus software, but the two of them work together to help protect your computer. You might say that a firewall guards the windows and doors against strangers or unwanted programs trying to get in, while an antivirus program protects against viruses or other security threats that can try to sneak in through the front door. Windows Firewall has three settings: On, On with no exceptions and Off.

1. ***On:*** Windows Firewall is turned on by default, and normally you should leave it that way. When you choose this setting, Windows Firewall blocks all unsolicited requests to connect to your computer, except for requests to programs or services selected on the Exceptions tab.

2. ***On with no exceptions:*** When you select the Don't allow exceptions check box, Windows Firewall blocks all unsolicited requests to connect to your computer, including requests to programs or services selected on the Exceptions tab. Use this setting when you need maximum protection for your computer,

such as when you connect to a public network in a hotel or airport, or when a dangerous virus or worm is spreading over the Internet. There is no need to keep Don't allow exceptions selected all the time, because when it is, some of your programs might not work correctly, and the following services are blocked from accepting unsolicited requests:

- File and printer sharing.
- Remote assistance and remote desktop.
- Discovery of network devices.
- Preconfigured programs and services on the exceptions list.
- Additional items that you have added to the exceptions list.

When you select Don't allow exceptions, you can still send and receive e-mail, use an instant messaging program, or view most Web pages.

3. ***Off:*** This setting turns Windows Firewall off. When you choose this setting, your computer is much more vulnerable to harm from unknown intruders or viruses from the Internet. This setting should only be used by advanced users for computer administration purposes, or if your computer is protected by another firewall.

Virus Protection Software

Viruses are destructive or deceptive programs that spread from computer to computer over the Internet or a network. Viruses can be attached to other files or disguised as files that look ordinary. You can help protect your computer from viruses and other security threats by:

- Installing and using up-to-date antivirus software.
- Setting up your e-mail and Internet software so that it is more difficult for files containing viruses to make their way onto your computer at all.

Antivirus software can help protect your computer against viruses and other security threats. Windows checks to see if your computer is using a full, up-to-date antivirus program.

Antivirus programs scan e-mail and other files on your computer for viruses, worms, and Trojan horses. If a virus, worm, or Trojan horse is found, the antivirus program either quarantines it or deletes it entirely before it damages your computer and files.

Some companies that make antivirus programs provide regular updates for viruses. Many antivirus programs have an automatic update capability. When your antivirus software is updated, new viruses are added to a list of viruses to check for, protecting your computer from new attacks. If your antivirus updates are not automatic, we recommend that you check for updates on a frequent basis because new viruses are identified every day. If the antivirus program you are using requires a subscription, we strongly recommended that you keep the subscription current to receive regular updates. If your list of viruses is out of date, your computer is vulnerable to new threats.

In addition to using up-to-date antivirus software, you should also make sure that it has a "real-time scanning" feature (depending on the brand of software, this feature might have another name). Real-time scanning checks files before they are opened or used.

Automatic Updates

For enhanced security, and to ensure that your computer always receives the latest updates in a timely manner, you should set up Automatic Updates so that it automatically downloads and installs critical updates as soon as they are released.

With automatic updates, Windows can routinely check for the latest important updates for your computer and install them automatically. These updates, which include critical updates and security updates, should be installed on your computer as soon as they are released, so that they can help protect your computer against viruses and other security threats.

Automatic updates finds all important updates for your computer, including security updates, critical updates, and service packs, and installs them automatically, so that you do not have to search for them or worry that some might be missing.

With automatic updates, windows can routinely check for the latest important updates for your computer and install them automatically. The Security Center can also help you to find out about the latest viruses or other security threats and get customer support from Microsoft for a security-related issue.

Microsoft Word

INTRODUCTION

A word processor is a package that processes textual matter and creates organized and flawless documents. Microsoft Word is a powerful tool to create professional looking documents. Microsoft Word is a word processing software package. You can use it to type letters, reports, and other documents. Microsoft Word is currently the most common word processor on the market. Because it is so common, the .doc format has become the de facto format for text documents. Word files can also be used to create other file formats, such as PDF and HTML. There are several things that can be done to make content created in Word more accessible. Millions of people use word processing software everyday to create documents such as letters, memos, reports, fax cover-sheets, mailing labels and news letters.

A number of features are available in Word Processing programs like MS Word:

1. ***Fast:*** Typing text in a word processor becomes speedy as there is no mechanical carriage movement associated.
2. ***Editing features:*** Text can be copied, deleted, added or modified very easily when required.
3. ***Formatting features:*** The typed text can be made to appear in any form or style (bold, italic, underline, etc.). Setting of paragraphs, left margin, right margin, line spacing, etc. can be done as per the choice of user.
4. ***Graphics:*** All word processors provide the facility of incorporating drawings in the documents, which enhances their utility.

5. ***Permanent storage:*** With word processors documents can be saved as long as desired. The saved document can be retrieved when desired.
6. ***Object linking and embedding (OLE):*** OLE is a program integration technology that you can use to share information. Objects are saved entrities of different types-charts, equations, video clips, pictures, etc.
7. ***Spell check:*** Facility of checking spellings and grammar is available in MS Word. Word processors can also suggest possible alternatives of incorrectly spelt words.
8. ***Mail merge:*** Mail merge facility enables you to send number of letters with more or less similar text. For example, same invitation letter has to be sent to invitees, only names and addresses are to be changed and in such cases mail merge proves useful.

STARTING MICROSOFT WORD

There are two ways for starting MS Word:

1. Double click on the Microsoft Word icon on the desktop.
2. Click the pointer on the Start button on the Windows taskbar. The start menu will appear. Click on Programs. The program menu will appear. Then click on Microsoft Word.

   Click on start → Programs → Microsoft Word

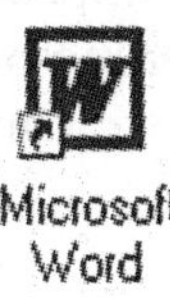

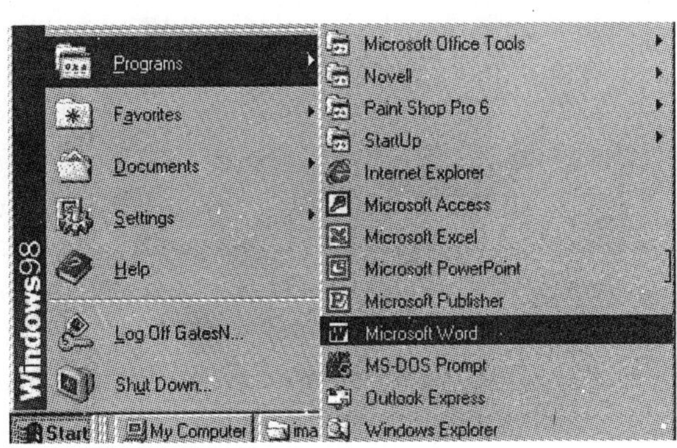

VIEWING TOOL BARS

Once the program is launched, a new, blank document is opened and is ready for you to start working. All of the commands in Word can be accessed through menus and toolbars. Menus contain lists of words that indicate the commands to be executed. Toolbars contain buttons that execute a particular command. Figure 4.1 shows the location of commonly used menus and toolbars.

The document window has following major components:

1. ***Title bar:*** Located at the top of the screen; it displays the name of the application (Microsoft Word) and the active document.
2. ***Menu bar:*** A collection of menus used to execute commands within the Word environment. Located below the Title bar, it lists Word menu options.
3. ***Format tool bar:*** This consists of tools frequently used for formatting documents. It contains command buttons that execute shortcuts associated with formatting text within a document. These include Font, Size, Bold, Italic, Underline, Left Justify, Center Justify, Right Justify, Lists and colors.
4. ***Standard toolbar:*** This toolbar consist of most frequently used commands and utilities. It contains command buttons that execute shortcuts to many common commands, such as Open a new document, Open an existing document, Save, Print, Print Preview, Spell Check, Cut, Copy, Paste and Format Painter (Table 4.1).
5. ***Ruler bar:*** Ruler bar allows formatting the vertical alignment of text in a document. It is used to get tab, margins and indents.
6. ***Status bar:*** Status bar displays information, which includes page number, the column and line number on which your cursor is present at any given point of time.
7. ***Scroll bar:*** Scroll bars are used to view different areas of the active window.

The toolbars in Microsoft Word provide easy access and functionality to the user. There are many shortcuts that can be

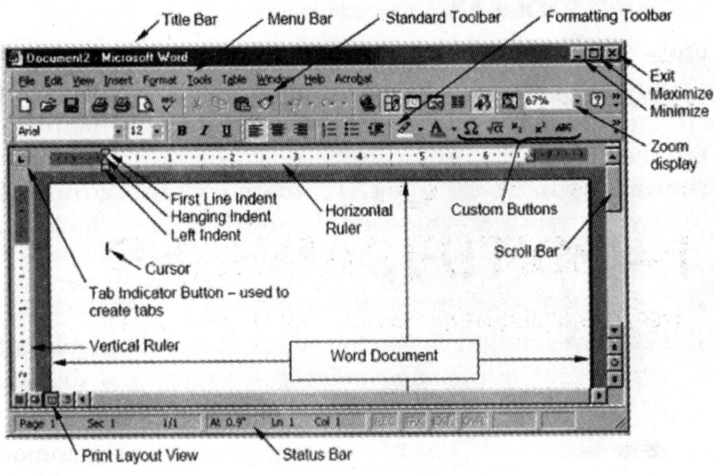

Fig. 4.1: Toolbars in MS Word

taken by using the toolbar. First, make sure that the proper toolbars are visible on the screen:

- Click view.
- Select toolbars.
- Select standard, formatting, and drawing.
- Other toolbars can be selected if you wish.

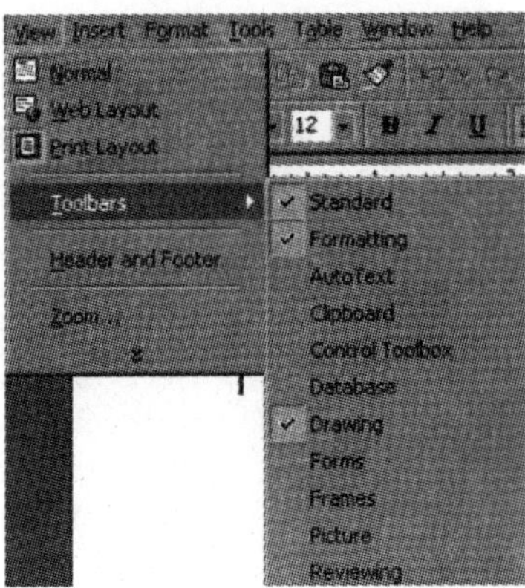

Table 4.1: Icons with their description

Name	*Icon*	*Description*
New blank document		Creates a new, blank file based on the default template.
Open (File menu)		Opens or finds a file.
Save (File menu)		Saves the active file with its current file name, location, and file format.
Mail Recipient		Sends the contents of the document as the body of the e-mail message.
Print (File menu)	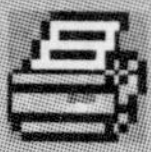	Prints the active file or selected items. To select print options, on the File menu, click Print.
Print Preview (File menu)		Shows how a file will look when you print it.
Spelling and Grammar (Tools menu)	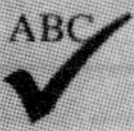 ABC✓	Checks the active document for possible spelling, grammar, and writing style errors, and displays suggestions for correcting them. To set spelling and grammar checking options, click Options on the Tools menu, and then click the Spelling and Grammar tab.
Cut (Edit menu)	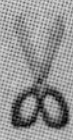	Removes the selection from the active document and places it on the Clipboard.
Copy (Edit menu)	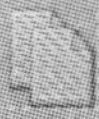	Copies the selection to the Clipboard.
Paste (Edit menu)		Inserts the contents of the Clipboard at the insertion point, and replaces any selection. This command is available only if you have cut or copied an object, text, or contents of a cell.

Contd..

Contd..

Format Painter (Standard toolbar)		Copies the format from a selected object or text and applies it to the object or text you click. To copy the formatting to more than one item, double-click , and then click each item you want to format. When you are finished, press ESC or click again to turn off the Format Painter.
Undo (Edit menu)		Reverses the last command or deletes the last entry you typed.
Redo (Edit menu)		Reverses the action of the Undo command.
Hyperlink		Inserts a new hyperlink or edits the selected hyperlink.
Tables and Borders		Displays the Tables and Borders toolbar, which contains tools for creating, editing, and sorting a table and for adding or changing borders to selected text, paragraphs, cells, or objects.
Zoom	75%	Enter a magnification between 10 and 400 percent to reduce or enlarge the display of the active document.
Office Assistant	?	The office assistant provides Help topics and tips to help you accomplish your tasks.

CREATING A DOCUMENT

Select the option File from the Menu bar. A drop down menu will be displayed. From this menu, choose the option New. The New dialog box will be displayed. Word will prompt you

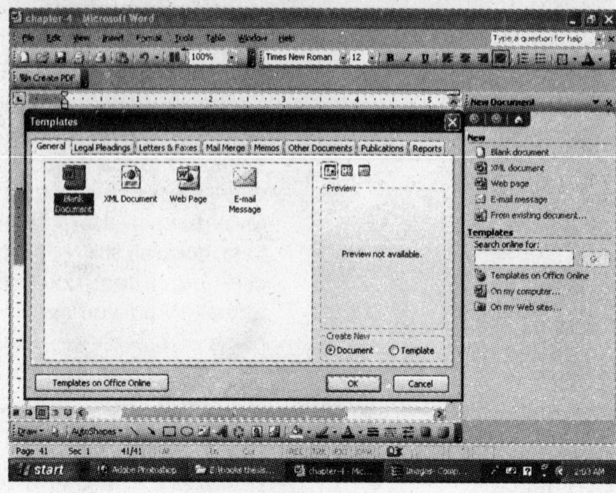

to choose a document template. Choose the default template—Blank Document under General option, for the time being and click OK. Alternatively you can either click new document icon on the standard toolbar or press Ctrl + N shortcut key. A new document window will be displayed for you to enter your text.

SAVING A DOCUMENT

Document created by you exists only in computer memory, which is a temporary storage area. For permanent storage you must save document as a file on hard or floppy disk/CD, etc.

1. Click on the option File on the menu bar.
2. Select the option Save from drop down menu. The Save As dialog box will be displayed.
3. Type the name of the new file in the File Name text box.
4. Click on Save to complete the process. The new document will be saved as word document with an extension .doc.

CLOSING A DOCUMENT

To close a document on which you are working, select Close from File drop down menu and the document will be closed. In case you have not saved the document, Word will prompt

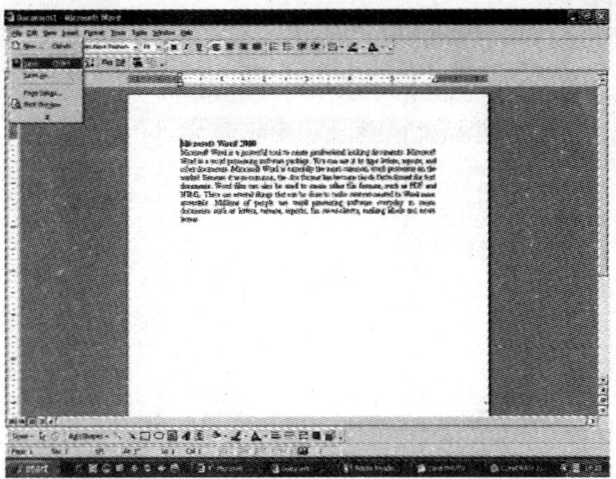

you to do so. Click Yes, if you want to save the document, No to quit without saving and Cancel to abort closing document and continue working.

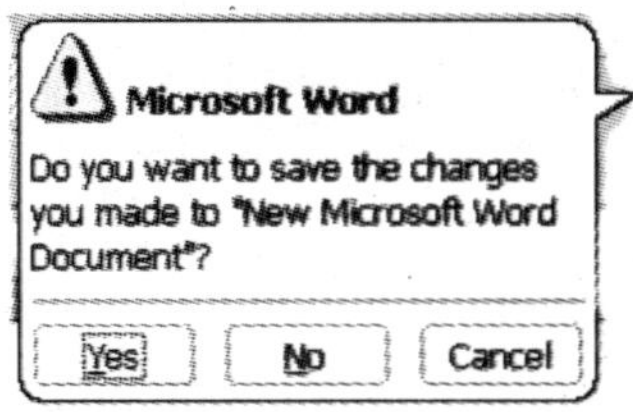

PAGE SETUP

Each page within a document can have its own page setup specified. Page setup refers to setting the margins for the sheet as well as the paper size, orientation, line numbers, headers and footers and borders.

1. Click on File. The File menu will appear.
2. Click on Page Setup. The Page Setup dialog Box will open (Fig. 4.2).
3. Click on Paper Size. The Paper Size tab will come to top. Click on the Paper Size down arrow. A list of Paper size will appear. The selected paper size will appear in the Paper-size drop-down box.

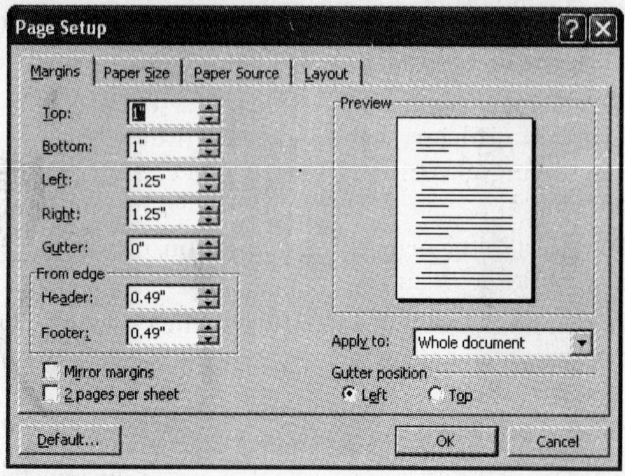

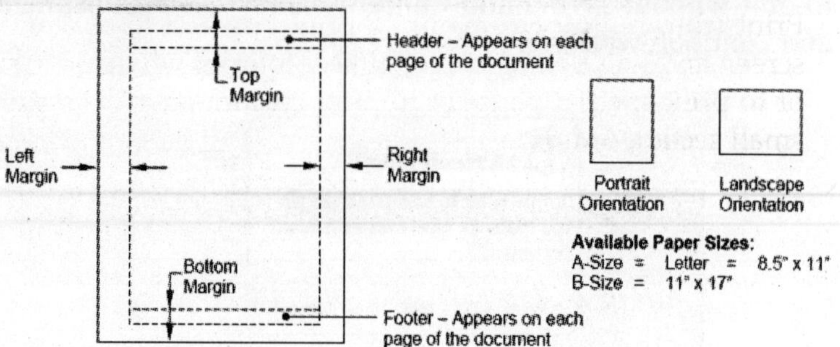

Fig. 4.2: Page setup in a document

4. Page Orientation can be chosen as Portrait (length-wise) or Landscape (width-wise) by clicking at one of the desired orientation buttons.
5. Click on OK. The Page Setup dialog box will close.

PRINTING THE DOCUMENT

Print Preview

To display each page, as it will look when printed, click Print Preview on the Standard toolbar. To edit text in print preview follow these steps:

1. In print preview, display the page you want to edit.
2. Click the text in the area you want to edit. Word zooms in on the area.
3. Click Magnifier. When the pointer changes from a magnifying glass to an I-beam, make your changes to the document.
4. To return to the original magnification, click Magnifier, and then click the document.
5. To exit print preview and return to the previous view of the document, click Close.

Printing Document

You can print the saved document or any of the page(s) of your document if printer is connected. Click on File option. Choose Print from pull-down menu. A print box will appear on the screen and will ask the choice of user to print whole document or to print specific pages or to print current page or to print a small section of text.

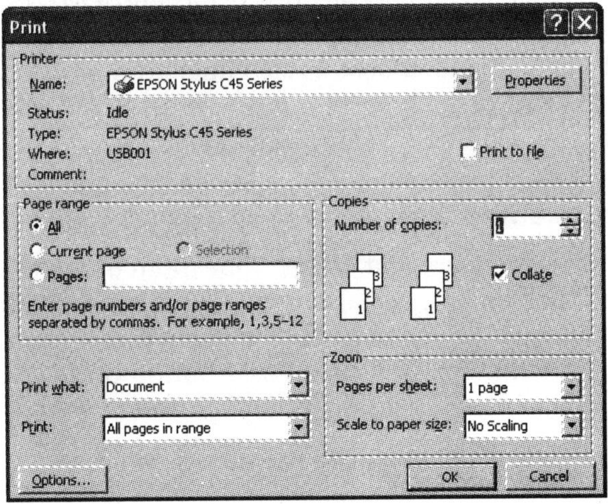

UNDO AND REDO

You can cancel the wrong portion, remove mistakes by using Undo button; you can also use Ctrl + Z keys. In this way you can even go many stages back. If you want to execute your operation again you can use Redo button; you can also use Ctrl + Shift + Back space key.

TEXT SELECTION

You can move an entire block to a new position or you may delete an entire block of text or may copy a block of text or even print it.

Selecting Text

You can select text by holding down Shift and pressing the key that moves the insertion point, i.e. arrow keys, page up, page down, etc. The keys used to extend selection are given in Table 4.2.

Copying Selected Text

Select the desired text using any of the keys given in Table 4.2. while holding Shift key. Now right-click on the mouse a short-cut menu is displayed, choose Copy from here or from Standard toolbar (you can also use Ctrl + C). Now place cursor at the desired position and choose Paste either from shortcut menu of selected text or click Paste button on the Standard toolbar. You can also use Ctrl + V for paste.

Moving Selected Text

Select the text, choose Cut either from shortcut menu or from Standard toolbar (you can also use Ctrl + X keys). Place cursor where text is to be moved. Click Paste either from shortcut menu of selected text (or click Paste button on the Standard toolbar).

Deleting Selected Text

You can delete unwanted text—a character, a word, a paragraph at a time or any combination of these. There are two common keys to delete text—Backspace key and Delete key. Pressing the Backspace key will delete one character at a

Table 4.2: Keys used to extend selection

To extend a selection	*Press*
One character to the right	Shift + Right Arrow
One character to the left	Shift + Left Arrow
To the end of a word	Ctrl + Shift + Right Arrow
To the beginning of a word	Ctrl + Shift + Left Arrow
To the end of a line	Shift + End
To the beginning of a line	Shift + Home
One line down	Shift + Down Arrow
One line up	Shift + Up Arrow
To the end of a paragraph	Ctrl + Shift + Down Arrow
To the beginning of a paragraph	Ctrl + Shift + Up Arrow
Once screen down	Shift + Page down
Once screen up	Shift + Page up
To the end of a window	Alt + Ctrl + Page down
To the beginning of a document	Ctrl + Shift + Home
To include the entire document	Ctrl + A
To a vertical block of a text	Ctrl + Shift + F8 and then use the arrow keys; press ESC to cancel selection mode.
To a specific location in a document	F8 + Arrow keys; press ESC to cancel selection mode.

time to the left of the insertion point; pressing the Delete key will delete one character at a time to the right of the insertion point. Select the text to be deleted, the text will be highlighted. Press Delete key, the text will be deleted.

FIND AND REPLACE

Find and Replace feature is a real-time saver in Word. Sometimes you need to search a particular text or word in the document. Or sometimes your situation requires replacement of word or text. All word processor provide Find and Replace utilities.

Find Text

Find command is useful to seek out text, which you may not locate easily visually. The sequence for finding text is:

- Click on Edit. The Edit menu will appear.
- Click on Find. The Find and Replace dialog box will open.
- Type the word or phrase that you want to search for. The typed text will appear in the Find what: text box.
- Click on Find Next. Word will take you to the first occurrence of the word or phrase that you are looking for. Click on Find Next again. Word will take you to the next occurrence of the word or phrase that you are looking for. You can continue till you have reached the last such occurrence.
- Click on OK. The message box will close.
- Click on cancel if you want to discontinue the search.

Replace Text

If you want to locate text and change it with something else, let Word do it for you with the Replace feature.

- Click on Edit. The Edit menu will appear.
- Click on Replace. The Find and Replace dialog box will open.
- Type the word or phrase that you want to search for. The typed text will appear in the Find what: text box.
- Click in the Replace with: text box. The blinking insertion point will appear.
- Type the replacement word or phrase. The text will appear in the Replace with: text box.

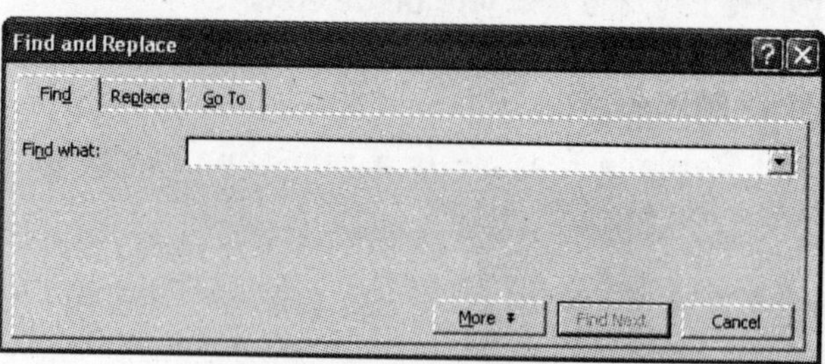

- Click Find Next. Word will highlight the first match.
- Choose one of the following:
  - Click on Replace, if this text you want to change. The text will be replaced and Word will highlight the next text match.
  - Click on Replace All. Word will replace all occurrences of the found text with the replace text and notify you the total number of replacements.
  - Click on the Find Next. Word will not make any changes and will locate the next occurrences of the text.
- Click OK. The message box will close.

DOCUMENT VIEWS

In Word 2007, you can display your document in one of five views: Draft, Web Layout, Print Layout, Full Screen Reading, or Online Layout (Table 4.3).

DISPLAYING DIFFERENT TOOLBARS

You can use menus and toolbars to give Microsoft Word instructions about what you want to do. A toolbar can contain buttons with images (the same images you see next to

Table 4.3: Types of document views

View/Layout	*Meaning*
Draft view	Draft view is the most frequently used view. You use Draft view to quickly edit your document.
Web layout	Web Layout view enables you to see your document, as it would appear in a browser such as Internet Explorer.
Print layout	The Print Layout view shows the document, as it will look when it is printed.
Reading layout	Reading Layout view formats your screen to make reading your document more comfortable.
Outline view	Outline view displays the document in outline form. You can display headings without the text. If you move a heading, the accompanying text moves with it.

corresponding menu commands), menus, or a combination of both. Word includes many built-in toolbars that you can show and hide as needed. By default, the Standard and Formatting built-in toolbars are docked side-by-side below the menu bar. You can customize or create your own toolbars by adding, reorganizing, and removing buttons and menus. You can also show, move, and hide toolbars.

While doing work in MS Word, sometimes you feel the necessity of some toolbars on the screen. You can display any of the toolbars available in MS Word.

1. Click over View option in menu bar.
2. Click over Tool bars in the View menu.
3. If you want to make the availability of Drawing toolbar (if not displayed already), you can click over Drawing checkbox means that the particular bar is displayed on the screen.

HEADERS AND FOOTERS

Headers and footers contain data that will appear at the top (header) or bottom (footer) of each page in the document. Using different sections, it is possible to change the header and footer throughout the document. The distance that the header and footer are spaced from the edge of the paper is specified in the Page Setup dialog box. To access the header and footer, use the menu sequence View → Header and Footer. From the Header and Footer toolbar shown below, it is possible to add page numbers, the date and time and other AutoText information. The toolbar opens automatically when you use the given menu sequence.

Text and graphics can be added to headers and footers. The toolbar closes automatically when you pick the Close button. The header and footer can also be edited by double clicking them once they are created.

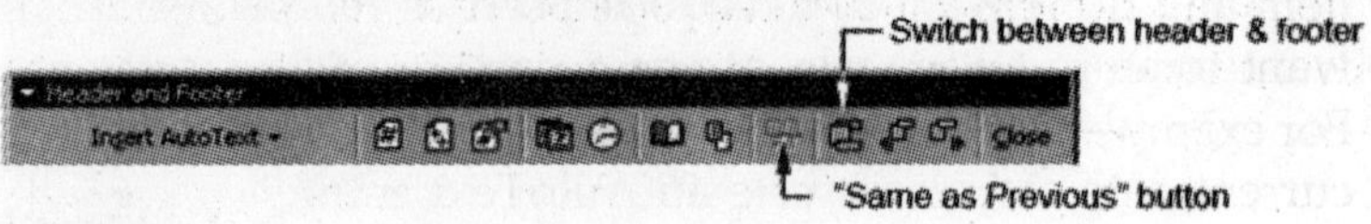

PAGE BREAKS AND SECTION BREAKS

If you come to a point in your document where you want to skip to the next page, you will need to insert a break. There are two kinds of breaks: Page Breaks and Section Breaks. Both are accessed by the menu sequence Insert → Break. A page break just skips down to the next page in the document. A section break does the same kind of thing, except that each section in a document can have its own header and footer. So, if you want to have different headers and footers throughout your document, insert Section Breaks. When changing the headers and footers, start from the END of the document and work forward. Be sure to turn OFF the "Same as Previous" button in order to change the header and footer for the individual section.

ADD PAGE NUMBERS

Page numbers help you keep your document organized and enable readers to find information quickly. You can add page numbers to the top, bottom, or margins of your pages, and you can choose where the numbers appear. For example, numbers can appear at the top of the page, on the left, right, or center of the page. Word also offers several number styles from which you can choose.

AUTOTEXT/AUTOCORRECT

AutoText offers a way to store and quickly insert text, graphics, fields, tables, bookmarks, and other items that you use frequently. Microsoft Word comes with a number of built-in AutoText entries that are divided into different categories. For example, if you are working on a letter, Word can offer letter-specific AutoText entries, such as salutations and closings.

In addition, you can create your own AutoText / AutoCorrect entries. This is useful if you often use the same large or complex item and don't want to have to reinsert or retype it, or if you want to store text that contains a particular style or format. For example, if a student needs a header on his paper with the current date, you can create an AutoText entry.

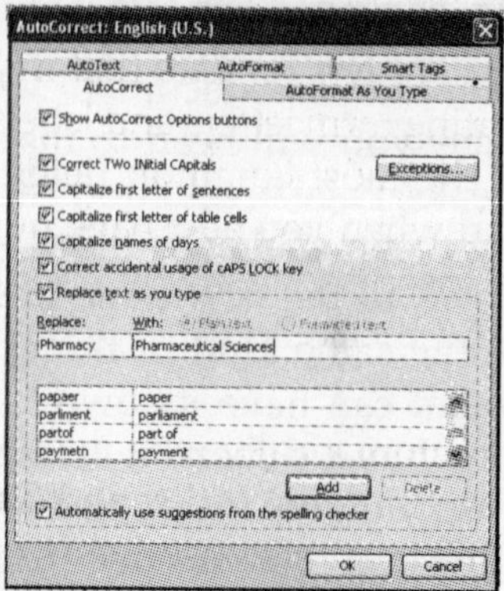

Cut and Copy both store information on the Clipboard. Information you store on the Clipboard is eventually lost. If you want to store information permanently for reuse, use AutoText. AutoText permanently stores information for future use. To create an AutoCorrect entry using these steps to store and automatically insert text and graphics:

- Create a header text (with or without graphic) that you want to store as an AutoCorrect entry. To store paragraph formatting with the entry, include the paragraph mark in the selection.
- On the Tools menu, click AutoCorrect.
- Make sure the Replace text as you type check box is selected.
- In the Replace box, type a name for the AutoCorrect entry (that is, the abbreviation or word that Microsoft Word replaces automatically as you type).
- Do one of the following:
  - To save the entry without its original formatting, click Plain text.
  - To save the entry with its original formatting, click Formatted text.
- Click Add.

When you are ready to automatically insert the AutoCorrect entry, type the abbreviation followed by a space or other punctuation.

FIELD

Fields are used as placeholders for data that might change in a document and for creating form letters and labels in mail-merge documents. Some of the most common fields are the PAGE field, which is inserted when you add page numbers, and the DATE field, which is inserted when you click Date and Time on the Insert menu and then select the Update automatically check box.

Fields are inserted automatically when you create an index or table of contents by using the Index and Tables command on the Insert menu. You can also use fields to automatically insert document information (such as the author or file name), to perform calculations, to create links and references to other documents or items, and to perform other special tasks.

SYMBOLS

It is often necessary to insert special characters and symbols into a document. Many sets of special characters are available for use in a document. To access the character sets, select Insert → Symbol for the menu bar. The dialog box opens. Select the character to insert and press the Insert button. The Cancel button changes to Close. Use it to close the dialog box.

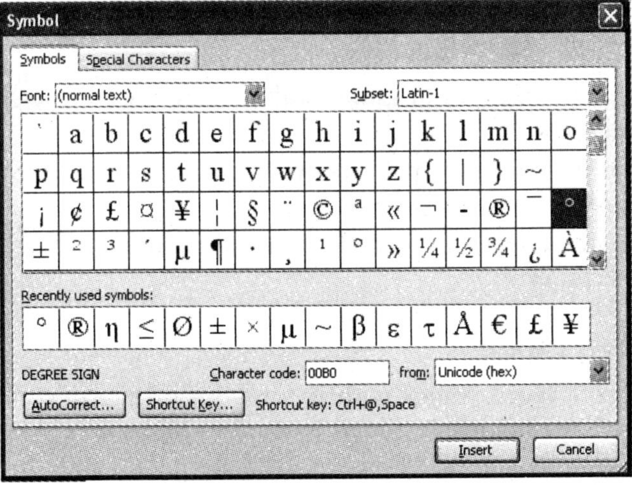

FOOTNOTE

Footnotes are used to cite sources within your written document. Any time you use information obtained from some other source, it should be cited. Footnotes are an automatic functionality of the software, which is more than just a superscript character. Use Footnotes by selecting Insert → Footnote... The Footnote function automatically keeps track of the footnote numbers and re-orders them as necessary if you move the reference. The function also creates a horizontal line at the bottom of the page.

CAPTION

A caption is a numbered label, such as "Figure 1," that you can add to a table, figure, equation, or other item. You can vary the caption label and number format for different types of items, for example, "Table II" and "Equation 1-A." If you later add, delete, or move captions, you can easily update the caption numbers all at once.

Create a new caption label as:

1. On the Insert menu, click Caption.
2. Click New Label.
3. In the Label box, type the label you want.

INSERTING GRAPHICS

There are two types of graphics that can be used to enhance your document:

a. *Drawing objects:* It includes AutoShapes, curves, lines and WordArt drawing objects.

b. *Pictures:* It includes bitmaps, scanned pictures, photographs and clip art.

Inserting Clipart

Microsoft Word comes with its own set of pictures in Clip Gallery. We can insert Clipart from clip gallery as:

1. Click on Insert. Insert menu will open.

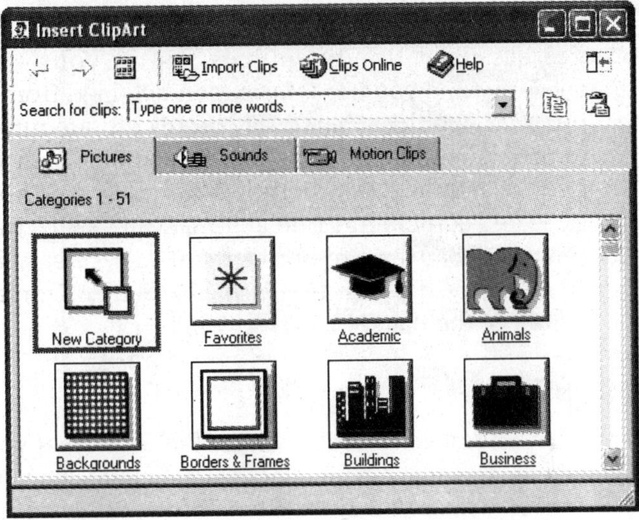

2. Click on Picture. Picture submenu will appear.
3. Click on Clip Art. Clip Art gallery window will open.
4. Choose the categories from which you like to insert clip art image into your document. Clipart images regarding that category will open.
5. Click on any picture. A pop menu will appear.
6. Click on Insert Clip button. The picture you have chosen will be inserted in your document.

Inserting WordArt

You can insert decorative text by inserting WordArt on the Drawing toolbar. You can create shadowed, skewed, rotated and stretched text, as well as text that has been fitted to predefined shapes. To insert WordArt follow these steps:

1. On the Drawing toolbar click Insert WordArt.
2. Click the type of WordArt drawing object you want and click OK.
3. In the Edit WordArt Text dialog box, type the text you want to format, select any other options you want and then click OK.

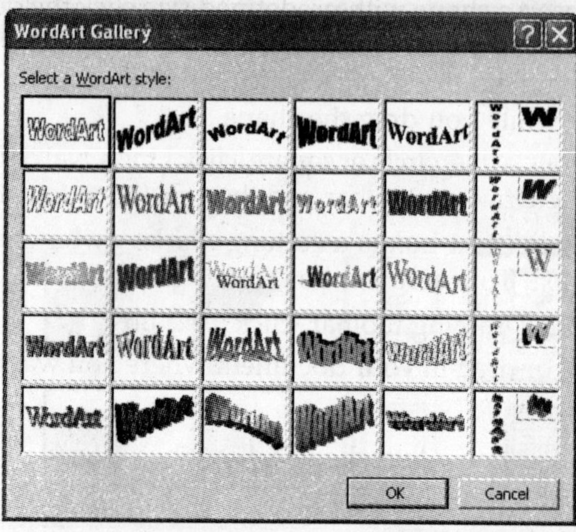

4. To add or change effects to the text, use the buttons on WordArt and Drawing toolbars. The WordArt toolbar appears when you click the WordArt special text.

Inserting Autoshapes and Text Box

a. ***Autoshapes:*** The Autoshapes menu on the Drawing toolbar contains several categories of shapes including lines, basic shapes, flow chart elements, stars and banners, and callouts.

   The autoshape can be inserted as:

   1. On the Drawing toolbar click Autoshapes, point to a category and then click the shape you want.

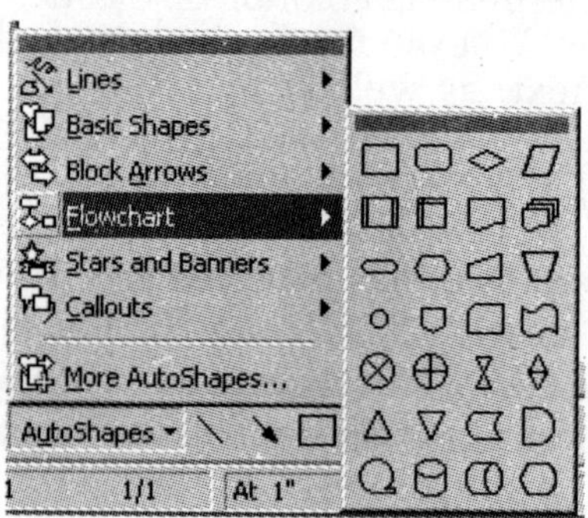

2. To insert a shape with predefined size click the document. To insert a different size, drag the shape to size you want. To maintain the shape's width-to-height ratio hold down Shift while you drag the shape.
3. To draw a line, circle or square, click Line, Oval or Rectangle on the Drawing toolbar and then click document.

b. ***Text box:*** A text box is a rectangular box wherein you can insert text. To insert text box follow the following steps:
1. On the Drawing toolbar, click Text Box.
2. Click or drag in your document where you want to insert the text box.

To insert text in an Autoshape follow these steps:

- Select Autoshape or Text box
- To add text for the first time right-click any shape (except a line or freeform), click Add Text on the shortcut menu and then type the text.
- To add text in existing text, right-click any shape (except a line or freeform), click Edit Text on the shortcut menu and then type the text.

c. ***Change fill color or line color in a drawing object:*** Once you have inserted a drawing object in the document, you can change its color or line color by following these steps:
1. Select the drawing object you want to change.
2. On the Drawing toolbar, click the arrow next to Fill color to bring out various fill colors available.
3. Click the desired Fill color or Line color.

EQUATIONS

Often times while writing, engineers have to refer to formulas and equations. So the ability to place equations in a document is important. Microsoft has included an equation tool, called the Microsoft Equation 3.0. An equation is an object that can be inserted into a Word document or other Microsoft products, such as Excel and PowerPoint. To insert an equation into a document, use the sequence:

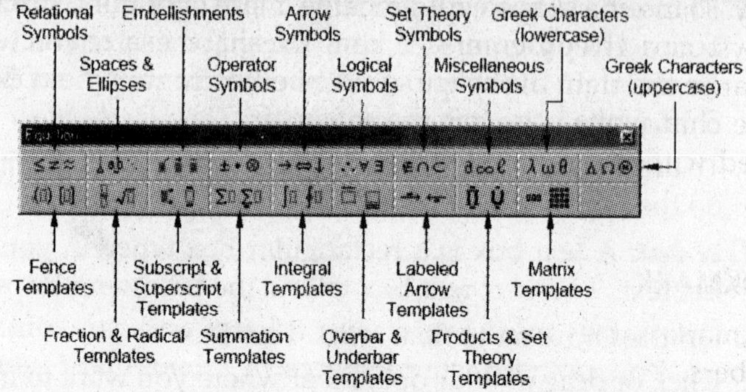

Fig. 4.3: Equation toolbar

1. Click where you want to insert the equation.
2. On the Insert menu, click Object, and then click the Create New tab.
3. In the Object type box, click Microsoft Equation 3.0.
4. Click OK.
5. Build the equation by selecting symbols from the Equation toolbar (Fig. 4.3) and by typing variables and numbers. From the top row of the Equation toolbar, you can choose from more than 150 mathematical symbols. From the bottom row, you can choose from a variety of templates or frameworks that contain symbols such as fractions, integrals, and summations.
6. To return to Word, click the Word document.

While the equation editor is open, Word switches to "edit mode". While in edit mode, all other Word functionality is suspended. The equation object is contained in a frame that automatically adjusts in size as the equation is built. To exit edit mode, click the mouse outside of the equation frame. Outside of edit mode, the frame surrounding the equation is not visible. Double-click on an existing equation to enter edit mode to edit the equation. In edit mode, all letters, numbers and keyboard characters can be typed into the equation as necessary. Special characters are available from the character menus on the first row of the equation toolbar, which is shown below. These characters could include, math operators, spaces, arrows, and Greek letters. When chosen, these characters appear to the right of the cursor (Embellishments are applied to the character to the left of the cursor). The cursor can be moved within the equation by pressing the keyboard arrow keys.

BOOKMARK

Bookmark names must begin with a letter and can contain numbers. You cannot include spaces in a bookmark name. However, you can use the underscore character to separate words, for example, "First_heading". To add a bookmark follow these steps:

1. Select an item you want a bookmark assigned to, or click where you want to insert a bookmark.
2. On the Insert menu, click Bookmark.
3. Under Bookmark name, type or select a name.
4. Click Add.

HYPERLINK

A hyperlink is a "hot spot" that allows you to jump to another location. The location can include another file on your hard

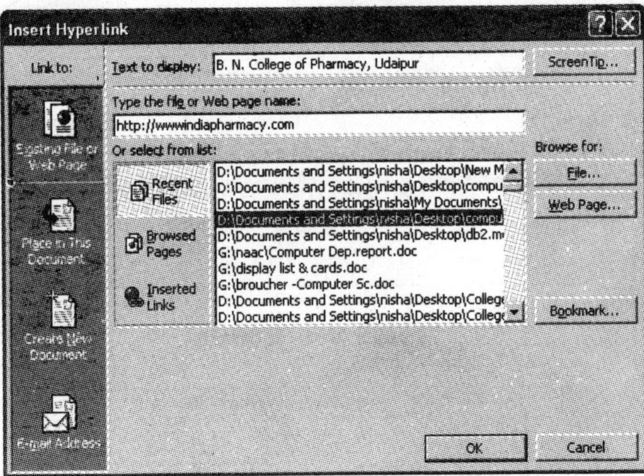

disk or company's network (such as a Microsoft Word document or a Microsoft Excel worksheet), an Internet address (such as http://www.microsoft.com), or a location such as a bookmark or slide. The field includes display text, which is often blue and underlined, that the user clicks to jump to the specified location. You can insert hyperlinks by clicking the Hyperlink command on the Insert menu.

FONT

Font is a set of characters (text) represented in a single typeface. Each character within a font is created by using the same basic style. The character formatting plays an important role in enhancing the appearance of your document. It is concerned with fonts (Times New Roman / Arial / Old Bookman Style, etc.), font size, text attributes (bold / italics / underline, etc.) and text positioning (subscript / superscript, etc.).

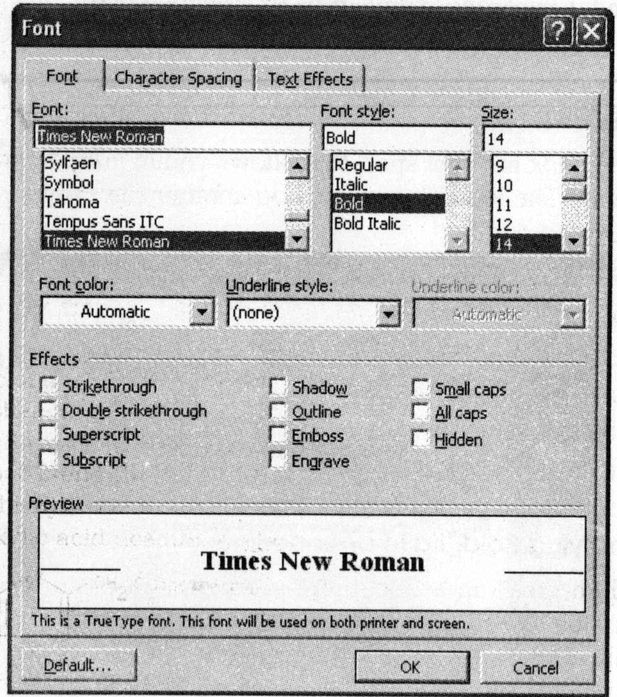

Set Default Font

The following steps are used for this:

1. If your document already contains text formatted with the properties you want to use, select that text.
2. On the Format menu, click Font.
3. Select the options you want to apply to the default font. If you selected text in step 1, the properties you want will appear in the dialog box.
4. Click Default. Any new document you open will use the font settings you selected.

Examples of English Fonts: Arial, Bookman Old Style, Courier New, Georgia, Impact, Lucida Bright, Park Avenue, Rockwell, Times New Roman, etc.

Changing a Font

The following steps are used for changing the font of a piece of writing:

1. Select the text to be formatted. The text will be highlighted.
2. Click on down arrow to right of Font drop down list. A list of fonts will appear.
3. Click on Font. The new font will be applied to your text.

Choosing Font Size

The following procedure is applied:

1. Select the text to be formatted. The text will be highlighted.
2. Click on down arrow to the right of Font Size drop down box. A list of available sizes will appear.
3. Click on a size. The new size will be applied to your text.

Applying Bold, Italic or Underline

When creating a document, you may need to emphasize particular words or phrases by bolding, underlining, or italicizing. Also, certain grammatical constructs require that you bold, underline, or italicize. You can bold, underline, and italicize when using Word. You also can combine these features, in other words, you can bold, underline, and italicize a single piece of text.

1. Select the text to be formatted. The text will be highlighted.
2. Click on appropriate toolbar button: either B for bold, I for italic or U for underline or any combination of these. The formatting will be applied.

Applying Text Effects

Font effects include shadowing, embossing, engraving and others; example of different text effects is shown in Table 4.4.

The following procedure is adopted for applying special effects:

1. Select the text to be formatted. The text will be highlighted.
2. Click on Format menu. The format menu will appear.
3. Click on Font. The font dialog box will open.

Table 4.4: Types of text effects available in MS Word

Effect	*Regular*	*Bold*	*Italic*	*Bold Italic*
Strikethrough	~~Text~~	**~~Text~~**	*~~Text~~*	***~~Text~~***
Double Strikethrough	~~Text~~	**~~Text~~**	*~~Text~~*	***~~Text~~***
Superscript	Text	**Text**	*Text*	***Text***
Subscript	Text	**Text**	*Text*	***Text***
Shadow	Text	**Text**	*Text*	***Text***
Outline	Text	**Text**	*Text*	***Text***
Emboss	Text	Text	Text	Text
Engrave	Text	Text	Text	Text
Small caps	TEXT	**TEXT**	*TEXT*	***TEXT***
All caps	TEXT	**TEXT**	*TEXT*	***TEXT***
Hidden				
Underline	Text	**Text**	*Text*	***Text***

4. Click on desired options in the Effect box. A check mark will appear in the selected effect.
5. Click OK. The dialog box will close and the effect will be applied to your text.

Applying Color to Text

You can add impact to the document by adding some color to text:

1. Select the text to be formatted. The text will be highlighted.
2. Click on down arrow to the right of font color button. A list of available colors will appear.
3. As you click on a color, the color palette box will close.
4. Now click anywhere in the document to deselect the text. The text will appear in selected color.

PARAGRAPH

When you type information into Microsoft Word, each time you press the enter key word creates a new paragraph. You can format paragraphs. For example, you can indent the first line of a paragraph, you can set the amount of space that

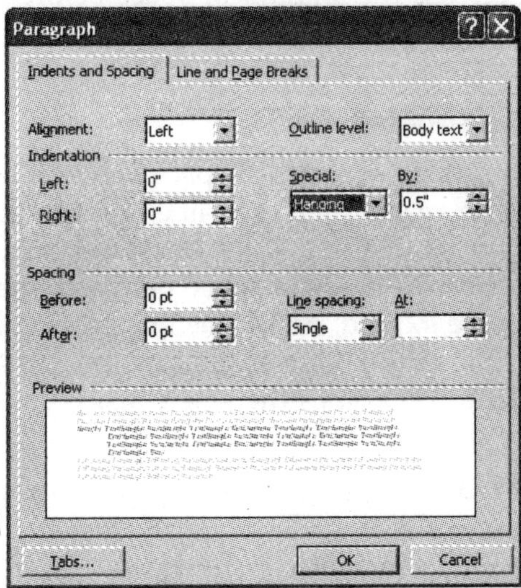

separates paragraphs, and you can align a paragraph left, right, center, or flush with both margins. Styles are a set of formats you can quickly apply to a paragraph. For example, by applying a style, you can set the font, set the font size, and align a paragraph all at once.

When you are formatting a paragraph, you do not need to select the entire paragraph. Placing the cursor anywhere in the paragraph enables you to format it. After you format a paragraph, pressing the Enter key creates a new paragraph in the same format.

Add Space Before or After Paragraph

When creating a document, space is often used to clearly identify where each paragraph begins and ends. By default, Word may place slightly more space between paragraphs than it does between lines in a paragraph. You can increase or decrease the amount of space that appears before and after paragraphs by entering amounts in the Before and After fields in the Paragraph section of the Page Layout tab. Use the up arrows next to the Before and After fields to increase the amount of space before or after each paragraph; use the down arrows to decrease the amount of space before or after each paragraph.

Change Line Spacing

Line spacing sets the amount of space between lines within a paragraph. The spacing for each line is set to accommodate the largest font on that line. If the lines include smaller fonts, there will appear to be extra space between lines where the smaller fonts are located. At 1.5, the line spacing is set to one-and-a-half times the single-space amount. At 2.0, the line spacing is set to two times the single-space amount (double space).

1. Place your cursor anywhere in the first paragraph of the sample text.
2. Click on Format. On the Format menu, click Paragraph.

3. Click the Line Spacing button in the Paragraph group. A menu of options appears.
4. Click the required spacing in the paragraph.

Create a Hanging or First Line Indent

The hanging indent feature indents each line except the first line by the amount specified in the By field. Some people and organizations delineate the start of a new paragraph by indenting the first line. If you want to indent the first line of your paragraphs, you can use the Paragraph dialog box to set the amount by which you want to indent. In the Special Field of the Paragraph dialog box, you tell Word you want to indent the first line by choosing First Line from the menu options. In the By field, you tell Word the amount, in inches by which you want to indent.

Indent Paragraphs

Indentation allows you to indent your paragraph from the left and/or right margin. You may find this necessary when you are quoting a large block of text.

Align Paragraphs

Microsoft Word gives you a choice of several types of alignments. Left-aligned text is flush with the left margin of your document and is the default setting. Right-aligned text is flush with the right margin of your document, Centered text is centered between the left and right margins, and Justified text is flush with both the left and right margins.

BULLETS AND NUMBERING

If you have lists of data, you may want to bullet or number them. When using Microsoft Word, bulleting and numbering are easy. In Microsoft Word, you can easily create bulleted or numbered lists of items. Several bulleting and numbering styles are available. You can select the one you wish to use.

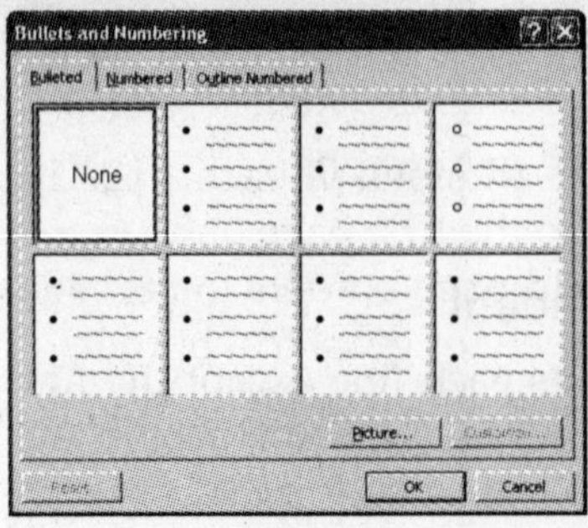

Bullets

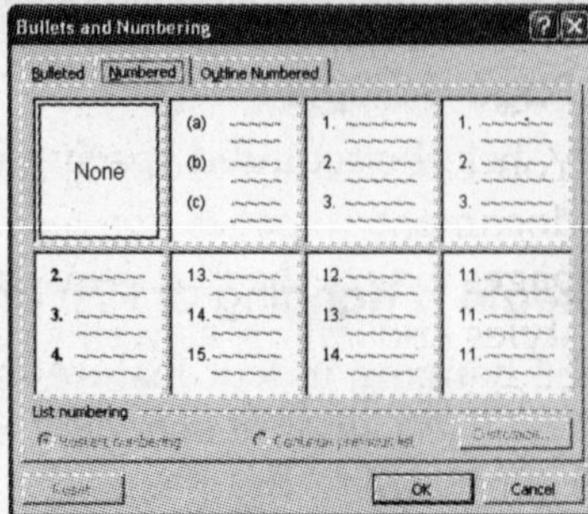

Numbering

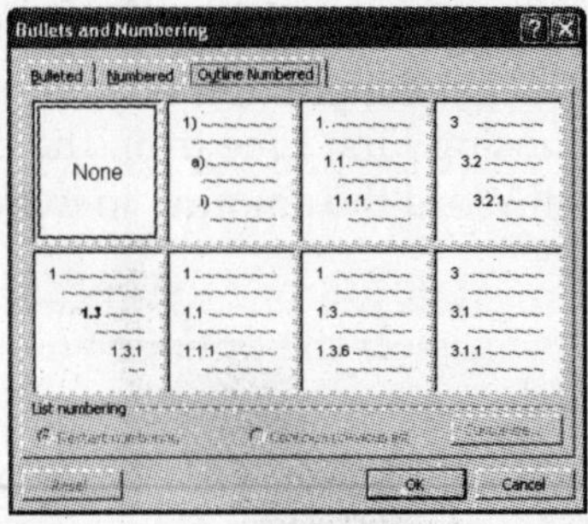

Outnumbered

To add bullets/numbers:

1. Type the list.
2. Select the words you just typed.
3. On the Format menu, click Paragraph.
4. In the Paragraph, click the down arrow next to the Bulleted/ Numbered button. The bullet/number library appears.
5. Click to select the type of bullet/number you want to use. Word adds bullets or numbers to your list.

To remove the bulleting/numbering:

1. Select the list again.
2. On the Format menu, click Paragraph.
3. In the Paragraph, click the down arrow next to the Bullets/ Number icon. The dialog box appears.
4. Click None. Word removes the bullets or numbers from your list.

BORDERS AND SHADING

Page Borders

You can add a border to any or all sides of each page in a document, to pages in a section, to the first page only, or to all pages except the first. You can add page borders in many line styles and colors, as well as a variety of graphical borders.

1. On the Format menu, click Borders and Shading, and then click the Page.
2. Select the options you want.
3. To specify that the border appear on a particular side of a page, such as only at the top, click Custom under Setting. Under Preview, click where you want the border to appear.
4. To specify a particular page or section for the border to appear in, click the option you want under Apply to.
5. To specify the exact position of the border on the page, click Options, and then select the options you want.

Text Borders and Shading

You can set apart paragraphs or selected text from the rest of a document by adding borders. You can also highlight text by applying shading.

Table Borders and Shading

You can add borders to a table or individual table cell, and you can use shading to fill in the background of a table. You can

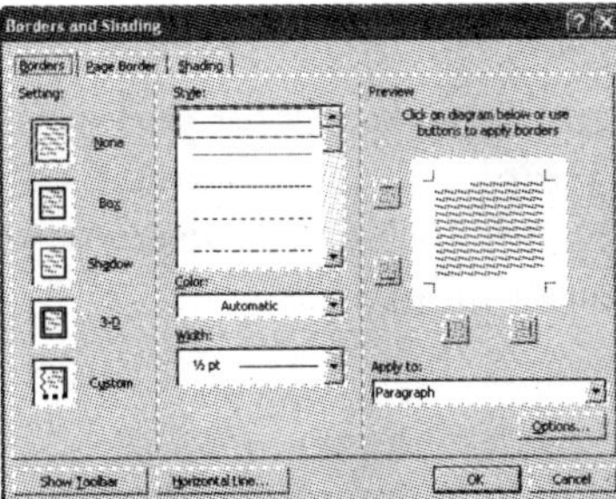

Border

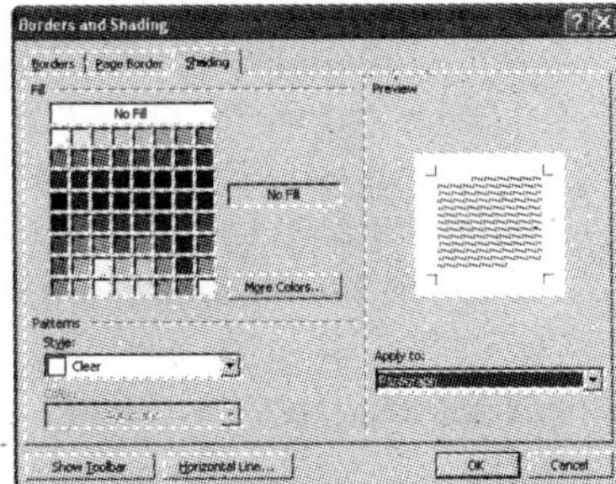

Shading

also use the Table AutoFormat command to quickly give a table a polished look with a variety of borders, fonts, and shading.

a. *Add a border to text:*

1. To add a border to a paragraph, click anywhere in the paragraph. To add a border only to specific text, select the text.
2. On the Format menu, click Borders and Shading, and then click the Borders tab.
3. Select the options you want, and make sure the correct option—Paragraph or Text is selected under Apply to.
4. To specify that only particular sides get borders, click Custom under Setting. Under Preview, click the diagram's sides, or use the buttons to apply and remove borders.
5. To specify the exact position of the border relative to the text, click Paragraph under Apply to, click Options, and then select the options you want.

b. *Add shading to a table, a paragraph, or selected text:* You can use shading to fill in the background of a table, a paragraph, or selected text.

1. To add shading to a table, click anywhere in the table. To add shading to specific cells, select the cells, including the end-of-cell marks.

   To add shading to a paragraph, click anywhere in the paragraph. To add shading to specific text, such as a word, select the text.
2. On the Format menu, click Borders and Shading, and then click the Shading tab.
3. Select the options you want.
4. Under Apply to, click the part of the document you want to apply shading to. For example, if you clicked a cell without selecting it in step 1, click Cell. Otherwise, Word applies the shading to the entire table.

Graphics Borders and Fills

You can add borders to drawing objects (including text boxes and AutoShapes) or to pictures, and you can enhance your drawing objects by adding a gradient (shaded), patterned, textured, or picture fill. Add or change a gradient (shaded), patterned, textured, or picture fill in a drawing object as:

1. Select the drawing object you want to change.
2. On the Drawing toolbar, click the arrow next to Fill Color, click Fill Effects, and then click the Gradient, Texture, Pattern, or Picture tab.
3. Select the options you want.

TAB STOPS

Tabs are basically used for aligning your paragraphs. The tabs are very useful keys that are used for faster movement of the text cursor or insertion. Tabs are the tools that are used to line text up vertically. You must use tabs if you want a vertical alignment. Estimating spacing by eye does not give a neat professional look to your document. By default, each line has a left tab at each 1/2" mark along its length. To add other tabs, click on the Tab Indicator Button to toggle between the different tab types available. Drag the tab indicator to the appropriate place on the ruler to set a new tab. All default tabs to the left of a new tab are deleted. The ruler is divided into 1/8" increments, so the ruler is marked every 8 divisions, which is one inch. The First Line Indent and Hanging Indent markers can also be dragged along the ruler to change indentation spacing. When the enter button is pressed, the cursor advances to the next line, carrying the tabs from the previous line. Unwanted tabs can be removed by dragging them off of the ruler. Use the Tab key to advance the cursor to the next tab location (Figs 4.4 and 4.5).

- *First line indent:* Indicates where the first line of a paragraph indents to.
- *Hanging indent:* Indicates where text lines up when it wraps from one line to the next.
- *Left tab:* Left justifies text at the tab point.
- *Center tab:* Center justifies text at the tab point.
- *Right tab:* Right justifies text at the tab point.
- *Decimal tab:* Aligns a decimal point with the tab point.
- *Line tab:* Draws a vertical line at the location of the tab.

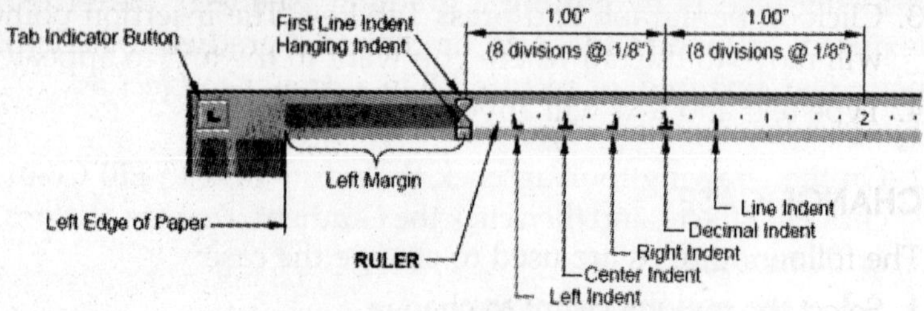

Fig. 4.4: Types of indents and tabs

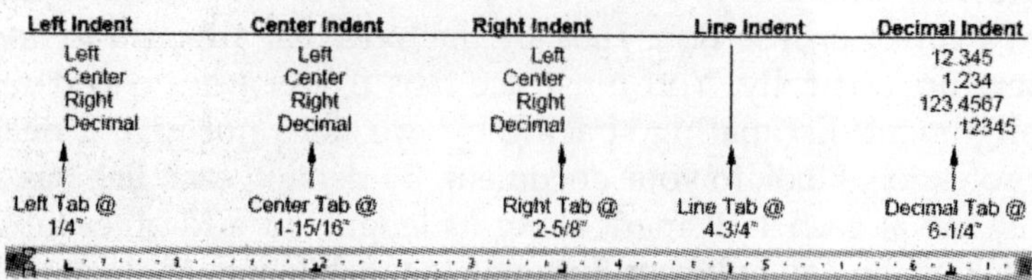

Fig. 4.5: Example of indents and tabs

The most common types of tab stops are:

a. *Left aligned tab stop:* Text or numbers are left aligned at the column specified by the tab stop.

b. *Right aligned tab stop:* Text or numbers are right aligned at the column specified by the tab stop.

c. *Center aligned tab stop:* Text or numbers are centered along the column position specified by the tab stop.

d. *Decimal tab stop:* The fractional figures are aligned in such a way so that all the decimal points are vertically aligned.

To set a tab follow the given below steps:

1. Place the mouse pointer on the Tab button at the left of the ruler to select any of the alignments.
2. Click on the Ruler to set the tab for current paragraph or any currently selected text. A left, center or decimal tab symbol will appear in the ruler at the spot you selected.

3. Click on paragraph and press Tab key. The insertion point will move to the tab where you want to the text to appear.
4. Type text and text will appear on the page.

CHANGE CASE

The following steps are used to change the case:

1. Select the text you want to change.
2. On the Format menu, click Change Case.
3. Click the capitalization option you want (Table 4.5).

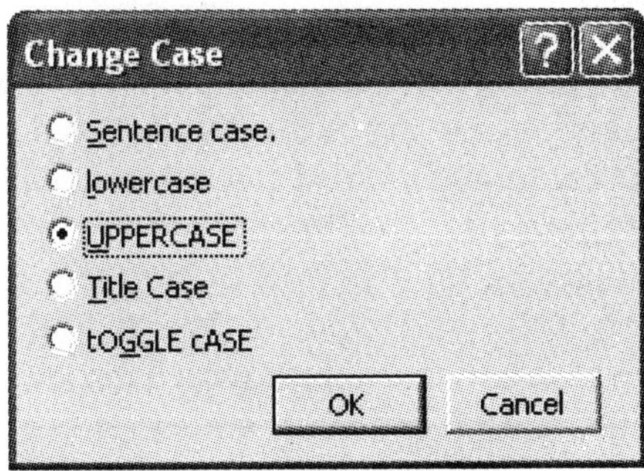

AUTOFORMAT

By using AutoFormat, you can quickly apply formatting such as headings, bulleted and numbered lists, borders, numbers, symbols, and fractions to your text. Microsoft Word can also:

- Automatically format Internet, network, and e-mail addresses as hyperlinks.
- Apply bold or italic character formatting to text surrounded by asterisks (*) or underscores (_).
- Replace two hyphens (--) with an em dash (–).

You can automatically format a document either as you type or after you have written it. Word analyzes each paragraph to see how it is used in the document; for example, as a heading or as an item in a numbered list and then applies a style that is appropriate for that item.

Table 4.5: Meaning of different cases

Case	Meaning
Sentence case	Capitalizes the first letter of the first word in the selected sentence.
Lowercase	Changes all selected text to lowercase letters.
UPPERCASE	Changes all selected text to capital letters.
Title Case	Capitalizes the first letter of each word in the selection.
tOGGLE cASE	Changes all uppercase letters to lowercase in the selection and vice-versa.

Word offers two ways to automatically format a document:

1. Format text automatically as you type. When you set options on the AutoFormat As You Type tab (Tools menu, AutoCorrect command), Word can automatically format text as you are typing your document. For example, if you type a number followed by a period or hyphen, followed by a space or tab, followed by text, Word makes the text a numbered list. You can select which types of automatic formatting changes Word does and does not make as you type. Turn on or off options for formatting a document automatically as you type.

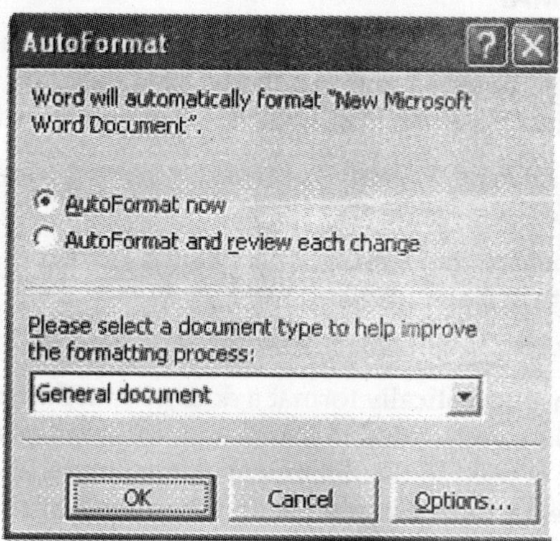

2. Format a document automatically after you have written it. When you use the AutoFormat dialog box (Format menu, AutoFormat command), Word can format text in one pass, enabling you to review all the changes Word makes and accept or reject each one. Automatically format a document in a separate pass.

In both cases, you can control which automatic changes Word makes. You can also turn off automatic formatting.

STYLE

When working with Word, you can use styles to quickly format your documents. A style is a set of formats consisting of such things as fonts, font colors, font sizes, and paragraph formats. Word 2007 supplies you with pre-designed style sets that contain styles for titles, subtitles, quotes, headings, lists and more.

You can see of all the styles available to you in the style set by clicking the launcher in the Styles group and opening the Styles pane. You can leave the Styles pane open and available for use by docking it. To dock the Styles pane, click the top of the pane and drag it to the left or right edge of the Word window. You do not need to select an entire paragraph to apply a style. If the cursor is anywhere in the paragraph, when you click on the style, Word formats the entire paragraph.

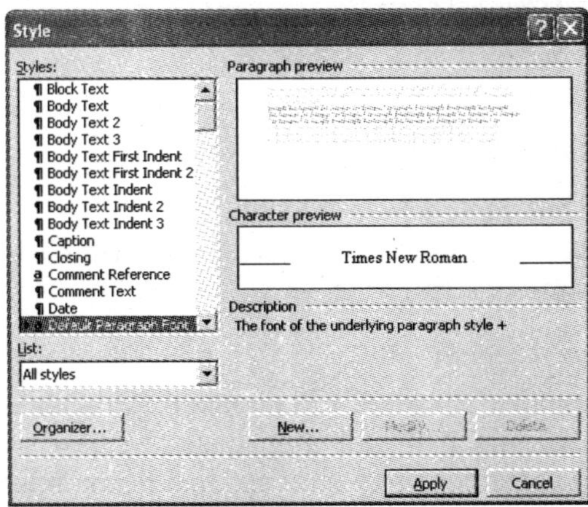

Once you have applied styles, changing to another style set is easy. You simply open the Style Set gallery. As you move your cursor down the menu, Word 2007 provides you with a live preview of the effect of applying the style set. To choose a style set, you click it.

A style is a set of formatting characteristics that you can apply to text in your document to quickly change its appearance. When you apply a style, you apply a whole group of formats in one simple task. When you start Microsoft Word, the new blank document is based on the Normal template, and text that you type uses the Normal style. This means that when you start typing, Word uses the font, font size, line spacing, text alignment, and other formats currently defined for the Normal style. The Normal style is the base style for the Normal template, meaning that it is a building block for other styles in the template.

There are a number of other styles besides Normal available in the Normal template. A few basic ones are shown in the Style list on the Formatting toolbar. You can preview and select others in the Style dialog box (Format menu, Style command).

When you want to change the style of text, you can apply an existing style, also known as a built-in style. If you do not see a style with the characteristics you want, you can create a new style, and then apply it.

Create a new character style:

1. On the Format menu, click Style.
2. Click New.
3. In the Name box, type a name for the style.
4. In the Style type box, click Character.
5. Select the other options you want, and then click Format to set attributes for the style.

Create a new paragraph style:

The quickest way to create a new paragraph style is to format a paragraph, select it, and then base the new style on the formatting and other properties applied to the selected text.

1. Select the text that contains the formatting you want to use for your style.
2. On the Formatting toolbar, click inside the Style box.
3. Type over the existing style name to create the name for the new style.
4. Press ENTER.

SPELLING AND GRAMMAR

Word checks your spelling and grammar as you type. Spelling errors display with a red wavy line under the word. Grammar errors display with a green wavy line under the error. In Word 2007, you can use the Review tab's Spelling and Grammar button to initiate a spell and grammar check of your document.

Use spell check as:

1. For example, type the following exactly as shown. Include all errors. Open thr door for Mayrala. She is a teacher from the town of Ridgemont.
2. Select: "Open thr door for Mayrala. She is a teacher from the town of Ridgemont".
3. Choose the Tools menu.
4. Click the Spelling and Grammar button. The Spelling and Grammar dialog box appears.
5. "The" is misspelled, so it is highlighted on the screen and noted in the Not in Dictionary box. Word suggests correct

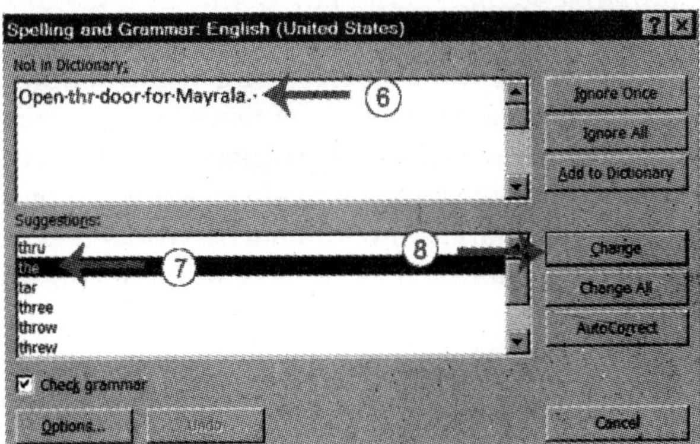

spellings. These suggestions are found in the Suggestions box.

6. Click "the" in the Suggestions box.
7. Click Change.

   Note: If the word is misspelled in several places, click Change All to correct all misspellings.

8. The name "Mayrala" is not in the dictionary, but it is correct. Click Ignore Once to leave "Mayrala" in the document with its current spelling.

   Note: If a word appears in several places in the document, click Ignore All so you are not prompted to correct the spelling for each occurrence.

9. "Ridgemont" is not found in the dictionary. If you frequently use a word not found in the dictionary, you might want to add that word to the dictionary by clicking the Add to Dictionary button. Word will then recognize the word the next time it appears. Click Add to Dictionary.
10. The following should appear on your screen: "Word finished checking the selection. Do you want to continue checking the remainder of the document?"
11. Click No. If you wanted Word to spell-check the entire document, you would have clicked Yes.

AUTOSUMMARIZE

AutoSummarize identifies the key points in a document for you to share with others or quickly scan. AutoSummarize determines key points by analyzing the document and assigning a score to each sentence. Sentences that contain words used frequently in the document are given a higher score. You then choose a percentage of the highest-scoring sentences to display in the summary. AutoSummarize works best on well-structured documents such as reports, articles, and scientific papers.

1. To create a summary for others to read, use AutoSummarize to have Word copy the key points and insert them into an executive summary or abstract.

2. To read a summary of an online document, you can display the document in AutoSummarize view. In this view, you can switch between displaying only the key points in a document (the rest of the document is hidden) and highlighting them in the document. As you read, you can also change the level of detail at any time.
3. To use AutoSummarize keywords and sentences outside of a document, you can have AutoSummarize copy high-scoring keywords and sentences to the Keywords and Comments boxes (respectively) on the Summary tab (File menu, Properties command). You can then use these file properties to search for files or to check the content of a file without opening the file.

You can summarize documents written in Chinese (simplified and traditional), English, French, German, Italian, Japanese, Korean, Portuguese (Brazilian), Spanish, or Swedish. AutoSummarize generates a summary based on the language in use when you install Word or Office. If a document is written in a language other than the default language, AutoSummarize uses that language instead. If a document contains text in more than one language, AutoSummarize generates a summary in the language used most frequently in the document. Word may attempt to automatically install the files it needs to create the summary.

PROTECT DOCUMENT

This feature prevents users from changing a form containing form fields. After creating a form that users will view and complete in Word, you must protect it so that users can enter information only in the designated areas.

1. On the Tools menu, click Protect Document.
2. Click Forms.
3. To assign a password to the form so that users who know the password can remove the protection and change the form, type a password in the Password box. Users who do not know the password can still enter information in the form fields.

4. To protect the entire form, click OK.
5. To protect only parts of a form, those parts must be in separate sections. Click Sections, and then clear the check boxes of the sections you do not want to protect.

MAIL MERGE

Many day-to-day applications require similar document containing similar text to be sent to a number of persons. These documents also have a typically common layout. Automation is desired when the number of letters to be generated is large. This task can be easily automated by use of mail merger feature of Word processor.

The three main components of the merge process include:

1. ***The main document:*** It contains normal text plus field names, which contain instructions for carrying out the merge. The basic information in the main document remains the same. Word would then insert the names and addresses in specific places in the merged document. Before you can instruct Word to merge documents, you must have inserted field names in your main document.
2. ***Field names:*** In the main document field names are used to indicate where variable information is to be inserted. In the data file, field name indicates the category of information in each column. The field names inserted into the main document must match the field names in the data file.
3. ***Data file:*** The data file stores information to be brought into the main document. You can think of the data file as a name and address list from which the program gets what you want to include in the main document. The data file table contains a column for each category of information or data field in the data file.

We can use the Mail Merge Helper to create form letters, mailing labels, envelopes, or catalogs. The Mail Merge Helper guides us through organizing the address data, merging it into a generic document, and printing the resulting personalized documents.

1. Open or create a main document, which contains the generic information that you want to repeat in each form letter, mailing label, envelope, or catalog.
2. Open or create a data source, which contains the data that varies in the merged documents; for example, the name and address of each recipient of a form letter. The data source can be an existing spreadsheet, database, or text file, or a Word table that you create by using the Mail Merge Helper.
3. In the main document, insert merge fields, which are placeholders that tell Microsoft Word where to insert data from the data source.
4. Merge data from the data source into the main document. Each row (or record) in the data source produces an individual form letter, mailing label, envelope, or catalog item. You can send the merged documents directly to a printer, or to e-mail addresses or fax numbers. Or you can collect the merged documents into a new document so you can review and print them later.

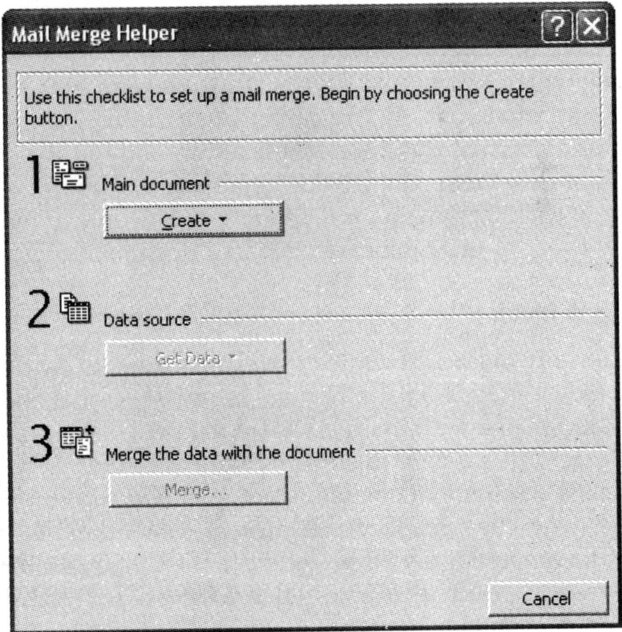

MACRO

If you perform a task repeatedly in Word, you can automate the task by using a macro. A macro is a series of Word commands and instructions that you group together as a single command to accomplish a task automatically. Instead of manually performing a series of time-consuming, repetitive actions in Word, you can create and run a single macro in effect, a custom command that accomplishes the task for you.

Uses for macros include:

- To speed up routine editing and formatting.
- To combine multiple commands; for example, inserting a table with a specific size and borders, and with a specific number of rows and columns.
- To make an option in a dialog box more accessible.
- To automate a complex series of tasks.

Word offers two ways for you to create a macro: The macro recorder and the Visual Basic Editor.

Creating a Macro

You can create a macro by using the macro recorder to record a sequence of actions, or you can create a macro from scratch by entering Visual Basic for Applications code in the Visual Basic Editor. When you are recording a macro, you can use the mouse to click commands and options, but the macro recorder does not record mouse movements in a document window.

Storing a Macro

You can store macros in templates or in documents. By default, Word stores macros in the Normal template so that they are available for use with every Word document. If you plan to use a macro in a single document, store it in that document. Individual macros in a document are stored in macro projects that you can copy from one document to another. To copy, delete, or rename a macro project, use the Organizer. On the Tools menu, point to Macro, click Macros, and then click Organizer.

TEMPLATES AND ADD-INS

Every Microsoft Word document is based on a template. A template determines the basic structure for a document and contains document settings such as AutoText entries, fonts, key assignments, macros, menus, page layout, special formatting, and styles. The two basic types of templates are global templates and document templates. Global templates, including the Normal template, contain settings that are available to all documents. Document templates, such as the memo or fax templates in the New dialog box, contain settings that are available only to documents based on that template. For example, if you create a memo using the memo template, the memo can use the settings from both the memo template as well as the settings in any global template. Word provides a variety of document templates, and you can create your own document templates.

Loading Templates and Add-ins

Templates can store styles, AutoText entries, AutoCorrect entries, macros, toolbars, custom menu settings, and shortcut keys. Loading a template makes it available as a global template. Add-ins are supplemental programs that you install to extend the capabilities of Word by adding custom commands and specialized features.

When you load a template or add-in, it remains loaded for the current Word session only. If you quit and then restart Word, the template or add-in is not automatically reloaded. To have a template or add-in available whenever you start Word, store the add-in or template in your startup folder. To locate or change your Startup setting, click Options on the Tools menu, and then click the File Locations tab.

Unloading Templates and Add-ins

To conserve memory and increase the speed of Word, it is a good idea to unload templates and add-in programs you do not often use. When you unload a template or add-in that is located in your startup folder, Word unloads the template for the current Word session but automatically reloads it the next time you start Word. When you unload a template or add-in located in any other folder, it is unavailable until you reload it. To delete a template or add-in from Word, you must remove the template or add-in from the Templates and Add-ins dialog box.

TABLE

Tables are used in a Word document to organize data or results. Most of the table functionality in Word can be accessed from the Table Toolbar. The Table toolbar can be turned on using the menu sequence View → Toolbars then selecting Tables and Borders from the list.

There are two methods for inserting a table: Use the Draw Table tool, or use the Insert Table tool, which is the same command as Table → Insert → Table. Using Insert → Table from the toolbar, the following dialog box opens:

When the cursor is placed over the table, the Table Anchor appears. The table can be dragged around the document by dragging the Table Anchor. Clicking on the Table Anchor also selects the entire table. When the table is selected, the menu sequence Table → Delete → Table will remove the table from

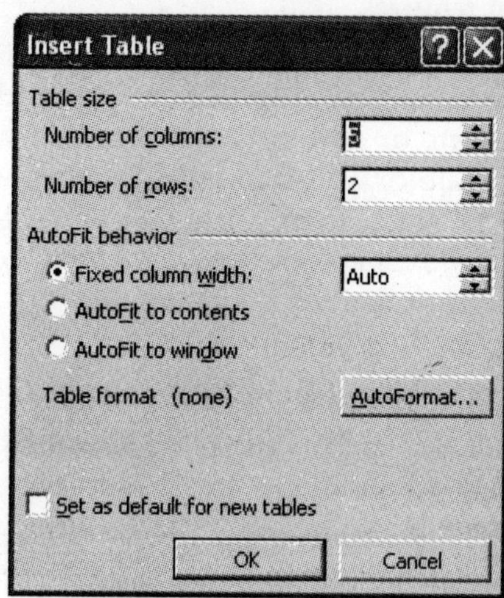

the document. Click in a cell and start typing to input data into the table.

Click on a line in a table and drag it to resize rows and columns. The preferred method for changing the size of a row or column is to right-click in a cell in the row or column and select "Table Properties..." from the menu. This action opens the Table Properties dialog box, which allows the user to specify the alignment of the table, the size of rows and columns as well as to indicate how text wraps around the table.

To change the fill of a cell:

1. Place the cursor in the cell or cells.
2. Pick the fill color from the tool on the Table toolbar.

To change a border of a cell:

1. Place the cursor in a cell or select multiple cells.
2. Select the line style from the list on the Table toolbar.
3. Select the line weight from the list on the Table toolbar.
4. Pick the appropriate template from the Border Template tool on the Table toolbar. The border is automatically applied.

To change the alignment of the text in a cell:

1. Place the cursor in a cell or select multiple cells or select the whole table.
2. Select the appropriate text alignment template from the Text Alignment tool of the Table toolbar.

To merge cells:

1. Select two or more cells to be merged.
2. Pick the Merge Cells tool from the Table toolbar.

To split a cell:

1. Select the cell to be divided.
2. Pick the Split Cells tool from the Table toolbar and specify the number of rows and columns to split the cell into.

To distribute rows evenly:

1. Select the rows to be distributed. Note that the whole row must be selected.

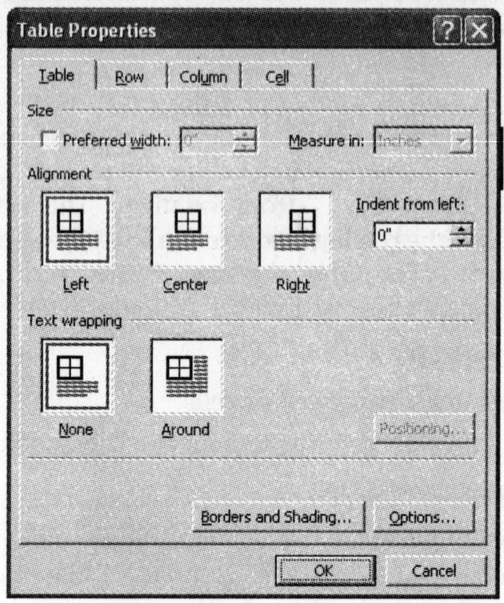

2. Pick on the Distribute Rows Evenly tool from the Table toolbar.

To distribute columns evenly:

1. Select the columns to be distributed. The whole column must be selected.
2. Pick on the Distribute Columns Evenly tool from the Table toolbar.

To delete a table:

1. Select the Table Anchor to select the table.
2. Use the menu sequence Table → Delete → Table.

To delete a row from a table:

1. Place the cursor in a cell in the row to be deleted.
2. Use the menu sequence Table → Delete → Rows.

To delete a column from a table:

1. Place the cursor in a cell in the row to be deleted.
2. Use the menu sequence Table → Delete → Columns.

To insert a row or column into a table:

1. Place the cursor in a cell in the row or column next to the one to be added. If more than one row or column is selected, the same number of rows or columns will be inserted.
2. Use the menu sequence Table → Insert and select:
   a. Columns to the left.
   b. Columns to the right.
   c. Rows above.
   d. Rows below.

Convert table to text:

1. Select the rows or table that you want to convert to paragraphs.
2. On the Table menu, point to Convert, and then click Table to Text.
3. Under Separate text with, click the option for the separator character you want to use in place of the column boundaries. Rows are separated with paragraph marks.

AutoFit:

- If you are working on a Web page or in Web layout view, you can set the table to automatically resize to fit in a window when you change the window size. Click in the table. On the Table menu, point to AutoFit, and then click AutoFit to Window.
- To make the columns in a table automatically fit the contents, click a table, point to AutoFit on the Table menu, and then click AutoFit to Contents.

FORMULA

Calculates a number by using a mathematical formula. You can use the Formula command (Table menu) to insert an = (Formula) field in a table or in regular text.

1. *Formula:* An expression that can contain any combination of numbers, bookmarks that refer to numbers, fields resulting in numbers, and the available operators and functions. The

expression can refer to values in a table and values returned by functions.

2. *Bookmark:* The name of a bookmark that refers to one or more values.
3. *Numeric picture:* Specifies how to display the result of the calculation the number of decimal places, how to display negative numbers, and so on. For more information.

FILE FORMAT CONVERTERS SUPPLIED WITH WORD

The file format converters supplied with word are shown in Table 4.6.

Table 4.6: File format converters

File format	*Comments*
Wordperfect for MS-DOS	Opens and saves versions 5.x and opens 6.x documents.
Wordperfect for Windows	Opens and saves versions 5.x and opens 6.x documents.
Microsoft Excel	Opens versions 2.x, 3.0, 4.0, 5.0, 95, and 97(or 97/2000).
Microsoft Word for Windows 2.x	Saves as version 2.x. No converter is needed to open Word 2.x documents.
Word 6.0/95	Saves as Word 6.0/95 binary file format with a .doc extension.
Word 97 and 6.0/95-RTF	Saves as Rich Text Format (RTF) with a .doc extension.
Microsoft Word	Opens Word 97/2000 documents in Word 6.0, Word 95, PowerPoint, Works, and Publisher.
Microsoft Word for the Macintosh	Saves as 4.x and 5.x. No converter is required for opening these formats in Word 2000.
Microsoft Works 4.0 for Windows	Opens and saves version 4.0 for Windows 95.

Contd...

Contd...

Lotus 1-2-3	Opens versions 2.x, 3.x, and 4.0.
Lotus Notes	Use to open Word 6.0, Word 95, Word 97, and Word 2000 in Lotus Notes 3.x and 4.x.
Recover Text from Any File	Recovers text from damaged documents.

PLAIN-TEXT FILE FORMATS SUPPLIED WITH WORD

The formats shown in Table 4.7 do not use a file converter.

Table 4.7: Plain-text formats

File format	*Comments*
Text only	Saves text without its formatting. Converts all section breaks, page breaks, and new line characters to paragraph marks. Uses the ANSI character set. Select this format only if the destination program cannot read any of the other available file formats.
MS-DOS text only	Converts files the same way as Text only format. Uses the extended ASCII character set, which is the standard for MS-DOS-based programs. Use this format to share documents between Word and non-Windows-based programs.
Text only with line breaks, MS-DOS text only with line breaks	Saves text without formatting. Converts all line breaks, section breaks, and page breaks to paragraph marks. Use this format when you want to maintain line breaks—for example, when transferring documents to an electronic mail system.
Text with layout, MS-DOS text with layout (uses a file converter)	Preserves line breaks. Inserts spaces in a converted document to approximate indents, tables, line spacing, paragraph spacing, and tab stops. Converts section breaks and page breaks to paragraph marks. Use this format to convert a document to a text

Contd...

Contd...

	file format while preserving the page layout.
Rich text format (RTF)	Saves all formatting. Converts formatting to instructions that other programs, including compatible Microsoft programs, can read and interpret.
Encoded text	Saves text without its formatting. Uses the encoding standard that you choose. Use this format when you share documents with people who use system software in another language.

Microsoft Excel

INTRODUCTION

Microsoft Excel is a spreadsheet program under Windows. It is commonly used for the purpose of calculations, recalculations and repetitive information. It is used in financial organizations. And is a very useful package for business applications—stocks, inventory control, investments, budgetary control and analysis. The features of MS Excel are as follows:

1. ***Workbooks:*** A document in MS Excel is called a workbook. Each workbook contains sixteen worksheets by default. A user can change this number by resetting the default options. Worksheets within workbooks make it easy to bind files of related information. When a user opens a workbook, he can use all the worksheets to perform a task. To create a workbook, a user will have to select the New command from the File menu. To open an existing workbook, a user will have to select the Open option from the File menu. A user can insert a worksheet between two worksheets by choosing the Worksheet option from the Insert menu.

2. ***Using keyboard:*** It provides different keyboard shortcuts for selecting a row, column, current cell, worksheet, etc. For example:

- *Entire column:* CTRL + Spacebar.
- *Entire row:* SHIFT + Spacebar.
- *Entire worksheet:* CTRL + SHIFT + Spacebar.

3. ***Entries in cell:*** A user can perform various kinds of entries in a cell. He can enter text, number, data, and time in a cell. He can also enter some special characters such as $ % + – / ( ). He can also enter date and time in a cell. He can select different formats for date and time according to his own requirements.

4. ***Entering data in series:*** A user can fill a range of cells either with the same value or with the series of values. This can be done using the AutoFill handle (small square on the bottom-right corner of the active cell).

5. ***Cell references:*** MS Excel provides three types of cell references: Relative, absolute, and mixed. Relative references refer to the cell relative to the given position. Absolute references refer to the specific cell irrespective of the position of the formula. The '$' sign is used to denote an absolute reference. Mixed references are a combination of both relative and absolute references. It has one absolute coordinate and one relative coordinate. $CI and C$1 are both examples of mixed references.

6. ***Searching and replacing data:*** MS Excel allows fast searching and instant replacing of data. To search or replace the data entered by a user, he can use the Find or Replace command from the Edit menu.

7. ***Inserting or deleting rows and columns:*** MS Excel provides the facility to insert rows or columns into the existing worksheet. Inserting a row of data shifts the rest of the rows down and removes the last row of the worksheet. Similarly, inserting a column shifts the rest of the columns to the right and deletes the rightmost column. This occurs because the total number of rows and columns remain the same in any case.

8. ***Formatting features:*** MS Excel provides several formatting features that enhance the appearance of the data, which is presented in the worksheets. Some of them are described as follows:

MS Excel allows setting up a page before printing. To set up a page, a user will have to open the File menu and click on the Page Setup. The Page Setup dialog box will appear that will allow the user to set the paper size, orientation of the data, scaling of the area, set the left, right, bottom, and top margin, set the header and the footer, etc.

MS Excel provides the Autofit selection that adjusts the width of the column according to the widest entry in that column. A user can hide or unhide certain rows or columns. He can also provide the default column standard width.

MS Excel allows a user to align the characters in different ways by using the Alignment tab page of the Format Cells dialog box. The dialog box provides a number of alignment options as given below:

Horizontal Alignment Options

- *General:* The text is left aligned and the numbers are right aligned. This is the default status.
- *Left:* Aligns the contents to the left of the cell.
- *Center:* Aligns the cell contents to the center of the cell.
- *Right:* Aligns the contents to the right of the cell.
- *Fill:* Fills the selected cells with the single character.
- *Justify:* This option is selected with multiple lines of text as it wraps the contents from left-to-right.

Vertical Alignment Options

- *Top:* Aligns the text at the top of the cell.
- *Center:* Places the text in the center of the cell.
- *Bottom:* Aligns the text on the bottom of the cell.
- *Justify:* Wraps the text from top-to-bottom.

9. ***Viewing of worksheets:*** MS Excel provides a facility of viewing the same worksheet simultaneously in more than one window. This is accomplished by selecting the New Window command in the Windows menu. A user can also create more than one window to arrange the workspace to promptly access the information needed. Using MS Excel, a window can be arranged in different ways by using the Arrange command from the Windows menu.

If a user wants to move between different windows, he can do so by pressing Ctrl+F6 to go to the next window or by pressing Ctrl+Shift+F6 to go to the previous window. He can temporarily hide or unhide windows by choosing the Hide command in Window menu to hide the active window or by choosing the Unhide command in the Window menu to unhide the hidden window.

When a user works on a very large worksheet with row and column headings, the row headings scroll off to the left when he moves towards the right. Similarly, when he moves down to see the data, the column headings scroll up. To overcome this problem, he can split the active window into two, with row or column headings in one window and the data on the other window.

10. ***Controls:*** The controls are the special objects, which enhance user interface and facilitate user input. MS Excel provides several custom controls such as list boxes, check boxes, and dialog boxes, etc. A large number of toolbars are found in the View menu. Users can add a toolbar or a number of toolbars into the working document depending upon the work involved and use different controls in their documents.

11. ***Functions and formulas:*** The built-in formulas are called functions. MS Excel provides analyzing data and manipulating text by using different functions. Users can easily calculate percentage, interest, average, etc. by using built-in functions. This can be done either by typing in the function-based formulas or by using function wizards. Formulas are widely used in simple computing (such as addition, subtraction, multiplication and division) and advanced computing. They provide the power to analyze data extensively.

12. ***Auto-calculation:*** MS Excel spreadsheet allows a user to automatically recalculate the whole worksheet every time a change is made in a single cell. There are basically two kinds of recalculations:

- *Automatic:* In this type of calculation, the change in the value of the cell automatically recalculates the whole worksheet.
- *Manual:* In this type of calculation, the recalculation of the complete worksheet is performed by pressing the F9 key. This option can be selected on the Calculation tab page of the Options dialog box, which is opened by choosing Options from the Tools menu.

13. ***Charts:*** One of the most important features of MS Excel is a chart. MS Excel allows users to view data entered as tables in a graphical form as charts, which helps a user to easily

understand, analyze, and compare data. Excel allows its users to create either two-dimensional charts or three-dimensional charts. A user can enhance the chart by adding chart items, such as data labels, a legend, titles, text, and gridlines. He can also do formatting on these items by using colors, alignment, fonts, and other formatting attributes. MS Excel also allows users to view charts along with the data by using embedded charts. These charts are included in the worksheet and can be copied, moved, and resized in the same way as can be done with any other graphical object.

14. ***Database:*** Data are raw facts, information is processed data, and a database is an organized collection of information. Every organization heavily depends upon databases to store, retrieve, and maintain different kinds of data. MS Excel provides all this in the form of its database feature.

With the above-described features of MS Excel, users can perform almost all the operations they want in a very efficient and easy way. Its advanced features have made it the first choice for professionals working in a financial organization to perform their lengthy tasks in an easy way and in a quick manner. Therefore, MS Excel has become the most preferred choice for most of the users as well as professionals throughout the world.

STARTING EXCEL

You can start Excel by:

1. Double-clicking on the Microsoft Excel application icon. This application is usually in a folder called Excel. An alias for this icon appears on the desktop of the computers. Or

Microsoft Excel

2. Click the pointer on the Start button on the Windows taskbar. The start menu will appear. Click on Programs. The program menu will appear. Then click on Microsoft Excel.

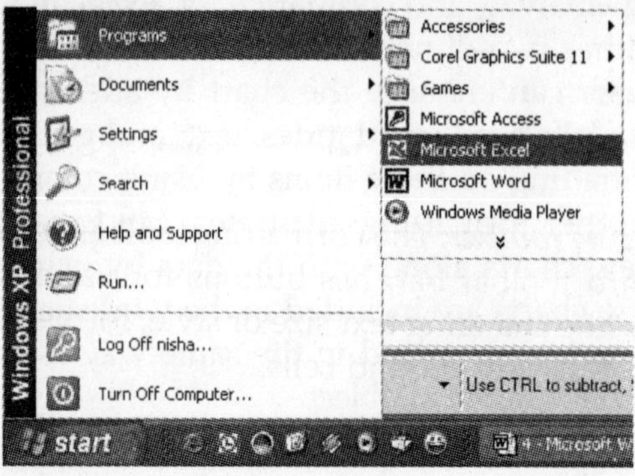

COMPONENTS OF EXCEL WINDOW

Besides the usual window components (close box, title bar, scroll bars, etc.), an Excel window has several unique elements identified as shown below:

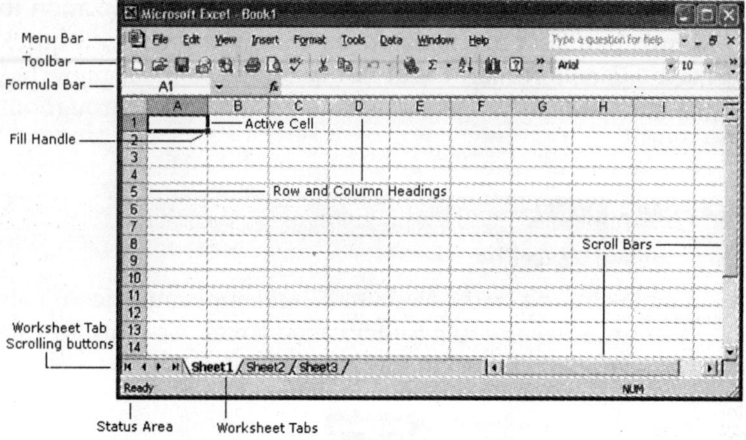

1. ***Standard toolbar:*** The Standard toolbar, located beneath the menu bar, has buttons for commonly performed tasks like adding a column of numbers, printing, sorting, and other operations. Excel let's you customize the toolbar or even display multiple toolbars at the same time. The Standard Excel XP toolbar appears.

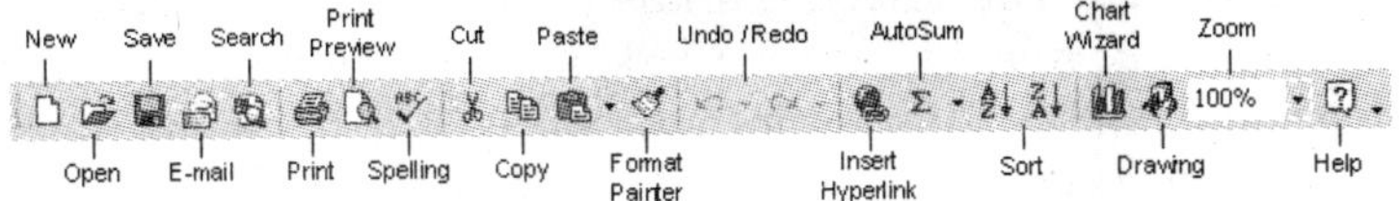

2. ***Formatting toolbar:*** The Formatting toolbar, located beneath the Standard toolbar bar, has buttons for various formatting operations like changing text size or style, formatting numbers and placing borders around cells.

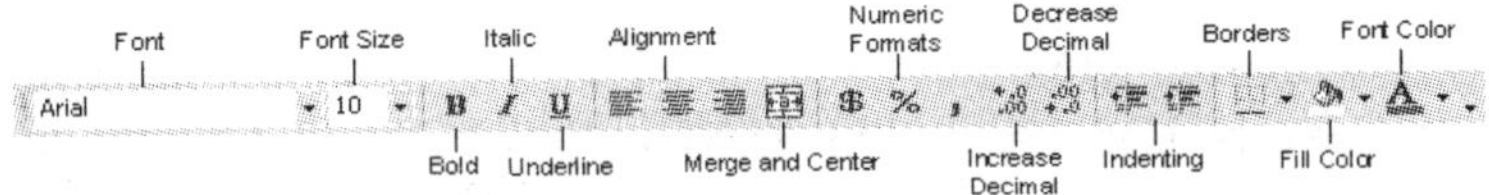

3. ***Formula bar:*** The Formula bar is located beneath the toolbar at the top of the Excel worksheet. Use the formula bar to enter and edit worksheet data. The contents of the active cell always appear in the formula bar. When you click the mouse in the formula bar, an X and a check mark appear. You can click the check icon to confirm and completes editing, or the X to abandon editing.

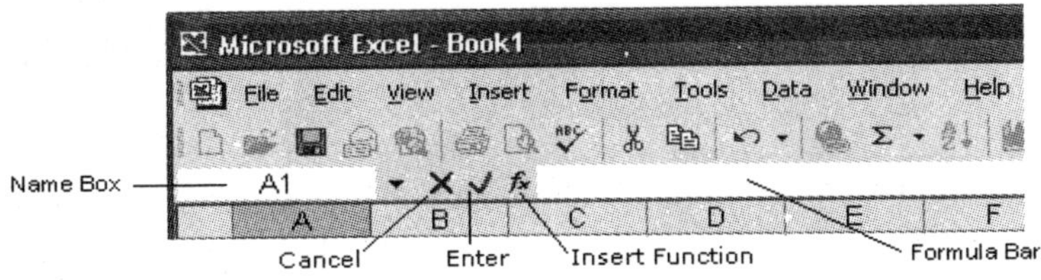

4. ***Name box:*** The Name box displays the reference of the selected cells.

5. ***Row and column headings:*** Letters and numbers identify the rows and columns on an Excel spreadsheet. The intersection of a row and a column is called a cell. Use row and column headings to specify a cell's reference. For example, the cell located where column B and row 7 intersect is called B7.

6. ***Active cell:*** The active cell has a dark border around it to indicate your position in the worksheet. All text and numbers that you type are inserted into the active cell. Click the mouse on a cell to make it active.

7. ***Fill handle:*** The lower right corner of the active cell has a small box called a Fill Handle. Your mouse changes to a cross-hair when you are on the Fill Handle. The Fill Handle helps you copy data and create series of information. For example, if you type January in the active cell and then drag the Fill Handle over four cells, Excel automatically inserts February, March, April and May.

8. ***Worksheet tabs:*** An Excel workbook consists of multiple worksheets. Use the worksheet tabs at the bottom of the screen to navigate between worksheets within a workbook.

WORKING WITH EXCEL DOCUMENTS

Opening and Closing Documents

To open an existing Excel workbook, choose Open from the File menu or click the Open tool on the toolbar. Excel will display the Open dialog box, which is similar in appearance and function to the Save As dialog box. It contains a File Name:

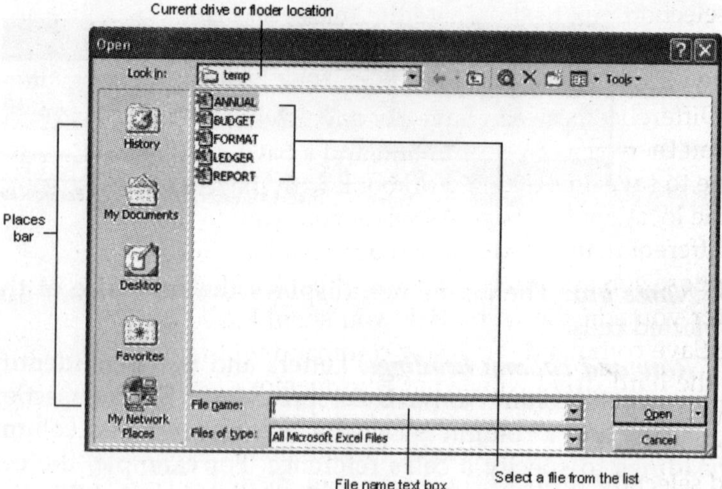

box for you to type a file name or file specification, a Look In: box to designate a location, and a drop-down menu of file types.

To open a file, select the appropriate location by clicking on the down pointing arrow next to the Look In: selection box. Excel will display all Excel files found there. Select the file you wish to open and click Open to open the file.

Saving a Document

The lower right corner of the active cell has a small box called a Fill Handle. Your mouse changes to a cross-hair when you are on the Fill Handle. The Fill Handle helps you copy data and create series of information. For example, if you type January in the active cell and then drag the Fill Handle over four cells, Excel automatically inserts February, March, April and May.

To save an untitled Excel workbook, from the File menu choose Save As or click the Save button on the toolbar (shown at right). The Excel Save As dialog box is the same as the Open dialog box above except it is labeled "Save As".

The Save As dialog box contains a text box for you to type a specific filename, a "Save File as Type:" box to save your workbook in a different format that other programs can read, a selection box to designate the folder and drive in which to save the file, and a "Places Bar" that offers other locations to save your file.

Difference between Save As and Save: Notice on the File menu there is a Save command and a Save As command. Use Save to save an existing workbook with the same name in the same location. Use Save As when you want to save a file with a different name or save it in a different location. For example, suppose you are working on a workbook called BUDGET.XLS. After you edit the workbook, you should save it again using the Save command. The Save command will replace the copy on the hard drive with what is in memory (what you see on your screen). At the end of the day, you might want to save a copy of the file on a diskette to take home. Choose Save As and select the proper drive in the Save As dialog box. This will create another copy of the file on your diskette.

Creating a New Workbook

The lower right corner of the active cell has a small box called a Fill Handle. Your mouse changes to a cross-hair when you are on the Fill Handle. The Fill Handle helps you copy data and create series of information. For example, if you type January in the active cell and then drag the Fill Handle over four cells, Excel automatically inserts February, March, April and May.

If you are already in Excel and you want to create a new workbook, choose New from the File menu or click the New tool on the toolbar. If you choose New from the file menu the Task Pane will open on the right side of the Excel worksheet. To create a blank workbook, click Blank Workbook in the Task Pane, and a new workbook opens.

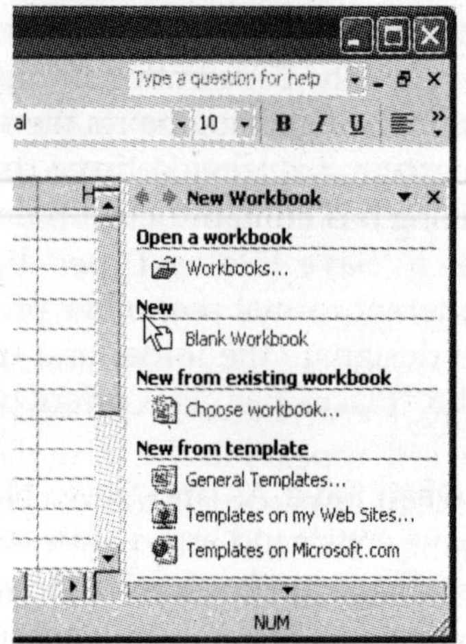

Managing Multiple Workbooks

Excel enables you to have more than one workbook open simultaneously. Each open workbook appears on the Window menu. The document with the check next to it is the active document. To switch to another document, simply choose that document from the Window menu. To navigate between worksheets within a workbook, click the worksheet tab you want to activate. Double-click a worksheet tab to change its name.

ENTERING AND EDITING DATA

Entering Data

You can enter text, numbers and dates in an Excel worksheet. In Excel's terminology, numbers and dates are called values and text is referred to as a label. To enter data of any type, click on the cell you want to contain that data, and then type the information you want in the cell. When you begin typing, your data also appears in the formula bar. When you have finished typing the data for the active cell, press the Return or Enter key.

Editing Data

The easiest way to edit the contents of a cell is to select the cell and then retype the entry. The new entry replaces the old contents. For example, to change the number in cell B6 to 199, select cell B6, type 199 and press Return. This method works well with numbers, but is more difficult when editing long text labels or formulas.

The formula bar gives you more flexibility while editing. When the mouse pointer moves into the formula bar, it changes shape to an I-beam, signifying that you can enter or edit text. Text in the active cell appears in the formula bar and you can edit it there. Use the mouse to select the text you want to change in the formula bar and then type the new text. Excel automatically replaces what is selected. Do not forget to press the Return key when you finish editing a cell.

You can also edit labels and values directly in cells. Double-click on the cell you want to edit. This puts an insertion point in the cell. Edit the contents of that cell the same way you would using the formula bar.

Moving the Active Cell

Cell selection and movement around the worksheet are similar operations in Excel. To select a given cell or make it active, simply click on that cell. Use the mouse or the arrow keys to move around the worksheet. For example, if you press the right arrow key twice you move two cells to the right. Refer to the table below for additional information on using the keyboard to navigate a worksheet.

To move	Press this key
One cell left	Left Arrow
One cell right	Right Arrow
One cell up	Up Arrow
One cell down	Down Arrow
To top of worksheet (cell A1)	Control Home
To last cell containing data	Control End
To end of data in a column	Control Down Arrow
To beginning of data in a column	Control Up Arrow
To end of data in a row	Control Right Arrow
To beginning of data in a row	Control Left Arrow

Go to Command

A quick way to move a large distance on a worksheet is with the Go To command on the Edit menu. When you select the Go To command, a dialog box prompts you to identify the cell. Enter the cell reference and click OK or press Return.

Clearing Cell Contents

To clear the contents of a cell choose Clear from the Edit menu. Then, select what you want to clear from the cell: All, Formats, Contents, or Notes. Most frequently you will want to clear the Contents of a cell. Pressing the Delete key also clears the contents of cells.

Undoing Mistakes

If you make a terrible mistake and you accidentally delete important data. Use the Undo command on the Edit menu or the Undo tool to correct the mistake.

Copying and Moving Data

Copy selected data from one cell to another with the Copy and Paste commands, or with the Drag and Drop procedure. If you want to move data instead, use the **Cut and** Paste commands, or the Drag and Drop procedure. These commands are described below:

- ***Cut:*** The Cut command extracts the selected data and puts it on the Clipboard, a temporary storage area. The contents of the Clipboard are overwritten with each copy or cut.
- ***Copy:*** The Copy command puts a copy of the selected data on the Clipboard.
- ***Paste:*** The Paste command inserts the Clipboard's contents into the active cell. Selected data is replaced by pasted text.
- ***Drag and drop:*** This procedure does not involve the Clipboard and works best when moving data a short distance. To move cells, position the mouse on the cell borders. Wait until the mouse changes to a left-pointing arrow. When the mouse is this shape, press and drag the data to the new location.

FORMATTING DATA

Changing Formats using Toolbar

In Excel, you can change text fonts and styles in the worksheet. Excel has a Formatting toolbar to simplify basic formatting tasks. The Formatting toolbar appears in the figure below.

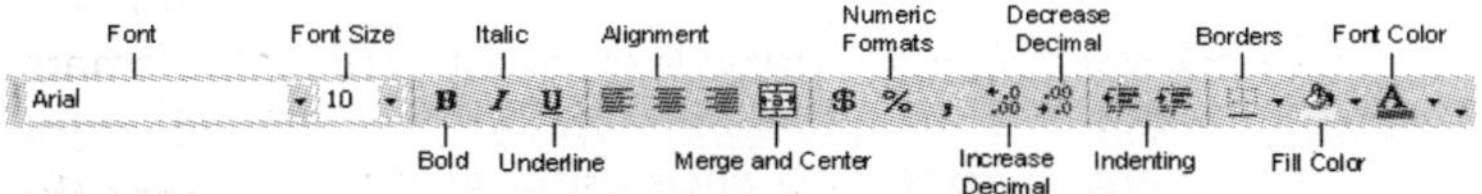

The formatting toolbar has several tools you can use to change formats. The B button makes cells bold, the I button italicizes cells and the U button underlines. Use these buttons to turn formats off as well as on. For example, if cells are bold and you want to turn off that format, select the cells and click the B button. The toolbar also has buttons to change font and size.

Font Tab in Format Cells

The formatting toolbar offers quick access to varying text formats. For a more complete selection of formatting options, use the Font tab in the Format Cells dialog box.

In the Font section you can select Font, Size, Style, Color and Effects. Notice the Preview area in the dialog box. This shows a preview of the font and style you select before you click the OK button.

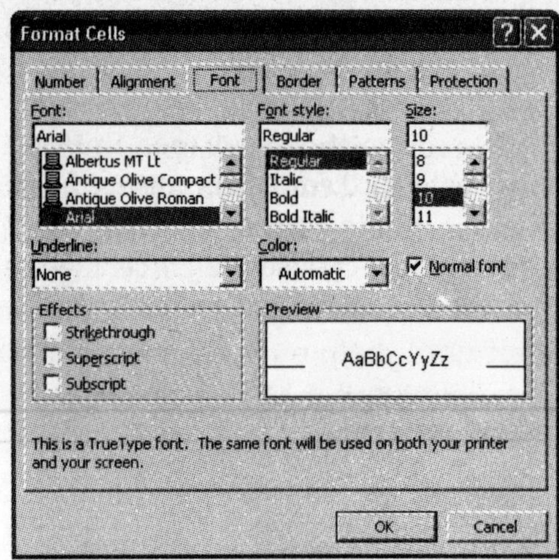

Alignment

By default, Excel left-aligns labels and right-aligns values in a worksheet. You can change cell alignment using the toolbar or the Format Cells command. The toolbar has text alignment icons next to the bold and italic icons. You can left-align, right-align, or center text within a cell using these buttons. Select the cell(s) you want to align and click the appropriate alignment button on the toolbar.

The toolbar also has a button that will center a label over a range of cells, for example, centering a title over a report. To center data over a range of cells, select the cell you want to center and the columns you want to center it over and click the Center over Cells button.

Format Alignment

You can also change the alignment of data within cells using the Alignment section of the Format Cells dialog. This dialog box also has options to change the orientation of text (i.e. sideways or vertical) and a box to wrap text within a cell.

Changing Numeric Formatting

To change the format of a number, choose the Cells command from the Format menu. In the Format Cells dialog box, Excel displays different tabs for various formatting types. To change numeric formats, click the Number tab. Select the category you want and then the actual format. For example, to display numbers as currency with two decimal places, select the Currency category, enter 2 for the number of decimal places, and select the appropriate currency symbol. Or to display a number as a percentage, choose the Percentage category and select the number of decimals you want to display.

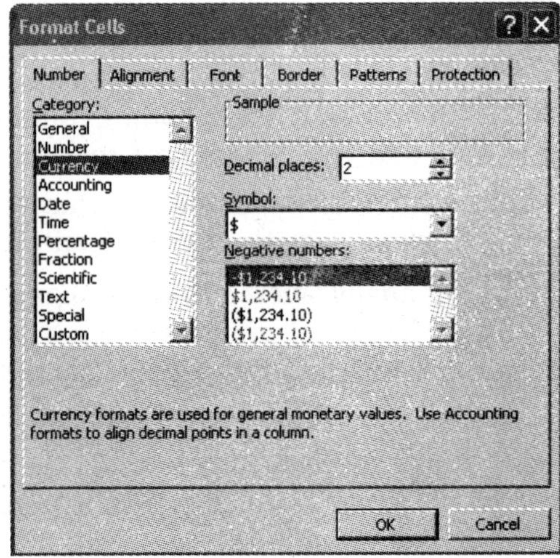

Placing Borders around Cells

The toolbar has a button for placing borders around cells. You can also use the Border section of the Format Cells dialog box, which provides more options. Select the cells you want a border on and choose the desired format from either the toolbar or the Format Cells dialog box.

Shading Cells

To apply a specific pattern or color to a range of cells, use the Patterns section of the Format Cells dialog box. The sample area in the Patterns dialog box displays what the selected colors and patterns will look like. You can also apply a solid color using the Fill Color tool on the Formatting toolbar.

Changing Column Width with Format Menu

To change column width using the Format menu, select the column or columns you wish to change and choose Column then Width. In the Column Width dialog box, type a number for the width of the column. The number represents the number of characters that can fit in the cell. The default column width is 10, which means a column is wide enough for ten, Helvetica 10-point characters. Choose Best Fit to automatically widen a column to accommodate the widest label, or click the Hide button to hide the column completely. Hiding columns is useful when you have data that you do not want to print.

Note: Changing row height is similar to changing column width. Select the row(s) you wish to change and choose Row then Height from the Format menu.

Changing Column Widths by Dragging Column Borders

You can change column widths by dragging column borders with the mouse. Move the mouse pointer to the right hand border of the column you wish to change. The mouse pointer will change shape to a left and right pointing arrow as seen below.

Click and drag the mouse to adjust the column width. Note that when you are adjusting the width in this way, a numeric width indicator appears in the upper left part of the formula bar.

ABC.XLS		
C	D ↔	E

FORMULAS AND FUNCTIONS

Formulas

In Microsoft Excel, you can enter numbers and mathematical formulas into cells. Whether you enter a number or a formula, you can reference the cell when you perform mathematical calculations such as addition, subtraction, multiplication, or division. When entering a mathematical formula, precede the formula with an equal sign. Use the following to indicate the type of calculation you wish to perform:

- + Addition
- – Subtraction
- × Multiplication
- / Division
- ^ Exponential

Mathematical calculations can be performed with the help of formulae. To build a formula, first select the cell in which you want the results to appear. In Excel, all formulas start with the = sign. After the = sign, type the cells you want to add or subtract along with the mathematical operation you wish to perform. For example, to add the January sales in the worksheet below, the formula would be = B3 + B4 + B5. If you want to subtract February Widget Sales from January Widget sales, the formula would be = B3 – C3.

	A	B	C	D	E	F	G	H
1								
2		**January**	**February**	**March**	**April**	**May**	**Totals**	**%'s**
3	**Widgets**	98	39	40	140	240		
4	**Figets**	122	18	50	150	250		
5	**Digets**	56	52	60	160	260		
6								
7	**Totals**							

Building many formulas can quickly become tedious. Fortunately, the Copy command described earlier also works with formulas.

Copying Formulas

The easiest way to copy a formula is with the Fill Handle in the lower right corner of the cell. Create your initial formula and then position the mouse on the Fill Handle. When the mouse changes shape to a cross-hair, press and drag over the adjacent cells you want to copy the formula to.

Functions

A function is a predefined formula that performs common calculations such as adding the values in a group of cells or generating a value such as the time or date. Few examples of different functions are shown in Table 5.1.

The integral parts of the function are:

1. ***Arguments:*** Arguments are values passes to the functions using which the function carries out some task. Arguments can be numbers, text, logical values, ranges or cell references. Arguments can also be constants, formulas or other functions.
2. ***Structure:*** The structure of a function begins with the function name, followed by an opening parenthesis, the arguments for the function separated by commas, and a closing parenthesis. If the function starts a formula, type an equal sign (=) before the function name.

To use functions, you need to understand reference operators. Reference operators refer to a cell or a group of cells. There are two types of reference operators: Range and union.

- A range reference refers to all the cells between and including the reference. A range reference consists of two cell addresses separated by a colon. The reference A1:A3 includes cells A1, A2, and A3. The reference A1:C3 includes cells A1, A2, A3, B1, B2, B3, C1, C2, and C3.

Table 5.1: Examples of functions in MS-Excel

Types of function	*Examples*
Statistical	AVERAGE
	COUNT
	MAX
	MIN
	MEDIAN, MODE, HAREMEAN
	Permutations (PERMUT)
	Trend Functions (FORECAST, GROWTH, TREND)
	Correlation coefficient functions (CORREL, FISHER, PEARSON)
Mathematical	SQRT
	ABS
	FACT
	LOG
	MOD
	ROUND
	Trigonometric and Degree functions (COS, DEGREES, PI, RADIANS, SIN, TAN)
	Algebraic functions (MULTINOMIAL)
	Summation functions (SUM, SUM PRODUCT, SUMSQ)
Financial	FV, NPV, IRR, RATE, PMT, PV.
	DISC, INTERATE, PRICE, YIELD
	Depreciation functions (DB, DDB, SLN, SYD, VDB)
Text	CHAR, LOWER, UPPER, FIND, LEFT, RIGHT
	LEN
	REPLACE, SUBSTITUTE
	CLEAN, TRIM
Logical	IF (logical test, value if true, value if false).
Day and Time	DATE
	NOW
	TIME

- A union reference includes two or more references. A union reference consists of two or more numbers, range references, or cell addresses separated by a comma. The reference A7, B8:B10, C9, 10 refers to cells A7, B8 to B10, C9 and the number 10.

  Here is an example of a function:

  = SUM (2, 13, A1, B2:C7)

In this function:

- The equal sign begins the function.
- SUM is the name of the function.
- 2, 13, A1, and B2:C7 are the arguments.
- Parentheses enclose the arguments.
- Commas separate the arguments.

Example: The SUM( ) function is probably the most common function in Excel. It adds a range of numbers. To build a SUM( ) function, begin by typing the = sign; all functions begin with the = sign. Next type the word SUM followed by an open parenthesis. You must now tell Excel which cells to sum. Using the mouse, click and drag over the range of cells you wish to add. A dotted outline will appear around the cells and the cell range will be displayed in the formula bar. When you have the correct cells selected, release the mouse button, type a closing parenthesis and press the <Enter> key. If you do not want to use the mouse, type in the references of the cells you want to sum. For example, to add cells B3 through B5, type = SUM(B3:B5). Excel interprets B3:B5 as the range of cells from B3 to B5.

a. ***AutoSum button:*** In Excel, the standard toolbar has a button that simplifies adding a column or row of numbers. The AutoSum button, which resembles the Greek letter Sigma automatically creates a SUM( ) function. When you click the AutoSum button Excel creates a sum function for the column of numbers directly above or the row of numbers to the left. Excel pastes the SUM( ) function and the range to sum into the formula bar. If the range is not correct, simply select the proper range with your mouse on the worksheet. When you have the correct range entered, press the <Enter> key to complete the function.

b. ***Using the insert function button:*** The Insert Function button is located by the Formula Bar. Click the Insert function button into activate the Insert Function dialog window. First, choose the Function Category you are interested in from the select a category drop down menu. Select function name and click OK as shown below.

Then the Function Arguments dialog box appears. Type the Number fields and click OK, the result appears.

Example: Add three numbers 150, 85 and 65 using function in MS Excel (The SUM function adds argument values).

1. Type 150 in cell A1.
2. Press Enter.
3. Type 85 in cell A2.
4. Press Enter.
5. Type 65 in cell A3.
6. Choose the Formulas tab.
7. Click the Insert Function button. The Insert Function dialog box appears.
8. Choose Math and Trig in the (or Select a category box).
9. Click Sum in the Function name box.

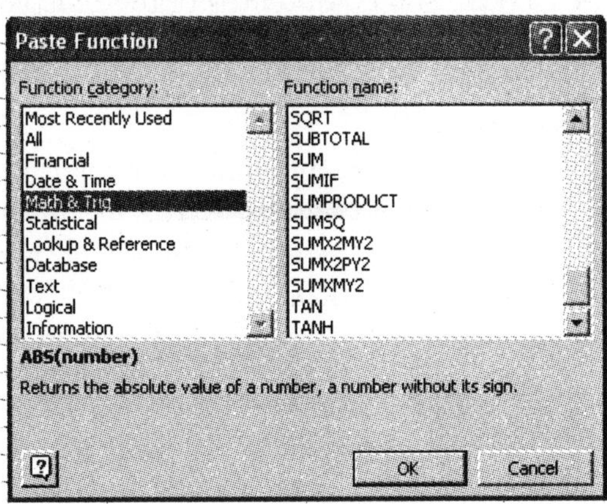

10. Click OK. The Function Arguments dialog box appears.
11. Type A1:A3 in the Number1 field, if it does not automatically appear.
12. Click OK. The sum of cells C1 to C3, which is 300, appears.

ADJUSTING PAGE SETUP SETTINGS

Before you actually print a worksheet, you should provide Excel information about margins, headers, footers, and page orientation. You change these settings using the Page Setup option on the File menu. The Page Setup dialog box, shown below, has controls for margins, page orientation, headers and footers and whether gridlines and row and column heading should be printed.

a. ***To change page margins:*** To change your margins, click the Margins tab, and enter the measurement for your margin, in inches, in the appropriate text box.

b. ***To change page orientation:*** If you want to change the orientation of the page from portrait (vertical) to landscape (horizontal) click the appropriate button in the Page Orientation section of the Page tab.

c. ***To change the header or footer:*** A header is text that prints at the top of each page. A footer is text that prints at the bottom

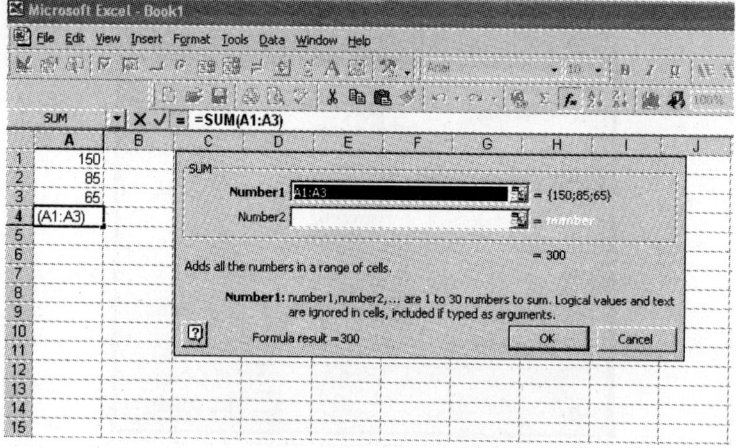

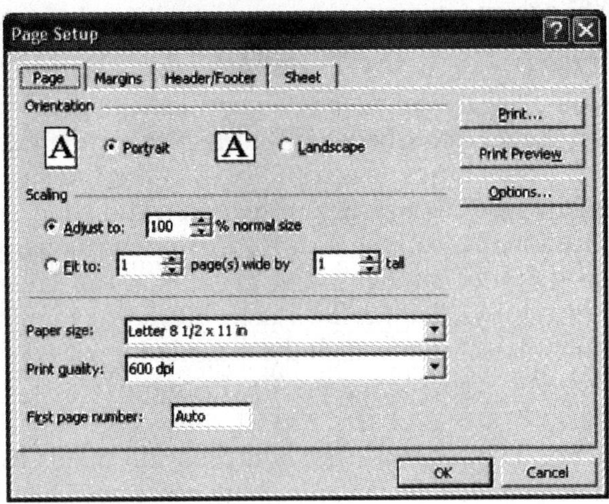

of each page. Headers and footers often include the name of the file being printed or an alternative title, the date, page number, or additional descriptive information. To change the header or footer, click on the Header/Footer tab in the Page Setup dialog box. The current header and footer will appear at the top and bottom of the dialog box respectively. Click the Custom Header or Custom Footer button to change the existing header or footer. The header and footer are divided into three sections (left, center and right). Press <Tab> or <Shift Tab> to move from section of the header or footer to another.

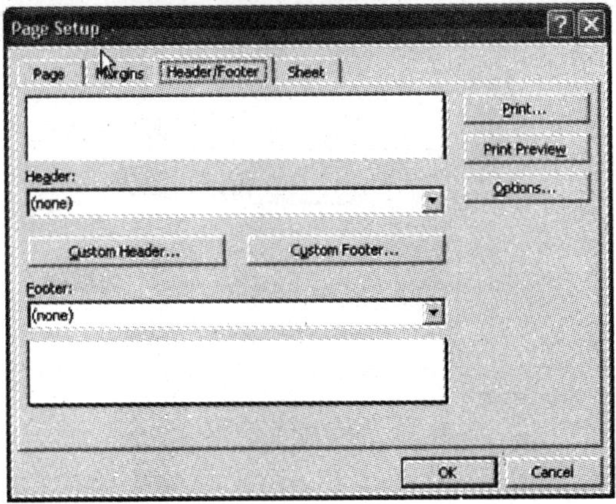

PRINTING

Print Preview

Before you actually print, it is a good idea to preview your output on the screen. Choose Print Preview on the File menu to preview your output on screen. Excel's Print Preview screen displays how the document will print on the page, but it is difficult to actually read the text. Notice that the mouse pointer takes the shape of a magnifying glass. You can enlarge the printed image by clicking the Zoom button or by using the magnifying glass. Simply click the magnifying glass on a part of the page you want to enlarge. The Print Preview screen also has several buttons at the top of the screen for making adjustments. For example, the Setup button opens the Page Setup dialog box and the Margins button lets you change page margin and column widths to fit more information on one page. If you are satisfied with how the output appears in the Print Preview screen, the Print button lets you send your output directly to the printer.

Sending Workbook to Printer

Choosing the Print option on the File menu or clicking the Print button on the toolbar opens a dialog box that lets you change print settings and specify the number of copies to print. The Print dialog box appears below.

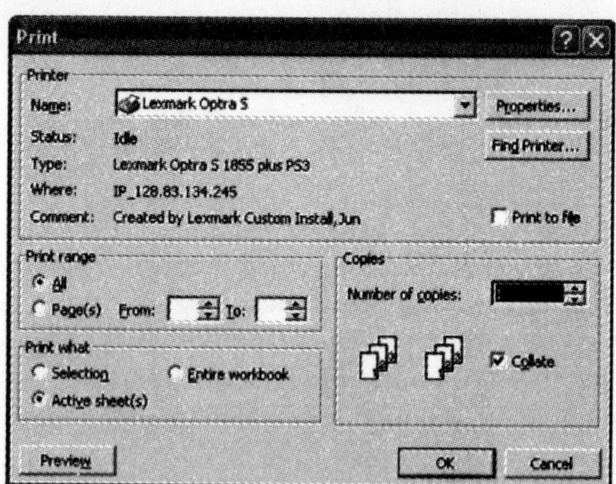

Within the Print dialog box, you can select what you want to print, how many copies and which pages. For example, if you only want to print the selected cells, or the entire worksheet you can choose those options.

CHARTS IN MS-EXCEL

Charts (or Graphs) are the pictorial representation of worksheet data. It allows you to display data in a chart that shows the relationship of data in graphical, rather than numerical form. A visual representation of data through charts often makes it easier to analyze and interpret information.

Types of Charts

MS-Excel support many types of charts as given below and shown in Figure 5.1.

1. ***Area chart:*** An area chart highlights the magnitude of change over time. It shows the relationship of parts to a whole.
2. ***Column chart:*** It shows data-changes over a period of time or comparisons among items.
3. ***Bar chart:*** It displays bars of various lengths to show relationship of data. The bars can be horizontal, vertical or stacked on top of one another.
4. ***Line chart:*** These charts are effective for showing a trend over a period of time, as indicated by a rising or falling line.
5. ***Pie chart:*** These charts have the shape of round pies cut into pieces or slices, are used to show the relationship of parts to a whole.
6. ***XY (Scatter) chart:*** An XY (scatter) chart either shows the relationships among the numeric values in several data series or plots two groups of numbers as one series of XY coordinates. This chart shows uneven intervals or cluster of data and is commonly used for scientific data.
7. ***Radar chart:*** It displays changes in values relative to center point.

8. ***Three-dimensional surface charts:*** It shows trends in values across two dimensions in a continuous curve.
9. ***Bubble chart:*** Like a scatter chart, with the third value displayed as the size of bubble.
10. ***Doughnut chart:*** It is like a pie chart but can contain multiple series.

Components of Chart

There are various components of a chart as given below:

1. ***X-axis:*** This is the horizontal axis known as category axis.
2. ***Y-axis:*** This is the vertical axis known as value axis.
3. ***Data series:*** This is the set of values you want to plot in the chart.
4. ***Chart area:*** This is the total region surrounding the chart.
5. ***Plot area:*** This is that area of chart in which your data is plotted.
6. ***Chart title:*** This is the descriptive text aimed at helping user identify the chart.
7. ***Axes titles:*** These are the titles given to three axis, i.e. X, Y and Z.
8. ***Legend:*** The legend helps you identify various plotted data series.
9. ***Gridlines:*** These are horizontal and vertical lines in the plot area. The gridlines are inserted in the chart to enhance its readability.
10. ***Data label:*** This is a label that provides additional information about a data marker, which represent a single data item or value coming from a worksheet cell.

Creating Charts in MS-Excel

1. Click and drag with the mouse arrow across the range that you want to chart. The cells will be highlighted.
2. Click on the Chart Wizard button. The Chart Wizard-step 1 of 4 dialog box will open.

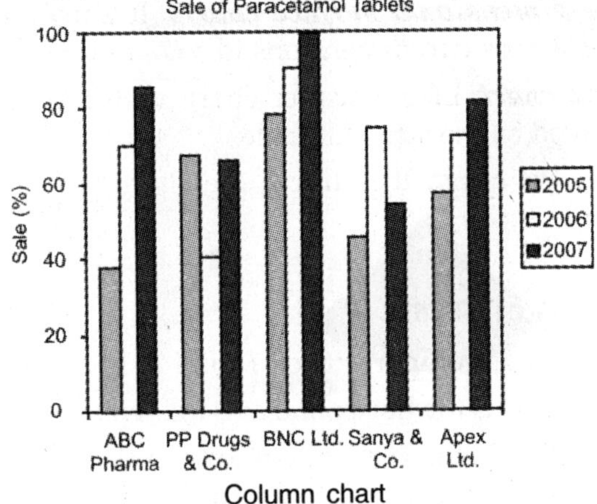

Column chart

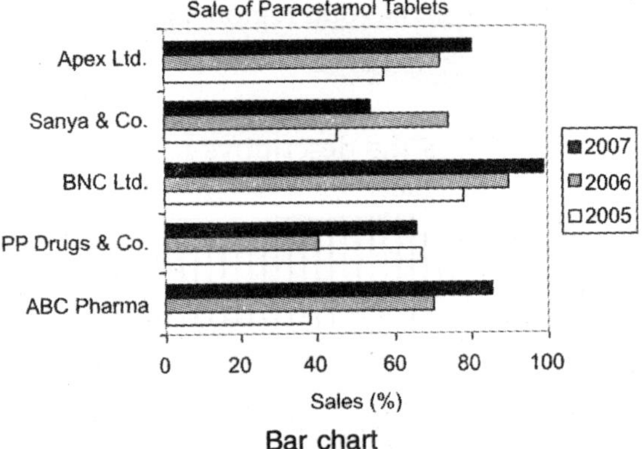

Bar chart

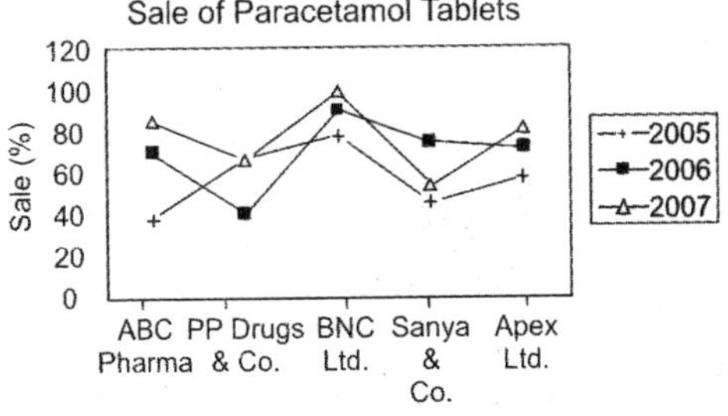

Line chart

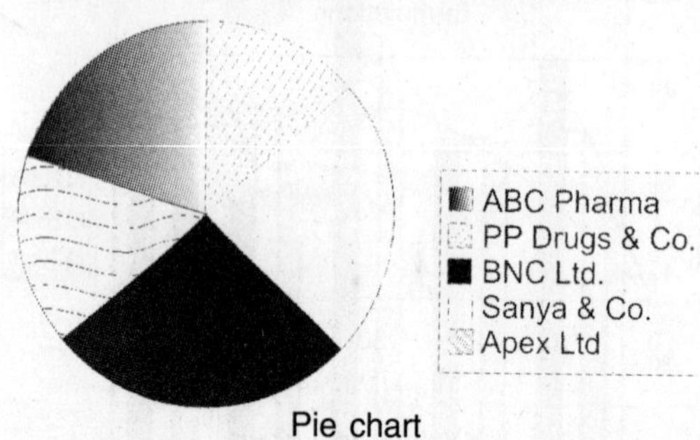

Pie chart

Sale of Paracetamol

100%
80%
60%
40%
20%
0%

Sale (%)

2007
2006
2005

ABC pharma
PP Drugs & Co.
BNC Ltd
Sanya & Co.
Apex Ltd

Area chart

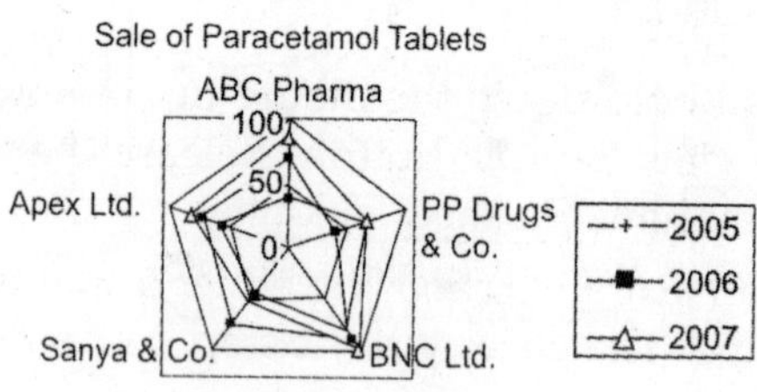

Radar chart

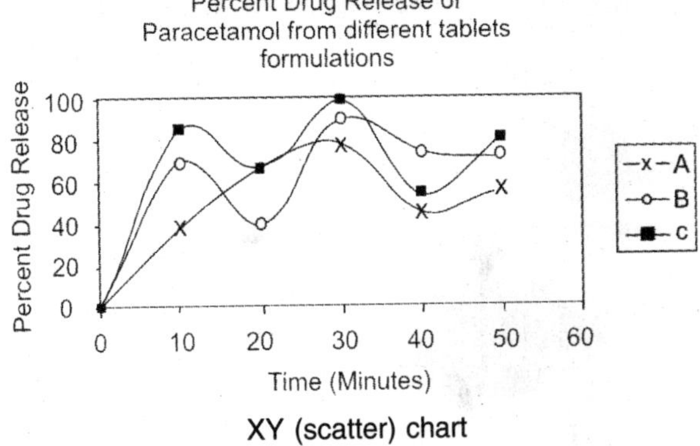

XY (scatter) chart

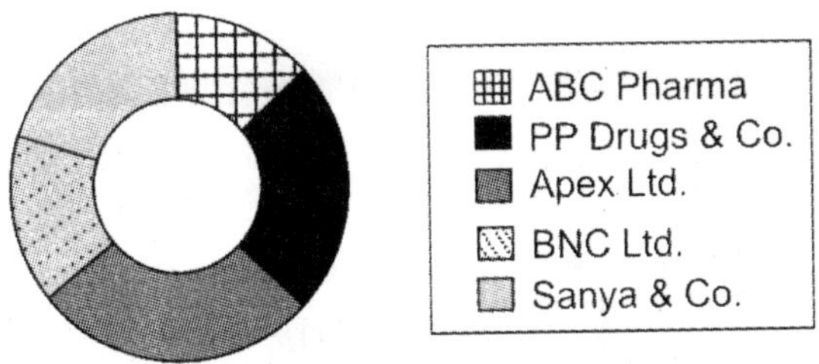

Doughnut chart

Fig. 5.1: Examples of different types of charts

3. Click on the Standard Types tab. The tab will come to the front.
4. Click on a chart type. The item will be highlighted.
5. Click on an option in the chart subtype area. The item will be highlighted.
6. Click and hold down the mouse button on the press and hold to view Sample button. Release the mouse button when you have finished looking.
7. Click on Next after choosing either a standard or custom chart type. The chart wizard step 2 of 4 dialog box will open.

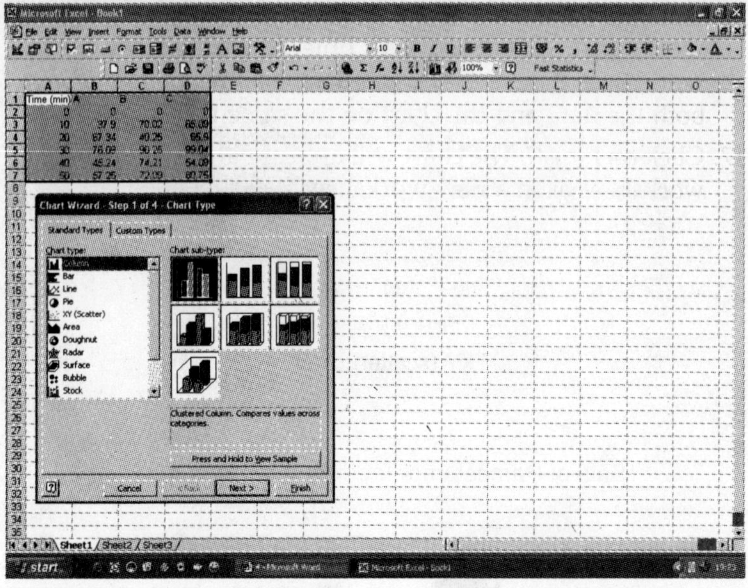

8. If you have selected your data before clicking on Chart Wizard in step 2, the data will appear in the Data range: box. You can change the data by typing a new range or by clicking on the Collapse Dialog button for the dialog box. Select the range in the worksheet and then click on the Expand Dialog button for the dialog box to return to the wizard.
9. Click on Next. The chart Wizard step 3 of 4 dialog box will open.
10. Click on the Title tabs. The tab will come to the front.
11. Type a title for your chart in the Chart title: text box.
12. Type titles for X and/Y axis, it is optional.
13. Click on the Data Labels tab. The tab will come to the front.
14. Click on one of the Data label options. Click None in the Data label box, if you want no option to be applied.
15. Click Next. The Chart Wizard step 4 of 4 dialog box will open.

16. Click on As new sheet to create your chart on a new worksheet, or click on As object in: to add it to the worksheet that contains the data, so that you can print both the data and the chart on the same page.
17. Click on Finish. The chart will appear either in the current worksheet or in a new worksheet.

Microsoft PowerPoint

INTRODUCTION

Microsoft PowerPoint is a proprietary presentation program developed by Microsoft. It is part of the Microsoft Office system, and runs on Microsoft Windows and the Mac OS computer operating systems. PowerPoint is widely used by business people, educators, students, and trainers and is among the most prevalent forms of persuasive technology. The current versions are Microsoft Office PowerPoint 2007 for Windows and 2008 for Mac.

PowerPoint presentations consist a number of individual pages or "slides". Slides may contain text, graphics, movies, and other objects, which may be arranged freely on the slide. PowerPoint, however, facilitates the use of a consistent style in a presentation using a template or "Slide Master". The presentation can be printed or displayed live on a computer and navigated through at the command of the presenter. For larger audiences the computer display is often projected using a video projector. Slides can also form the basis of webcasts.

PowerPoint provides three types of movements:

1. Entrance, emphasis, and exit of elements on a slide itself are controlled by what PowerPoint calls Custom Animations.
2. Transitions, on the other hand are movements between slides. These can be animated in a variety of ways.
3. Custom animation can be used to create small story boards by animating pictures to enter, exit or move.

Presentations can be saved and run in any of the file formats: the default .ppt (presentation), .pps (PowerPoint Show) or .pot (template). In PowerPoint 2007 and Mac OS X 2008 versions, the XML-based file formats .pptx, .ppsx and .potx have been introduced, along with the macro-enabled file formats .pptm, .potm, .ppsm.

STARTING POWERPOINT

Microsoft PowerPoint is a powerful tool to create professional looking presentations and slide shows. PowerPoint allows you to construct presentations from scratch or by using the easy to use wizard. There are two ways as described below; either could be used to start PowerPoint:

1. Double-click on the Microsoft PowerPoint icon on the desktop.

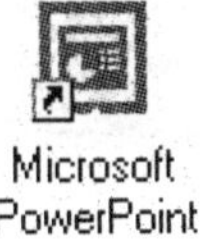

2. Click on Start → Programs → Microsoft PowerPoint.

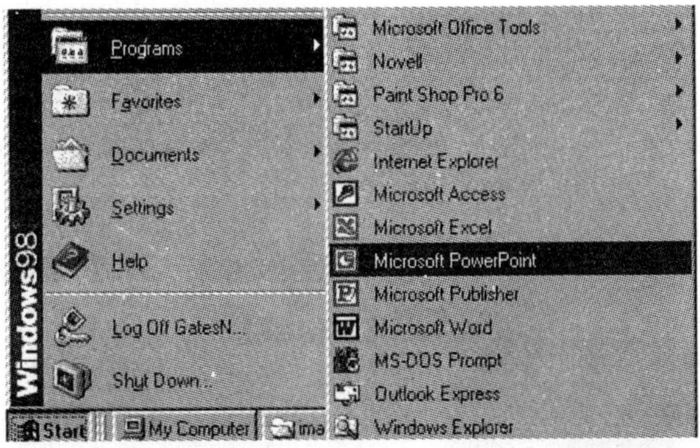

CREATING NEW PRESENTATION

Open PowerPoint and you will be prompted by a dialog box with four choices. Each of these options are explained on this page. If PowerPoint is already open or this box does not appear, select File | New from the menu bar.

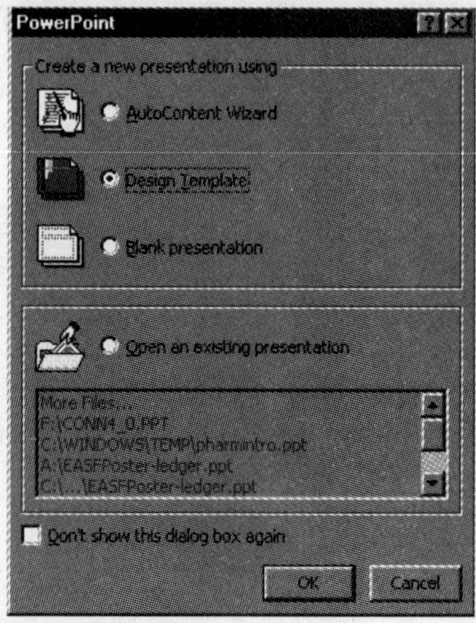

1. ***Autocontent wizard:*** The AutoContent Wizard provides templates and ideas for a variety of presentation types. Page through the wizard by clicking the Next button on the bottom of each page after making necessary choices. Creates a new presentation by prompting you for information about content, purpose, style, handouts, and output. The new presentation contains sample text that you can replace with your own information. Simply follow the directions and prompts that are given by Microsoft PowerPoint.

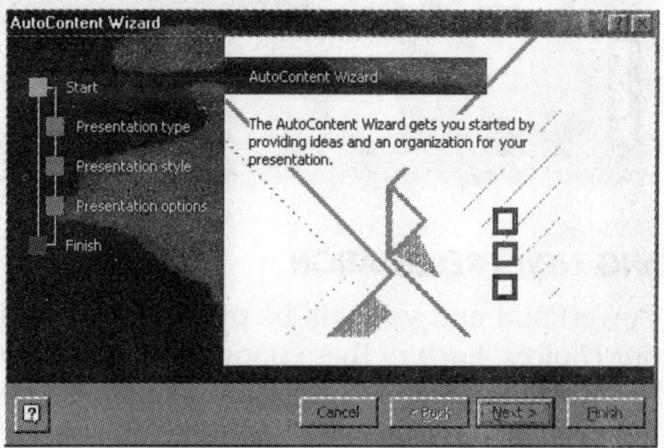

2. ***Design template:*** PowerPoint provides many templates with different backgrounds and text formatting to begin your presentation. Preview each design by highlighting the template name on the list. Press OK after you have chosen the design.

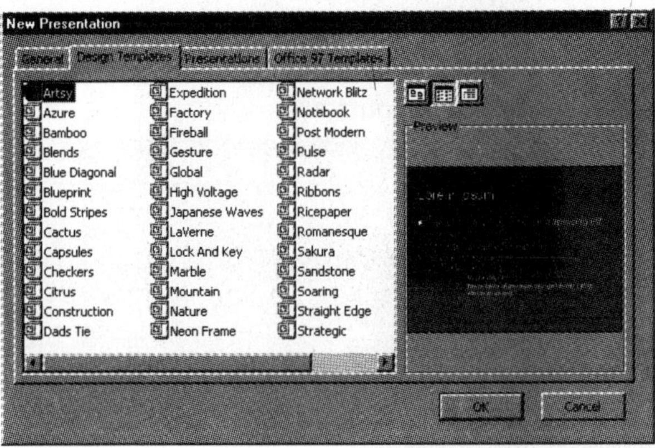

3. ***Blank presentation:*** Select Blank Presentation to build the presentation from scratch with no preset graphics or formatting.

4. ***Open an existing presentation:*** Select this option to open a PowerPoint presentation that already exists. Select the folder the file is located in from the Look in: drop-down menu and

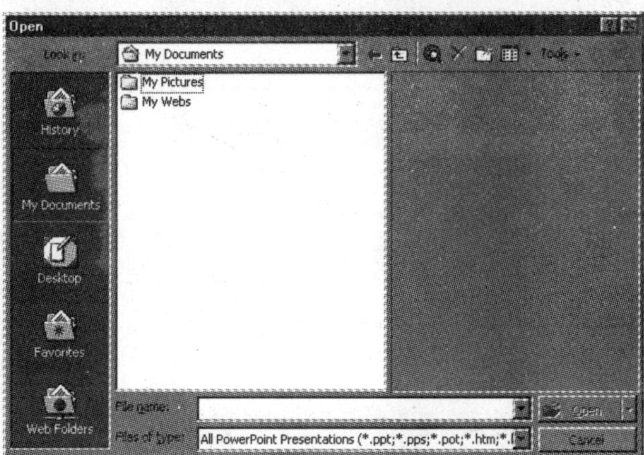

highlight the file on the list. Click Open to open the presentation.

After selecting the presentation type, you will be prompted to choose the layout of the new slide. These layouts include bulleted lists, graphs, and/or images. Click on each thumbnail image and a description will be printed in the message box. Highlight the layout you want and click OK.

Pre-designed slide layouts are:

- Title Slide
- Bulleted List
- Two Column Text
- Table
- Text and Chart
- Chart and Text
- Organizational Chart
- Chart
- Text and Clip Art
- Clip Art and Text
- Title Only
- Blank Slide.

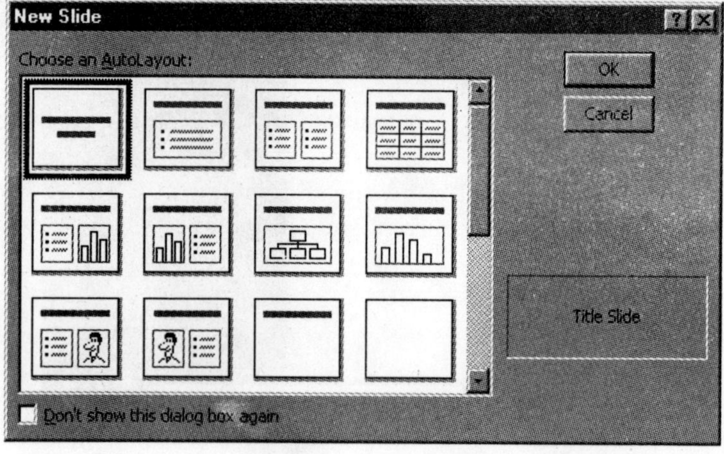

POWERPOINT VIEWS

There are different views within Microsoft PowerPoint that allow you to look at your presentation from different perspectives. PowerPoint gives you four screen layouts for constructing your presentation in addition to the Slide Show. You can select the page view by clicking the buttons just above the formatting toolbar and the bottom of the page.

1. ***Normal view:*** This screen is split into three sections showing the presentation outline on the left, the slide in the main window, and notes at the bottom. Switches to normal view, where you can work on one slide at a time or organize the structure of all the slides in your presentation.
2. ***Outline view:*** The presentation outline is displayed on the majority of the screen with small windows for the slide and notes. This view is recommended for editing text. Switches to outline view, where you can work with the structure of your file in outline form. Work in outline view when you need to organize the structure of your file.
3. ***Slide view:*** The slide view displays each slide on the screen and is helpful for adding images, formatting text, and adding background styles. Switches to slide view, where you can work on one slide at a time.
4. ***Slide sorter view:*** A small image of each slide is displayed in Slide Sorter view. Slides can easily be ordered and sorted from this screen. Displays miniature versions of all slides in a presentation, complete with text and graphics. In slide sorter view, you can reorder slides, add transitions, and animation effects. You can also set the timings for electronic slide shows.
5. ***Slide show view:*** Runs your slide show in a full screen, beginning with the current slide if you are in slide view or

Normal View	Outline View	Slide View	Slide Sorter View	Slide Show View

the selected slide if you are in slide sorter view. If you simply want to view your show from the first slide:

a. Click slide show at the top of the screen.

b. Select view show.

WORKING WITH SLIDES

1. ***Insert a new slide:*** Follow these steps to insert a new slide into the presentation:
   a. In the Outline window, select the slide you want the new slide to appear after by clicking the slide's number.
   b. Select Insert | New Slide from the menu bar or click the new slide button on the standard toolbar.
   c. Choose the page layout from the window and press OK.
2. ***Applying a design template:*** To add a design template or changing the existing one, selection Format | Design Template from the menu bar. Select the template and click Apply.
3. ***Changing slide layouts:*** To change the layout template of the slide select Format | Slide Layout from the menu bar. Select one of the layout thumbnail images and click Apply.
4. ***Reordering slides:*** To reorder a slide in Slide Sorter View, simply click on the slide you wish to move and drag it to the

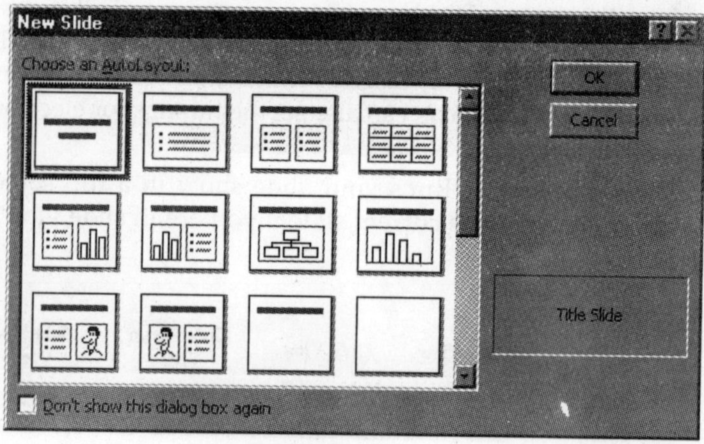

new location. In Normal or Outline View, click the slide icon beside the number of the slide you want to move and drag the icon to a new location.

5. ***Hide slides:*** If you do not want a slide to appear during the slide show, but do not want to delete the slide as it may be used later, the slide can be hidden by selecting Slide Show | Hide Slide from the menu bar. To add the slide back to the slide show, select Slide Show | Hide Slide again.
6. ***Create a custom slide show:*** The Custom Slide Show feature allows you to select the slides you want to display in the slide show if not all the slides should be used.
   a. Select Slide Show | Custom Slide Show from the menu bar.
   b. Click the New... button in the Custom Shows window.
   c. In the Define Custom Show window, type a name for the slide in the Slide show name field.
   d. Add slides to the custom show by highlighting them in the Slides in presentation window and clicking the Add >> button. Those slides will then appear in the Slides in custom show window.
   e. To remove slides from the custom show, highlight their names in the Slides in custom show window and click the Remove button.

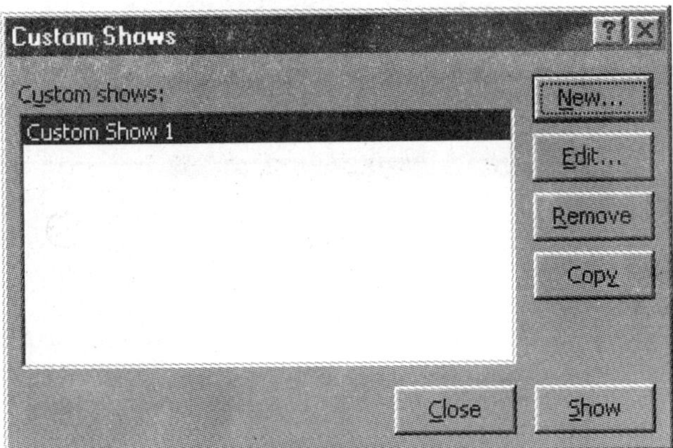

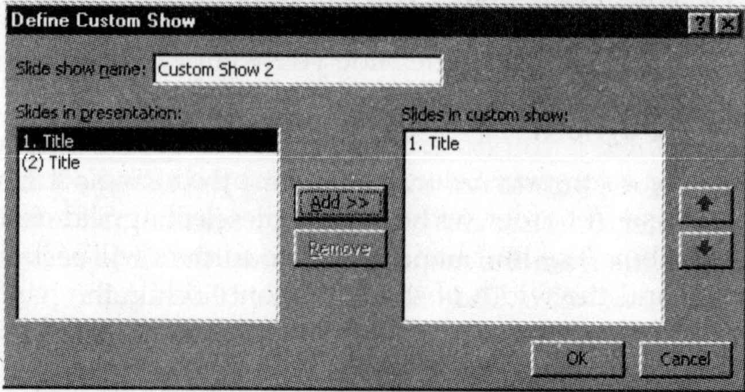

f. To reorder slides in the custom show, highlight the slide that should be moved and click the up and down arrows to change its order in the show.

g. Click OK when finished.

h. Click the Show button on the Custom Shows window to preview the custom slide show and click Close to exit.

7. ***Edit a custom slide show:***

a. Select Slide Show | Custom Slide Show from the menu bar.

b. Edit the show by highlighting the name in the Custom shows box and clicking the Edit... button.

c. To delete a show, highlight the name and click Remove.

d. Create a copy of a show by clicking the Copy button. The copy can then be renamed by clicking the Edit... button.

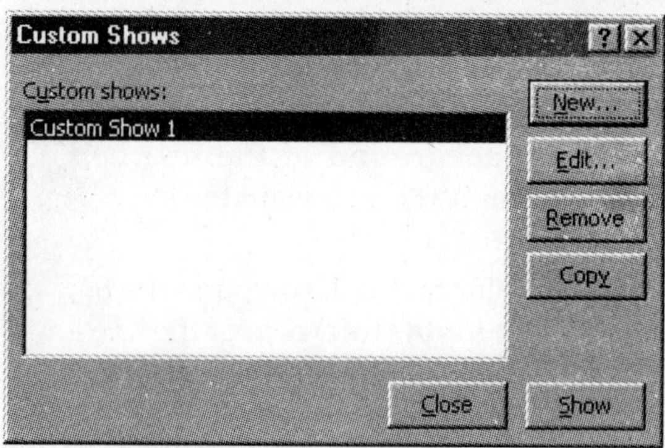

e. Click the Show button to preview the custom slide show and click Close to exit.

ADDING CONTENT

1. ***Resizing a text box:*** Select a text box by clicking on it with the mouse. A border with nine handles will appear around the text box. The four handles on the corners will resize the length and the width of the box at once while the handles on the sides will resize only in one direction. Click one of the handles and drag it with the mouse. Release the mouse button when it is the size you want it to be. Move the text box by clicking and dragging the thick, dotted border with the mouse.

2. ***Text box properties:*** Change the colors, borders, and backgrounds of a text box from the Format AutoShape dialog box.
   a. Activate the text box by clicking on it and select Format | Colors and Lines from the menu bar.
   b. Under the Colors and Lines tab, select a Fill color that will fill the background of the text box. Check the Semitransparent box if you want the slide background to show through the color.
   c. Select a Line color that will surround the box as well as a Style or Weight for the thickness of the line and a Dashed property if the line should not be solid.
   d. Click the Text Box tab.

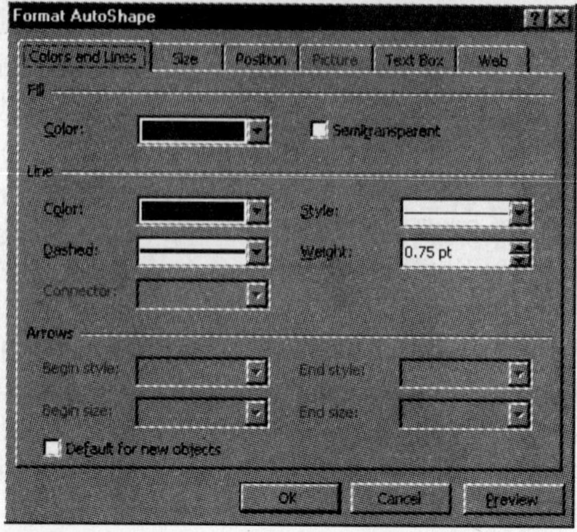

e. Change the Text anchor point to reposition the text within the text box.

f. Set Internal margins to the distance the text should be to the text box edges.

g. Click OK to add the changes to the text box.

3. ***Delete a text box:*** To delete a text box from a template, simply click the border of the text box and press the Delete key on the keyboard.

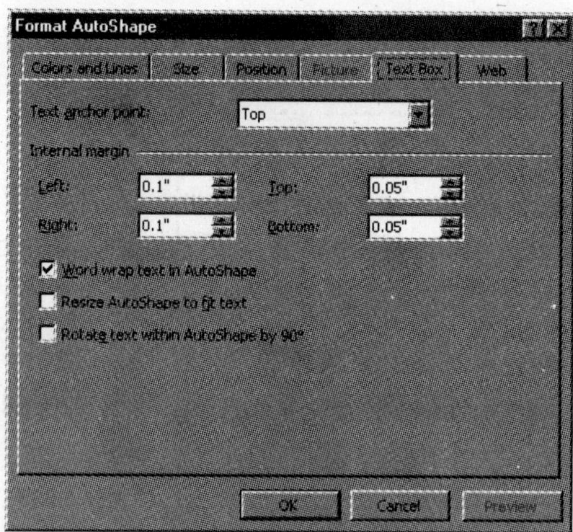

Bulleted Lists

1. ***Bulleted lists on design templates:*** Bulleted lists allow you to clearly display the main points of your presentation on slides. The text boxes on design templates already include bulleted lists. Click the place holder on the slide to begin adding text and press the Enter key to return to the next line and add a new bulleted item. To go to the next line without adding another bullet, hold down the Shift key while pressing Enter.
2. ***Bulleted list from a text box:*** If you are not creating a bulleted list from an existing placeholder on a design template, or if you would like to add an additional bulleted list, follow these steps to create a new list:
   a. In slide view, create a text box by selecting Insert | Text Box from the menu bar.
   b. "Draw" the text box on the slide by holding down the left mouse button while you move the mouse until the box is the size you want it.
   c. Choose Format | Bullets and Numbering from the menu bar.
   d. Change the Size of the bullet by changing the percentage in relation to the text.

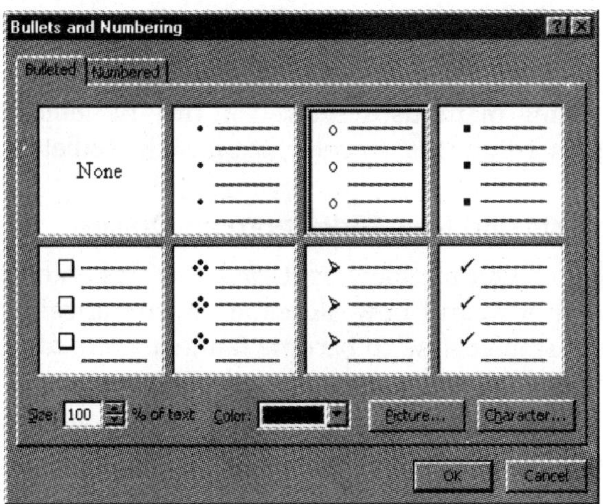

e. Choose a color for the bullet from the Color menu. Click More Colors for a larger selection.

f. Select one of the seven bullet types shown and click OK.
OR

Click the Picture button to view the Picture Bullet window. Select one of the bullets and click OK.

OR

Click the Character button to select any character from the fonts on the computer. Select a symbol font such as Wingdings or Webdings from the Bullets from drop-down menu for the best selection of icons. Click on the characters in the grid to see them larger. Click OK when you have chosen the bullet you want to use.

g. Click OK on the Bullets and Numbering window and use the same methods described in the "Bulleted Lists on Design Templates" to enter text into the bulleted list.

Bulleted Lists and New Slides from an Outline

In Normal or Outline view, text can easily be entered in the outline window and new slides are automatically added. Follow the steps below to become familiar with adding slide content in outline view:

1. Next to the Slide 1 icon, type the title of the slide. The text you type beside the slide icons will be the large-type titles on each slide.

2. Press ENTER to type the next line. This will automatically create a new slide. To create a bulleted list for the first slide, press the TAB key or click the demote button on the More Buttons menu accessible by clicking the "triple arrow" button at the end of the formatting toolbar.

   OR

   Press ALT+SHIFT+Right Arrow to demote the selection to a bulleted list item.

3. Continue entering text for the bulleted list, pressing ENTER at the end of each line to create a new bullet.

4. Create a multilevel list by executing the demote action again to create a bulleted sublist. Press the promote button on the More Buttons menu or press ALT+SHIFT+Left Arrow to return to the original list.

5. Create a new slide by executing the promote action until a new slide icon appears.

6. Continue creating new slides and bulleted lists by using the demote and promote actions until the presentation is completed. Use the formatting instructions below to format the lists.

If there is more than one bulleted list on the slide, the lists will be designated by numbers enclosed in black boxes. The example below shows the slide created from the outline on the left. The bulleted list on the left side of the slide is labeled list "1" on the outline and the list on the right is labeled list "2". When typing the outline, begin typing in the new list by pressing CTRL+ENTER. In this example, CTRL+ENTER was pressed after typing "Access".

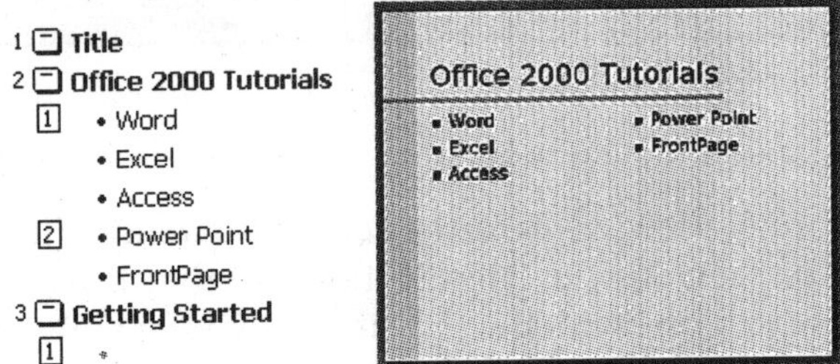

Numbered List

Follow these steps to create a numbered list:

1. Create a text box.
2. With the text box selected, choose Format | Bullets and Numbering from the menu bar.
3. Click the Numbered tab at the top of the Bullets and Numbering window.
4. Change the size of the numbers by changing the percentage in relation to the text.
5. Choose a color for the numbers from the Color menu. Click More Colors for a larger selection.
6. Change the Start at value if the numbers should not begin with 1.
7. Select one of the seven list types shown and click OK.

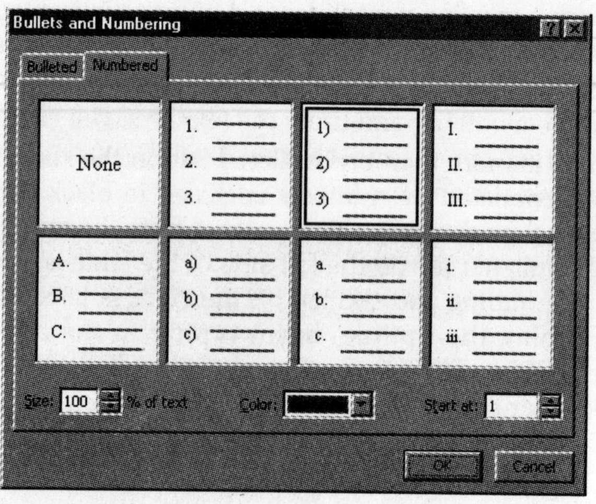

Adding Notes

From Normal View, notes can be added to the slide. These notes will not be seen on your presentation, but they can be printed out on paper along with the slide the notes refer to by selecting Print What: Notes Pages on the Print menu.

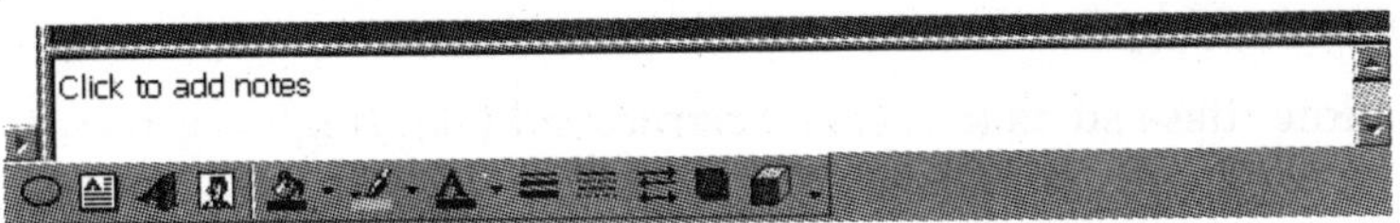

Audio and Video

1. ***Audio:*** To add sound to your presentation select Insert | Movies and Sounds | Sound from Gallery or Sound from File. Select a sound file and click OK.
2. ***Video:*** To add a video to your presentation select Insert | Movies and Sounds | Movie from File or to insert an animation from Microsoft's gallery choose Insert | Movies and Sounds | Movie from Gallery. Select the video file and click OK.

WORKING WITH TEXT

Adding Text

If the slide layout includes text boxes, simply click on the text box to add text. To add a text box to the slide, select Insert | Text Box from the menu bar and draw the text box with the mouse. Set text editing options by selecting Tools | Options from the menu bar and clicking the Edit tab.

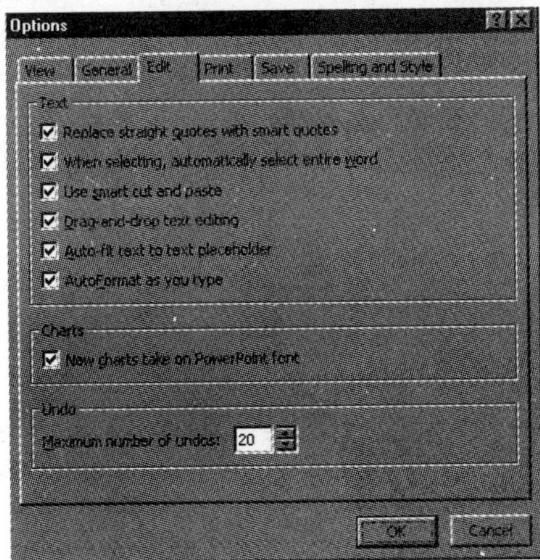

Formatting Text

Select the text that will be formatted by highlighting the text either on the outline or on the slide. Choose Format | Font from the menu bar or right-click on the highlighted selection and select Font from the popup shortcut menu or. Select a font face, size, style, effect, and color from the Font dialog box. Click the Preview button to see how the changes will appear on the slide before making a decision.

Replace Fonts

Design templates have a preset font that you may want to change or you may want to change the font used on for the entire presentation for a number of reasons. This can be accomplished quickly using the Replace Fonts feature. Select Format | Replace Font from the menu bar. Choose the font you want to Replace from the first drop-down menu and the font it should be replaced With from the second menu, and click the Replace button.

Line Spacing

Change the amount of space between lines in a text box by selecting Format | Line Spacing from the menu bar.

- ***Line spacing:*** Select the amount of vertical space between lines. A value of "1" is equal to single spacing and "2" is double spacing. Values between and above these numbers are valid as well.

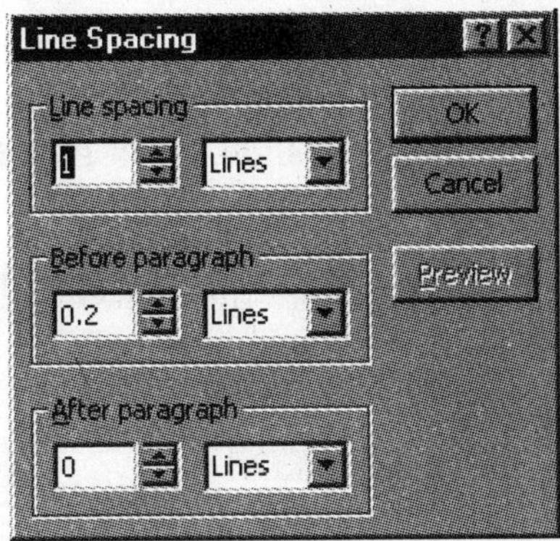

- ***Before paragraph and after paragraph:*** This value will determine the amount of vertical space before and after each paragraph in a text box.

Change Case

Change the case of the characters in a paragraph by selecting Format | Change Case from the menu bar without having to retype the text.

- ***Sentence case:*** Capitalizes the first letter of the first word in each sentence.
- ***Lowercase and uppercase:*** Changes the case of all the letters.
- ***Title case:*** Capitalizes the first letter of every word and reduces the rest to lowercase.
- ***Toggle case:*** The opposite of Title case, it makes the first letter of every word lowercase and capitalizes the remaining letters.

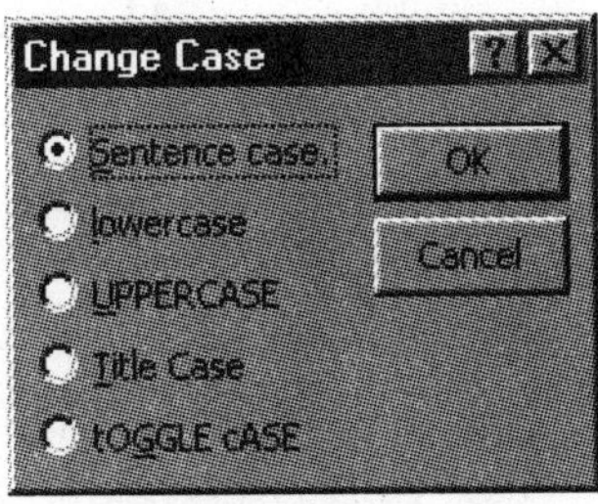

Spell Check

Correct the spelling in the presentation by selecting Tools | Spelling from the menu bar or by pressing the F7 key on the keyboard.

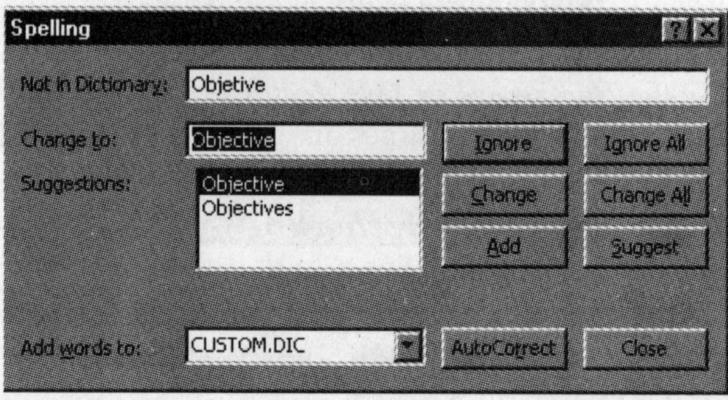

1. The spell checker will prompt you to make corrections of the first word that is spelled wrong.
2. If the word is spelled correctly, click Ignore or Ignore All if the same word appears several times during the presentation. If this word will appear in many presentations (such as your name), click Add to add the word to the dictionary and you would not be prompted by a misspelling again.
3. If the word is spelled wrong, highlight one of the Suggestions or type your own revision in the Change to box. Click Change to correct this occurrence of the word or Change All to correct all occurrences of the word in the presentation.
4. Click Close to abort the spelling check early.
5. When the spell checker has read through the entire presentation, you will be prompted by a window telling you that the spelling check is complete. Click OK.

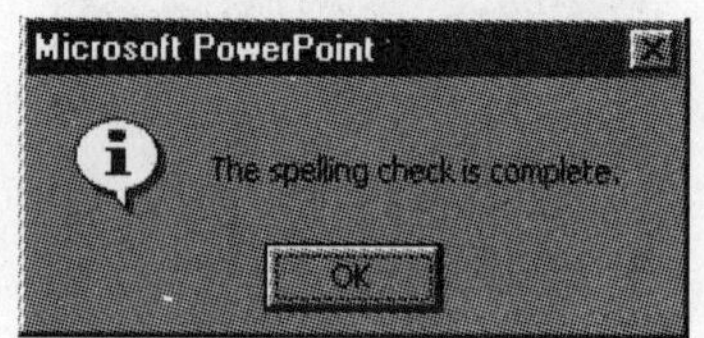

Spelling Options

Select Tools | Options from the menu bar and click the Spelling and Style tab.

- ***Check spelling as you type:*** If this box is checked, PowerPoint will check the spelling of every word as you type. Misspelled words will be underlined with wavy red lines.
- ***Hide spelling errors in this document:*** Check this box to remove the wavy red lines from words that are spelled wrong.
- ***Always suggest corrections:*** If this box is checked, suggestions for misspelled words will appear when you activate the spell checker.
- ***Ignore words in uppercase:*** PowerPoint recommends that you do not type slide titles in all uppercase letters so it will treat words like this and other all uppercase acronyms as misspelled. Check this box to ignore this suggestion and acronyms that are typically typed in all caps.
- ***Ignore words with numbers:*** Check to ignore words that are combinations of letters and numbers.

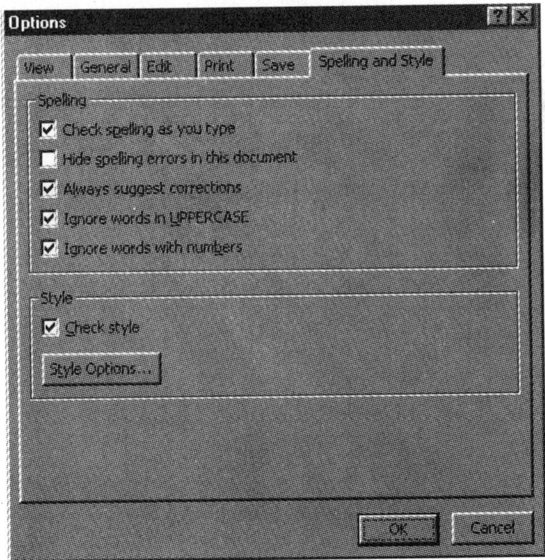

COLOR SCHEMES AND BACKGROUND

Color Scheme

The colors of predesigned slide templates can be changed and a color scheme can be added to blank presentations.

1. Select Format | Slide Color Scheme from the menu bar.
2. Click one of the preset color scheme thumbnail images in the Color schemes box.

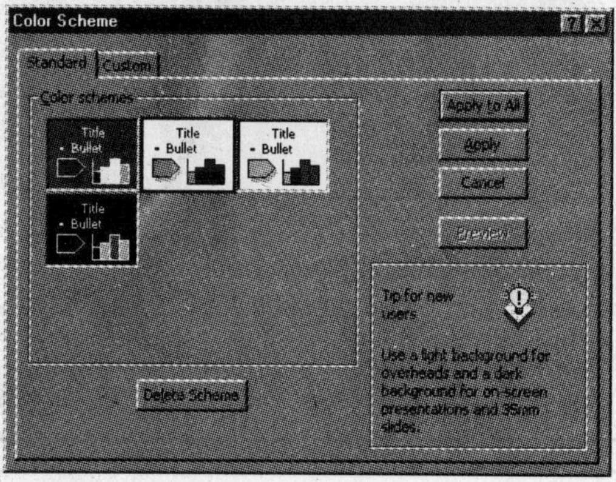

3. Click the Preview button to see how the scheme will appear on the slide.
4. To make changes to the color scheme, click the Custom tab on the dialog box.

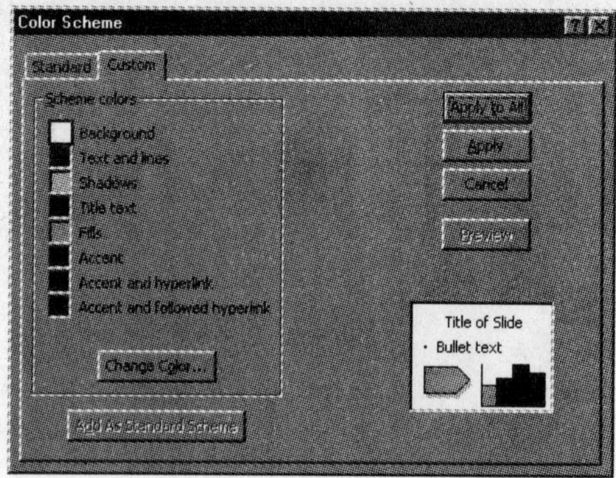

5. Change the colors of the slide elements by selecting the color swatch beside the name of the element and clicking the Change color button.
6. Highlight one of the colors from the Text and Line Color window or select the Custom tab to view more color choices and click OK when finished.

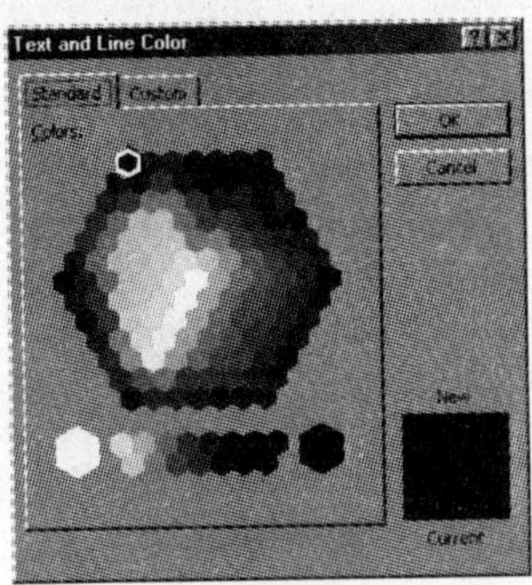

7. When you have finished all color formatting, click Apply to All to apply the color scheme to all the slides in the presentation or Apply to add the scheme only to the current slide.

Backgrounds

Follow these steps to add background colors and patterns to a slide:

1. Select Format | Background from the menu bar.

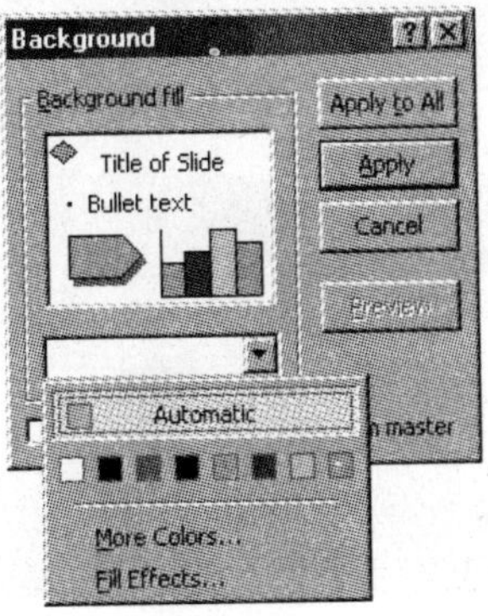

2. Select a color from the drop-down menu below the Background fill preview or choose More Colors... for a larger selection.
3. Select Fill Effects from the drop-down menu to add gradients, texture, patterns, or a picture to the background.

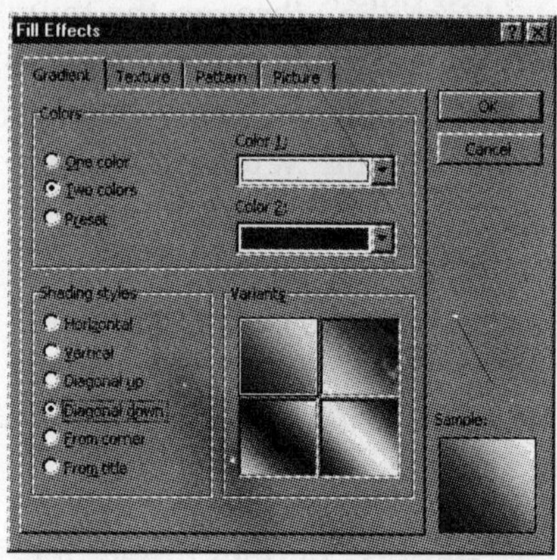

4. ***Gradient tab:***

   a. Select One color if the color chosen will fade into the background and select the color from the Color 1 drop-down menu. Choose Two colors if the gradient will use two colors and select those colors from the Color 1 and Color 2 drop-down menus. Preset provides a selection of

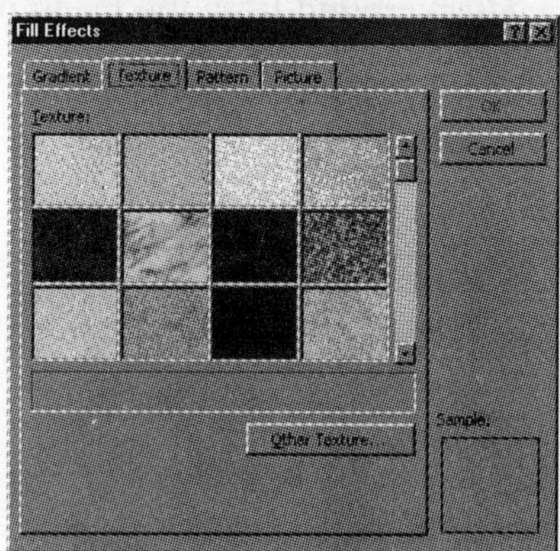

color combinations. Select one from the Preset colors drop-down menu.

b. Select the type of gradient from Shading styles.

c. Click one of the four Variants of the styles chosen.

5. ***Texture tab:*** From the Texture window, select a repeating background by scrolling through the thumbnail images or click Other Texture... to select an image from a file.

6. ***Pattern tab:*** Select a two-tone pattern by clicking one of the pattern swatches and selecting the Foreground and Background colors.

7. ***Picture tab:***

   a. Click the Select Picture button to choose a picture from a file. After the picture is selected, a preview and description will be shown in this window.

   b. Click OK to apply the changes made from the Fill Effects windows.

   c. Click Apply to All to add the changes to every slide or Apply to make changes only to the current slide.

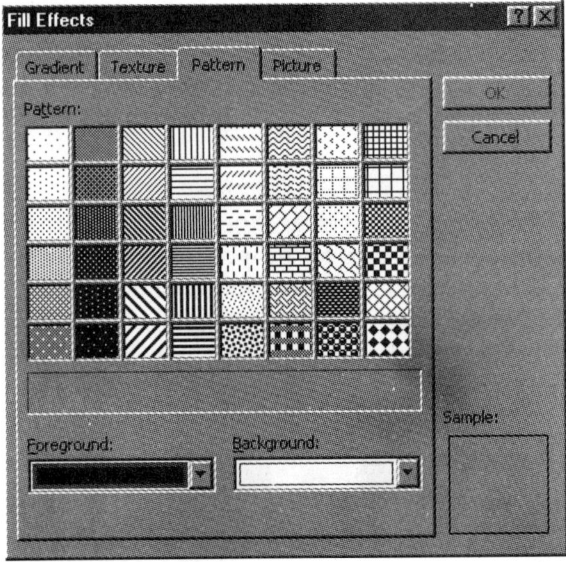

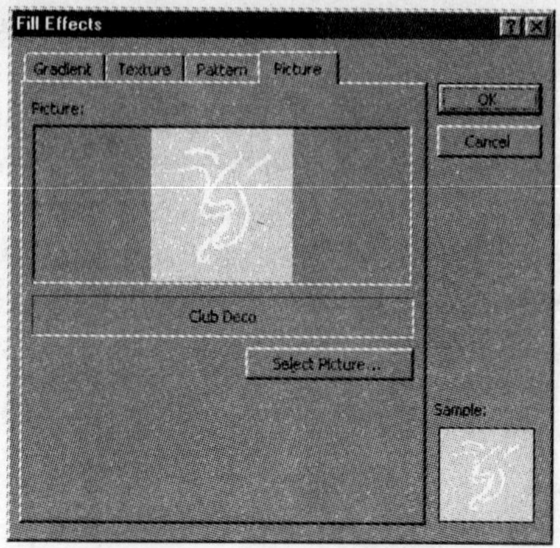

GRAPHICS

Drawing Toolbar provides many commands for creating and editing graphics. The toolbar is located at the bottom of the PowerPoint screen or it can be activated by selecting View | Toolbars | Drawing from the menu bar.

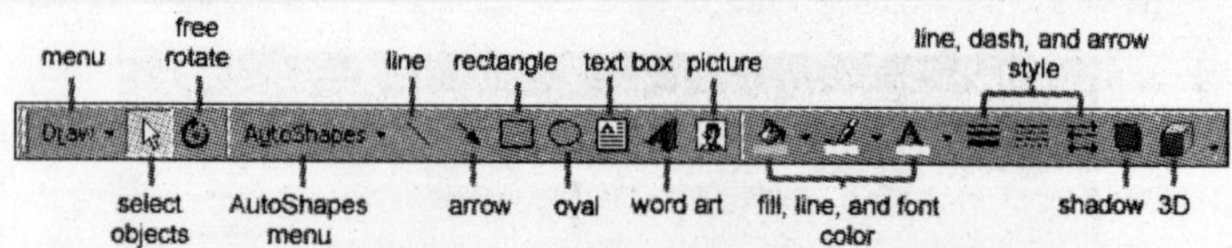

Menu

1. ***Grouping:*** Images can be grouped together so they become one image and can be moved together or the same formatting changes can be applied to both at once. Select all the images that will be grouped by holding down the SHIFT key and clicking once on each image. Then select Group from the Draw menu. The images can be

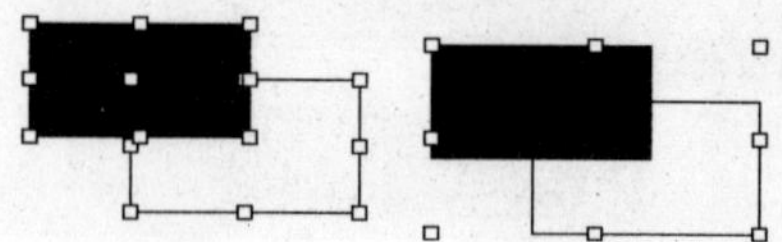

ungrouped by selecting Ungroup from the same menu. The rectangles in the image to the left are separate images with their own sets of handles and they are grouped together in the image to the right.

2. ***Order:*** The order of overlapping images can be changed using this feature. In the example of two rectangles below, the green rectangle is selected and the Send Backward command was used to move the image below the blue rectangle. Send Backward and Bring Forward will move elements by one layer. Send to Back and Bring to Front move the elements to the back or top of a series of several overlapping graphics.

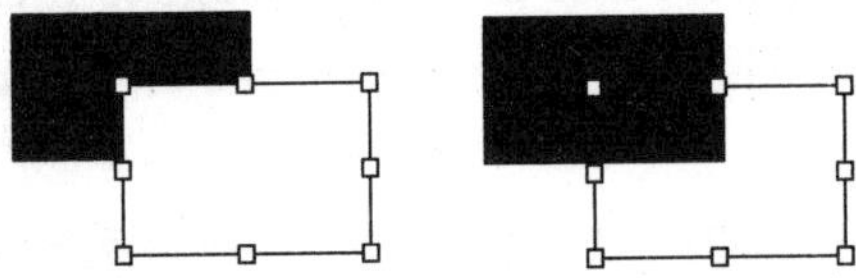

3. ***Nudge:*** Use the nudge actions to move an object slightly in one direction.
4. ***Align or distribute:*** Select a group of objects and choose one of the the commands from the Align or Distribute menu to change the position of the objects in relation to one another.
5. ***Rotate or flip:*** Rotate an object 90 degrees or flip the object over its x- or y-axis.
6. ***Select objects:*** Deactivate all drawing functions.
7. ***Free rotate:*** This button will place green handles on certain objects so they can be arbitrarily rotated. Click and drag the handles to rotate the objects.

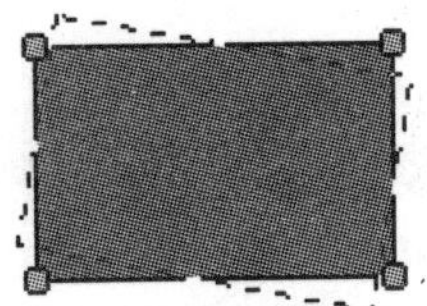

8. ***AutoShapes menu:*** Click the small down arrow to the right of the "AutoShapes" text to select a shape.
9. ***Line and arrow:*** Click and drag the mouse on the slide to add lines. Hold down the SHIFT key to draw a straight line. Use the end points of the completed line to stretch and reposition the line.
10. ***Rectangle and oval:*** Click and drag the mouse on the slide to add rectangles and ovals. Hold down the SHIFT key to add squares and circles.
11. ***Text box:*** Click to draw a text box on the slide.
12. ***Word art:*** Click to add WordArt.
13. ***Picture:*** Click to add a clip art image to the slide.
14. ***Fill color:*** Choose a fill color for rectangles, ovals, and clip art.
15. ***Line color:*** Select a border color for shapes and pictures.
16. ***Font color:*** Highlight text on the slide and click the small down arrow next to the Font color icon to select a color.
17. ***Line style:*** Highlight a line or arrow that has been drawn and click this button to select a thickness or style for the line.
18. ***Dash style:*** Highlight a line or arrow and select a dash style.
19. ***Arrow style:*** Change the arrow head style for an existing arrow or change a line to an arrow.
20. ***Shadow:*** Select a text box to add shadow to text or choose any other object on the slide to add a drop shadow.
21. ***3D:*** Add a three-dimensional effect to text and other objects.

Adding Clip Art

To add a clip art image to a slide, follow these steps:

1. Select Insert | Picture | Clip Art from the menu bar or click the Picture button on the Drawing toolbar.

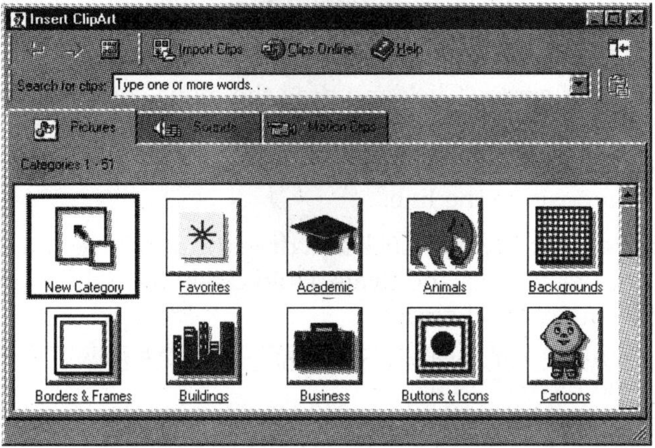

2. To find an image, click in the white box following Search for clips and enter keywords describing the image you want to find. OR

   Click one of the category icons.

3. Click once on the image to want to add to the slide and a selection bar will appear.

4. Click once on the image you want to add to the slide and the following popup menu will appear:

   a. Insert Clip to add the image to the slide.

   b. Preview Clip to view the image full-size before adding it to the slide. Drag the bottom, right corner of the preview window to resize the image and click the "x" close button to end the preview.

   c. Add Clip to Favorites will add the selected image to your favorites directory that can be chosen from the Insert ClipArt dialog box.

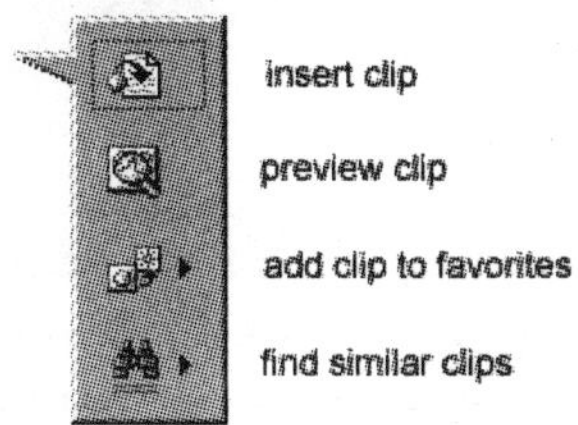

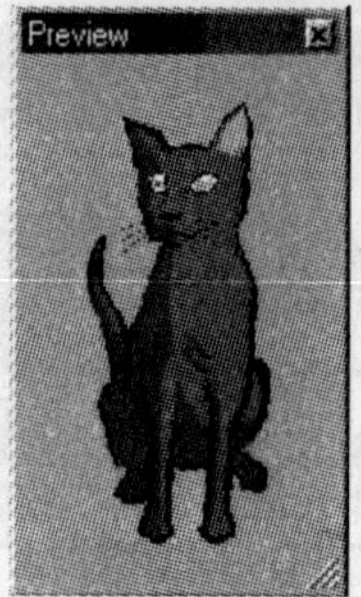

d. Find Similar Clips will retrieve images similar to the one you have chosen.

5. Click the Close button in the top, right corner of the Insert Clip window to stop adding clip art to the slide.

Add an Image from a File

To add a photo or graphic from a file:

1. Select Insert | Picture | From File from the menu bar.
2. Click the down arrow button on the right side of the Look in: window to find the image on your computer.
3. Highlight the file name from the list and click the Insert button.

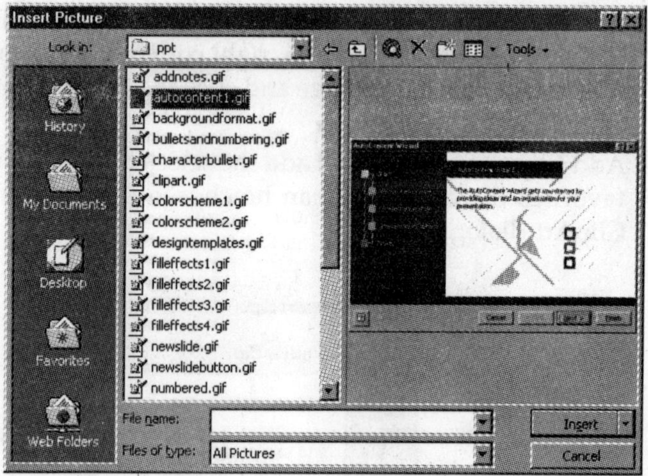

Editing a Graphic

Activate the image you wish to edit by clicking on it once with the mouse. Several handles will appear around the graphic. Click and drag these handles to resize the image. The handles on the corners will resize proportionally while the handles on the straight lines will stretch the image. More picture effects can be changed using the Picture toolbar.

AutoShapes

The AutoShapes toolbar allows you to draw a number of geometrical shapes, arrows, flow chart elements, stars, and other graphics on a slide. Activate the AutoShapes toolbar by selecting Insert | Picture | AutoShapes or View | Toolbars | AutoShapes from the menu bar. Click the buttons on the toolbar to view the options for drawing each shape.

1. ***Lines:*** After clicking the Lines button on the AutoShapes toolbar, draw a straight line, arrow, or double-ended arrow from the first row of options by clicking the respective button. Click in the slide where you would like the line to begin and click again where it should end. To draw a curved line or freeform shape, select curved lines from the menu (first and second buttons of second row), click in the slide where the line should appear, and click the mouse every time a curve should begin. End creating the graphic by clicking on the starting end or pressing the ESC key. To scribble, click the last button in the second row, click the mouse in the slide and hold down the left button while you draw the design. Let go of the mouse button to stop drawing.

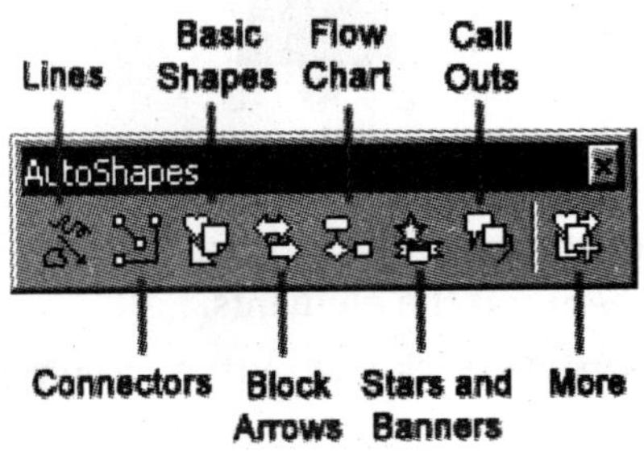

2. ***Connectors:*** Draw these lines to connect flow chart elements.
3. ***Basic shapes:*** Click the Basic Shapes button on the AutoShapes toolbar to select from many two- and three-dimensional shapes, icons, braces, and brackets. Use the drag-and-drop method to draw the shape in the slide. When the shape has been made, it can be resized using the open box handles and other adjustments specific to each shape can be modified using the yellow diamond handles.

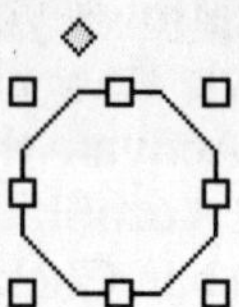

4. ***Block arrows:*** Select Block Arrows to choose from many types of two- and three-dimensional arrows. Drag-and-drop the arrow in the slide and use the open box and yellow diamond handles to adjust the arrowheads. Each AutoShape can also be rotated by first clicking the Free Rotate button on the drawing toolbar. Click and drag the green handles around the image to rotate it. The tree image below was created from an arrow rotated 90 degrees.

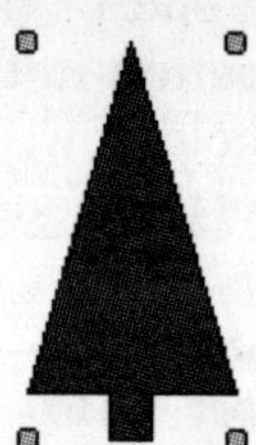

5. ***Flow chart:*** Choose from the flow chart menu to add flow chart elements to the slide and use the line menu to draw connections between the elements.
6. ***Stars and banners:*** Click the button to select stars, bursts, banners, and scrolls.

7. ***Call outs:*** Select from the speech and thought bubbles, and line call outs. Enter the call out text in the text box that is made.
8. ***More autoShapes:*** Click the More button to choose from a list of clip art categories.

Each of the submenus on the AutoShapes toolbar can become a separate toolbar. Just click and drag the gray bar across the top of the submenus off of the toolbar and it will become a separate floating toolbar.

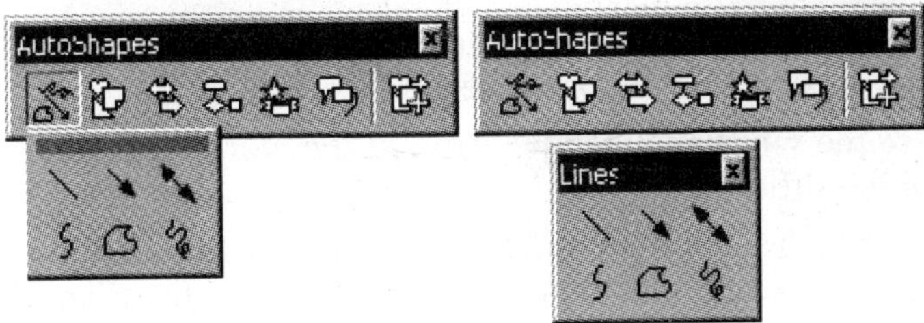

WordArt

Add headlines in striking colors and shapes to your presentation using WordArt.

1. Select Insert | Picture | WordArt from the menu bar or click the WordArt button on the Drawing toolbar.
2. Choose a WordArt style from the listing and click OK.

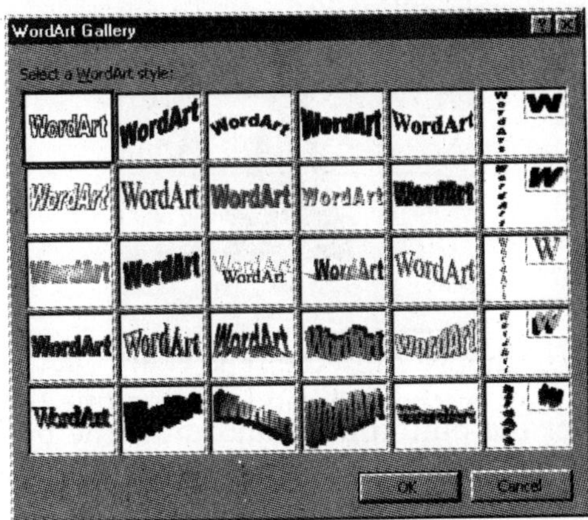

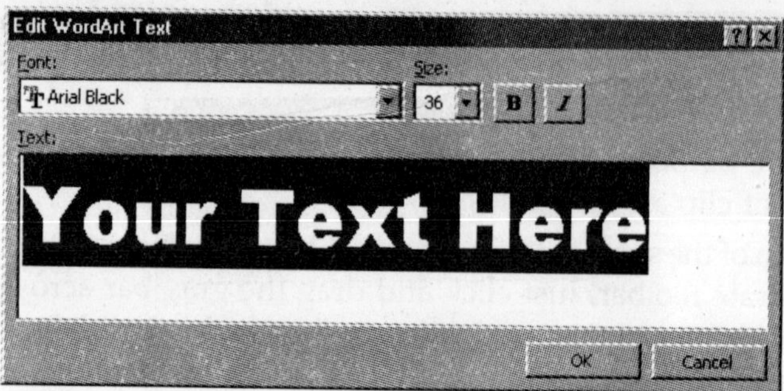

3. Enter the text in the Edit WordArt Text box and choose the font, size, and style for the text. Click OK.
4. Use the white box handles around the wordart to resize it on the slide.
5. Drag the yellow diamond handle to change the shape of the text. To revert back to no shape, double-click the diamond.

Slide Effects

Use the action button toolbar to add functioning buttons to slides in a presentation.

1. Select Slide Show | Action Buttons from the menu bar. Click the bar across the top of the button menu and drag it off the menu so it becomes a floating toolbar.

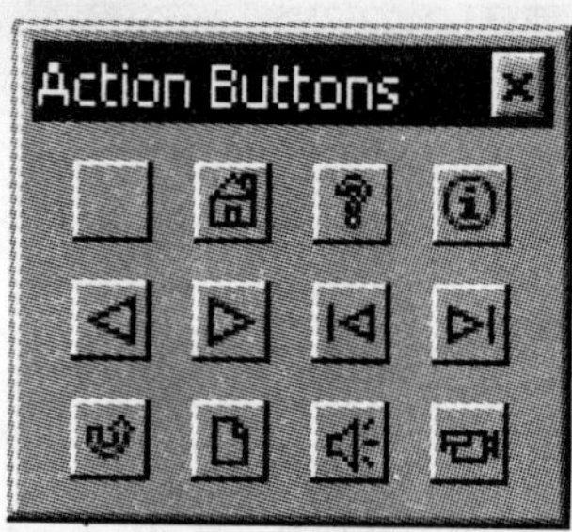

2. Click one of the button faces and draw the button on the slide using the mouse. The Action Settings menu will then appear.

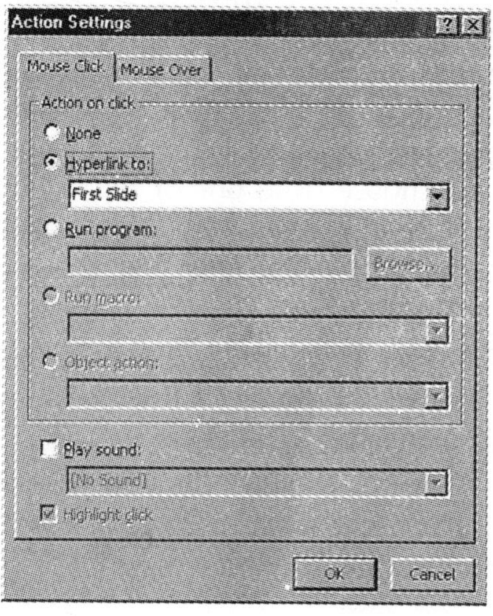

3. Set the actions under either the Mouse Click or Mouse Over tabs. Actions specified for Mouse Click will execute when the button is clicked on the slide while actions for Mouse Over will occur when the mouse pointer hovers over the button.
4. Select an action for the button by choosing a Hyperlink to destination.
5. If you want a sound to be played when the button is clicked, check the Play sound box and choose a sound from the drop-down menu.
6. Click OK when finished.

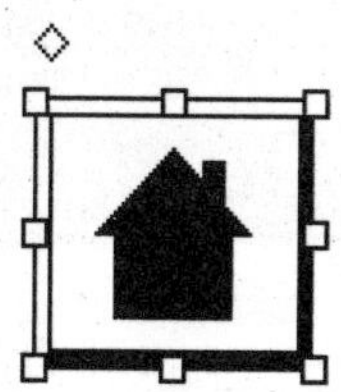

7. The button on the slide can be resized using the white box handles and the depth of the button can be changed by dragging the yellow diamond.

Slide Animation

Several animations for slide objects are available through the drop-down menus on the menu bar. First, select the text box or graphic that will be animated. Select Slide Show | Preset Animation and choose from one of the options. To select a different animation or turn the animation off, select the appropriate choice from the same menu. For more options, follow the procedure below:

1. Select Slide Show | Custom Animation from the menu bar.
2. Select the object on the slide that will be animated from the Check to animate slide objects list.
3. Under the Effects tab, select the animation type (or select "No Effect" to turn an animation off) and direction from the drop-down menus and select a sound if you wish.
4. Select an After animation effect if the text should change colors after the animation executes.
   a. ***Color palette:*** Select one of the color swatches or click More Colors for a larger selection. The text will change to the selected color when the mouse is clicked during the slide show.
   b. ***Don't Dim:*** This option erases all After Animation effects.

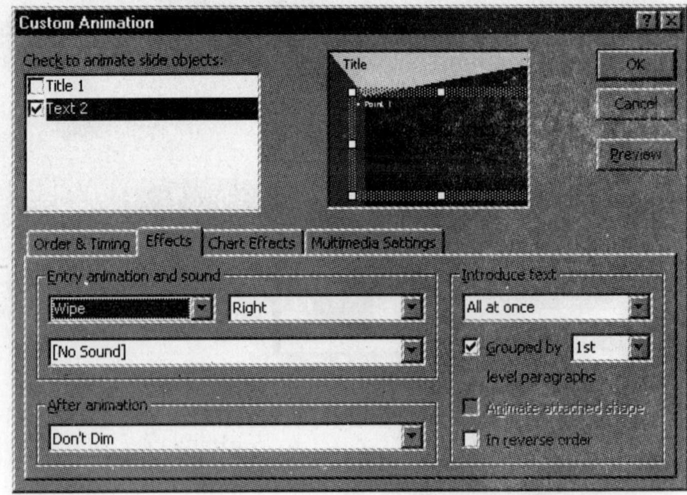

c. ***Hide after animation:*** Text will be immediately erased after the animation is completed.

d. ***Hide on next mouse click:*** The text will be erased when the mouse is clicked.

5. Choose the style of displaying the text under the Introduce text section. The drop-down menu provides options for displaying the characters for each bulleted item. Select "All at once" for the text to appear immediately, "by Word" for the text to appear one word at a time, or "by Letter" for a typewriter effect that displays one letter at a time.
6. Click the Order and Timing tab to alter the order that the objects appear on the slide. Highlight the object in the Animation order box and click the Move arrows to move the object's position within the animation sequence. Under Start animation, choose "On mouse click" to activate the animation by clicking the mouse or "Automatically" for the animation to execute after a set number of seconds.
7. Click the Preview button at any time.

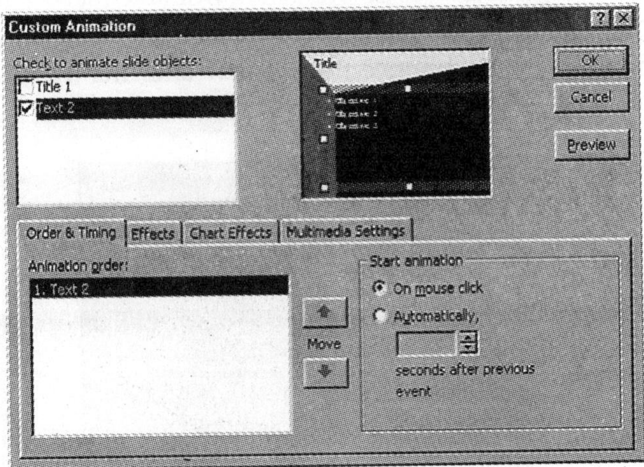

Animation Preview

Select Slide Show | Animation Preview from the menu bar to view the Animation Preview window. Click anywhere within this window with the mouse to preview the animations that

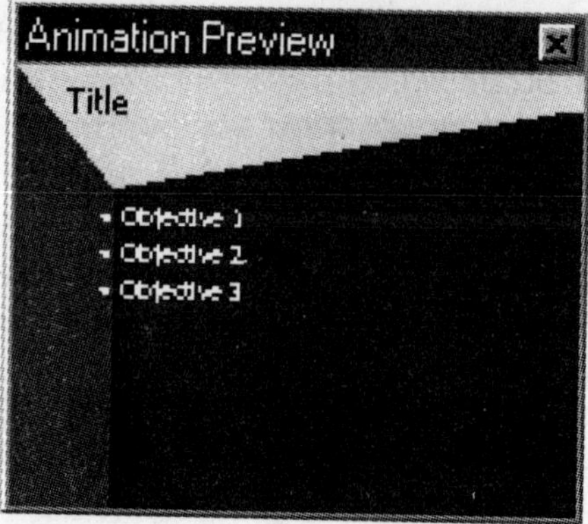

have been set. To hide the window, click the x close button in the top, right corner.

Slide Transitions

Add transition effects when changing slides by following these steps:

1. Select Slide Show | Slide Transition from the menu bar.
2. From the Effect section, choose a transition from the drop-down menu and notice the preview after the transition is selected. Select a speed for the transition as well.

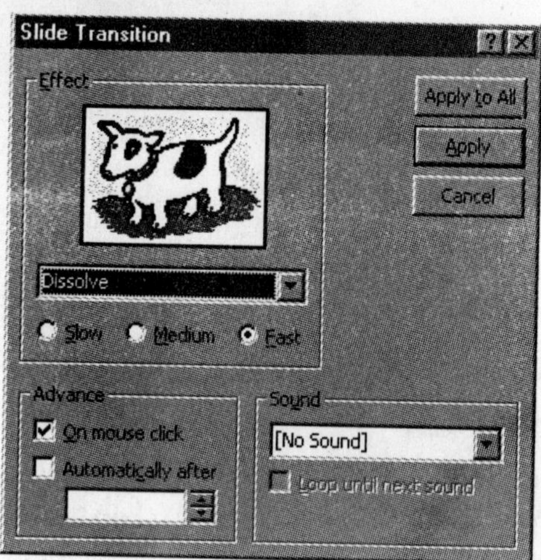

3. Under Advance, check "On mouse click" for the slide transition to occur by clicking the mouse or using keystrokes or check "Automatically after" and a number of seconds if the transition should occur automatically.
4. Select a Sound if necessary and check the Loop until next sound if it should keep repeating until the next sound is played.
5. Click Apply to All if the transition effects should be added to every slide or Apply if the effects should be added only to the current slide.

Slide Show Options

Select Tools | Options and click the View tab to choose from several more slide show options.

1. Popup menu on right mouse click: Check this box if you want to be able to access the shortcut menu during a presentation.
2. Show popup menu button: Check this box to activate the menu button that appears in the bottom, left corner of the screen during a presentation.
3. End with black slide: Insert a blank, black slide to the end of the presentation.

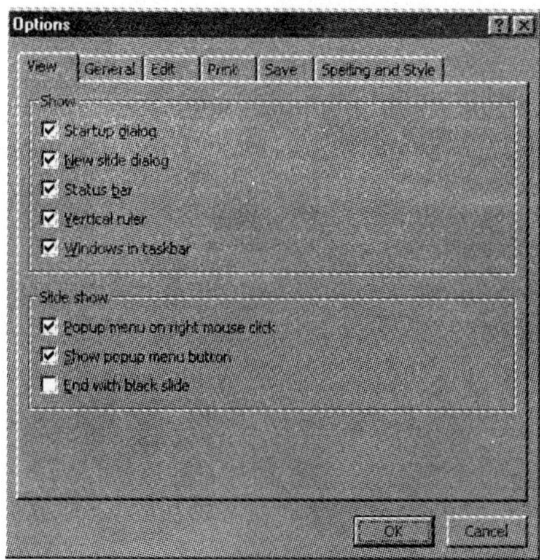

MASTER SLIDES

Slide Master

Change the style of all slides in the presentation by changing the properties on the Slide Master. Each Design Template has its own Slide Master that can be altered. If you create slides from scratch, a consistent style can be added to the presentation by formatting the Slide Master.

1. Select View | Master | Slide Master from the menu bar.
2. Format the master slide just as you would format a regular slide by formatting text, formatting lists, adding background patterns and effects, and setting footers.
3. Click the Close button on the Master toolbar to quit editing the master slide and return to the presentation.

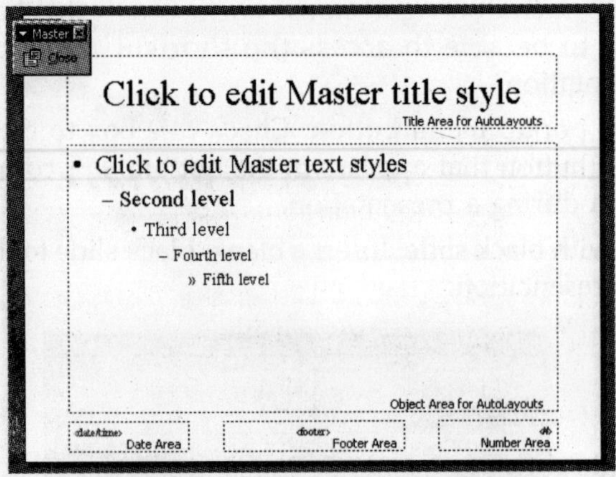

Headers and Footers

Add the date and time, slide numbers, and other footer text to the master slide from the Header and Footer window.

1. Select View | Header and Footer from the menu bar.
2. Check the Date and time box to add this feature to the slide. Select Update automatically to always display the current date and time or click Fixed and enter a date that will not change in the text field provided.

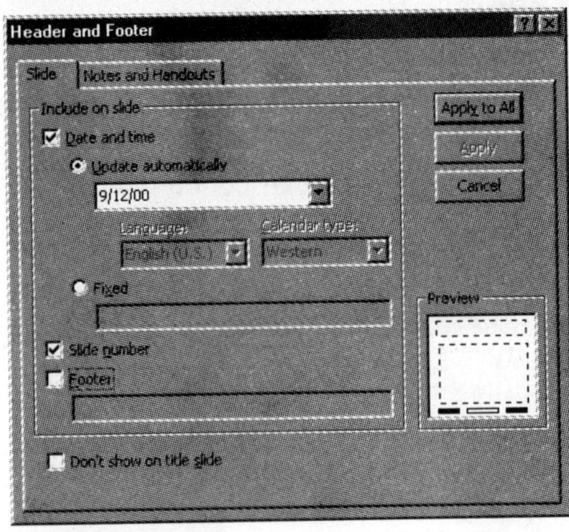

3. Check the Slide number box to add this feature to the slides.
4. Click the Footer box and add other text to the footer area of the slide.
5. Check the Don't show on title slide box to hide these features on the title slide of the presentation.
6. Click the Notes and Handouts tab to make the same changes to notes and handouts pages.
7. Click Apply to All to add the changes to every slide or Apply to add only to the current slide.

Slide Numbers

To add the slide numbers in a fixed position on the slide, use the Header and Footer window detailed above. The slide number can otherwise be added anywhere on the slide by placing the cursor where the slide number should appear and selecting Insert | Slide Number from the menu bar. The text of the slide number can the formatting just as regular text style is changed.

Date and Time

A date and/or time can also be added using the Header and Footer window or anywhere else on the slide. Place the cursor where the date and time should appear on the slide and select Insert | Date and Time from the menu bar. Select a format from the Available formats box and click Update automatically if this feature should always be updated to reflect the current date and time. Click OK to finish.

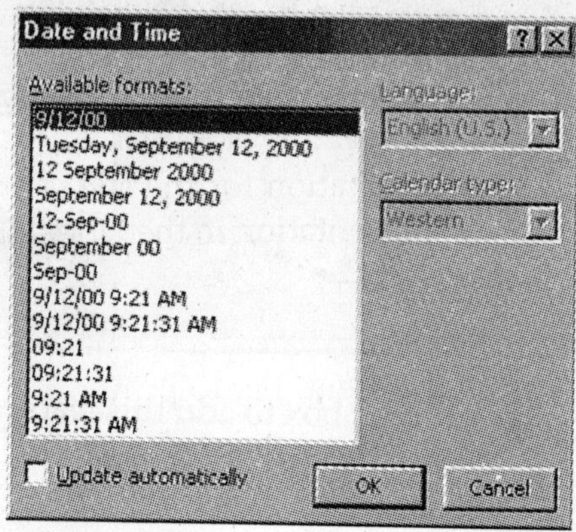

SAVING AND PRINTING

Save as Web Page

Presentations can be saved by selecting File | Save from the menu bar. However, if you want to post Power Point presentations on the Internet, you may want to save them as web pages so students and other visitors to your web site can view the presentation even if they do not have Power Point installed on their computers. Select File | Save As Web Page from the menu bar. Choose your web page directory on the network from the Look in: drop-down menu and name the file in the File name: box. Click Save to save the presentation in web format.

Page Setup

Select File | Page Setup from the menu bar to access options for printing the presentation slides. Select the format the printed slides will be used for from the Slides sized for drop-down menu or enter a specific print size using the Width and Height

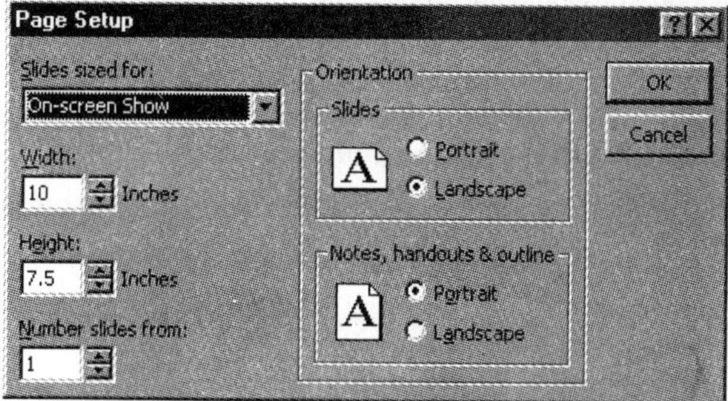

boxes. Select the page orientation for the slides and for other print material from the presentation in the Orientation section.

Print

Select File | Print from the menu bar to print the presentation.

1. ***Print range:*** Select All to print all the slides in the presentation, Current slide to print only the current slide,

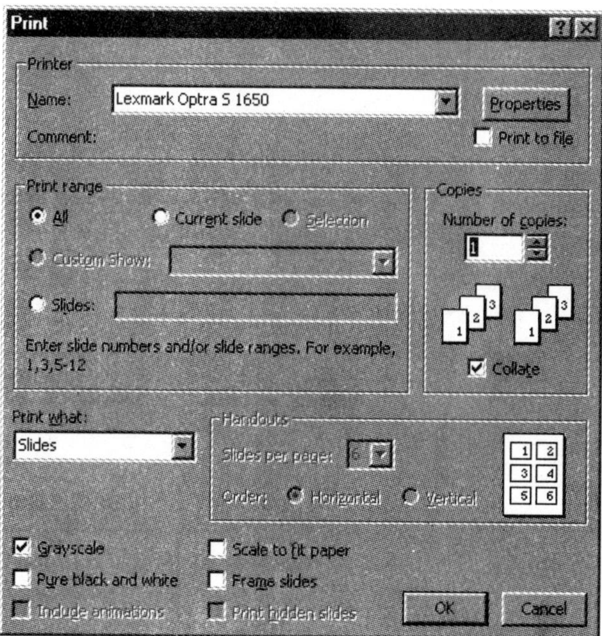

or enter slide numbers in the Slides field to print only certain slides.

2. ***Copies:*** Enter the number of copies of each slide specified in Print range and check the Collate box if necessary.
3. ***Print:***
   a. Slides prints a full-page slide on each page.
   b. Handouts prints as many slides as you designate on each page.
   c. Notes Page prints one slide with that slide's notes on each page.
   d. Outline view prints the outline of the presentation.

Microsoft Access

INTRODUCTION

Microsoft Access is a computer application used to create and manage computer-based databases on desktop computers and/or on connected computers (a network). Microsoft Access can be used for personal information management (PIM), in a small business to organize and manage data, or in an enterprise to communicate with servers.

Microsoft Access is a powerful program to create and manage your databases. It has many built in features to assist you in constructing and viewing your information. Access is much more involved and is a more genuine database application than other programs such as Microsoft Works.

First of all you need to understand how Microsoft Access breaks down a database. Some keywords involved in this process are: Database File, Table, Record, Field, Data-type.

- ***Database file:*** This is your main file that encompasses the entire database and that is saved to your hard-drive or floppy disk.

  Example: Student Database.mdb

- ***Table:*** A table is a collection of data about a specific topic. There can be multiple tables in a database.

  Example #1: Students

  Example #2: Teachers

- ***Field:*** Fields are the different categories within a Table. Tables usually contain multiple fields.

  Example #1: Student LastName

  Example #2: Student FirstName

- ***Datatypes:*** Datatypes are the properties of each field. A field only has 1 datatype.

  FieldName: Student LastName

  Datatype: Text

STARTING MICROSOFT ACCESS

Like any other computer application, in order to use Microsoft Access, you must first install it. After installing Microsoft Access, then you can open it. There are two ways as described below; either could be used to start MS Access:

1. Double click on the Microsoft Access icon on the desktop.

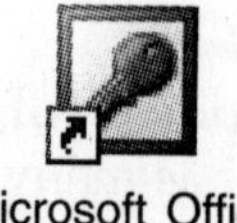

2. Click on Start → Programs → Microsoft Access.

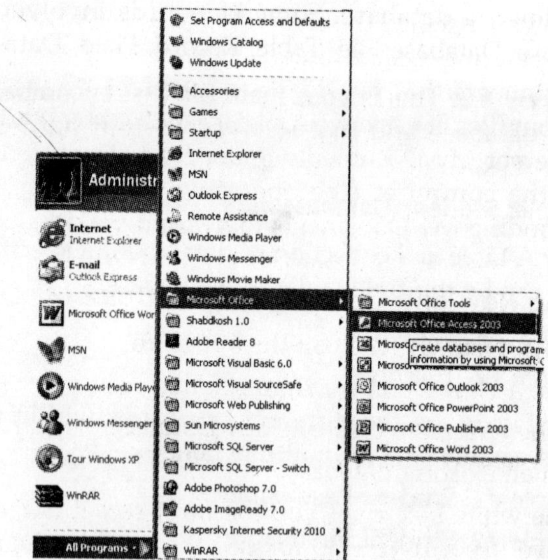

If you have a Microsoft Access database such as an e-mail attachment, a file on a floppy disk, on the network, or in any other means, once you see its icon, you can double-click it. Not only will this action launch Microsoft Access, but also it will open the file.

If you are working on a network of related computers, your database may be located in another computer. In this case the network or database administrator would create a link or shortcut to the drive that is hosting the database. You can then click or double-click this link or shortcut to open the database and, as a result, launch Microsoft Access.

A MICROSOFT ACCESS DATABASE FILE

The Database as a File

A Microsoft Access database is primarily a Windows file. It must have a location, also called a path, which indicates how the file can be retrieved and made available. Although you can create a database on the root directory such as the C: drive, it is usually a good idea to create your files, including your databases, in an easily recognizable folder.

When you installed the computer (or when it was installed), it (the operating system) might have created a folder called My Documents that provides a convenient place for you to create your files. If various people use the same computer, there is a different My Documents folder for each one. When you log in, the computer (the operating system) locates your corresponding My Documents folder and makes it available.

Creating New and Opening Existing Databases

The above picture gives you the option to:

1. Create a New Database from scratch.
2. Use the wizard to create a New Database.
3. Open an existing database.
   - The white box gives you the most recent databases you have used. If you do not see the one you had created, choose the More Files option and hit OK. Otherwise

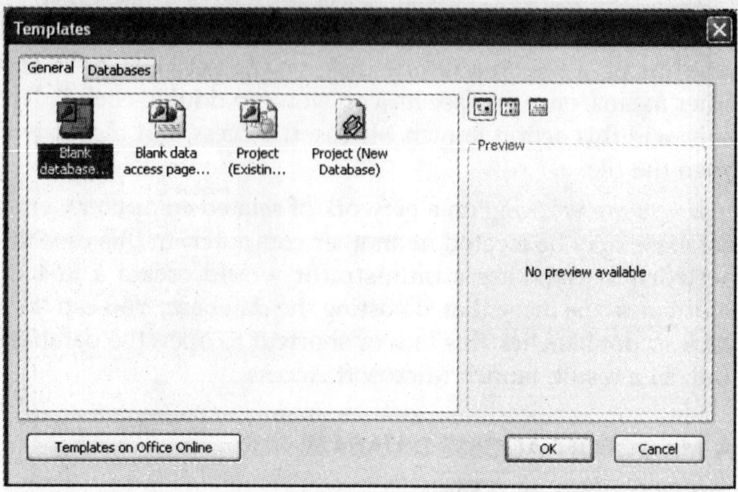

choose the database you had previously used and click OK.

Create a database using the Database Wizard:

1. When Microsoft Access first starts up, a dialog box is automatically displayed with options to create a new database or open an existing one. If this dialog box is displayed, click Access Database Wizards, pages, and projects and then click OK.

   If you have already opened a database or closed the dialog box that displays when Microsoft Access starts up, click New Database on the toolbar.

2. On the Databases tab, double-click the icon for the kind of database you want to create.
3. Specify a name and location for the database.
4. Click Create to start defining your new database.

Create a database without using the Database Wizard:

1. When Microsoft Access first starts up, a dialog box is automatically displayed with options to create a new database or open an existing one. If this dialog box is displayed, click Blank Access Database, and then click OK.

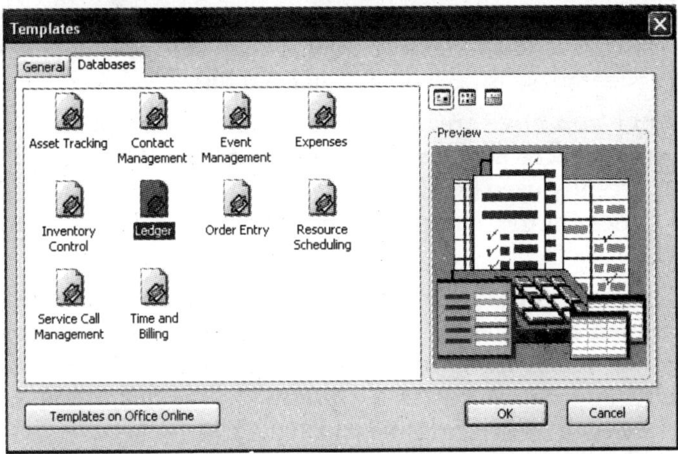

If you have already opened a database or closed the dialog box that displays when Microsoft Access starts up, click New Database on the toolbar, and then double-click the Blank Database icon on the General tab.

2. Specify a name and location for the database and click Create (below is the screen that shows up following this step).

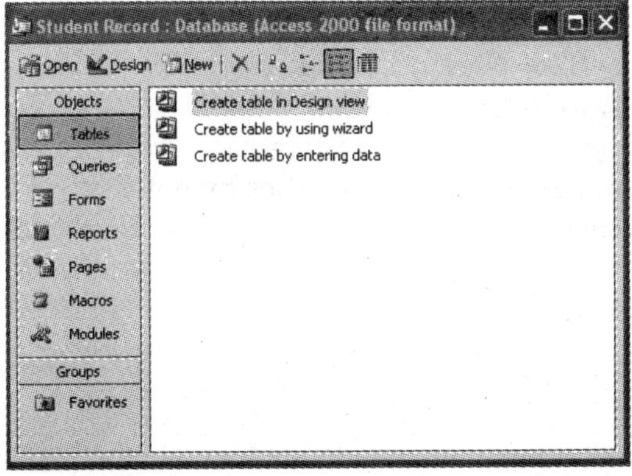

DATABASE MANAGEMENT

Unlike some other programming environments, Microsoft Access considers a database as a single Windows file with a name. We will eventually learn that this file can contain various objects that actually make up a database. Therefore, a Microsoft Access database is opened as a normal file.

After you have created a database, as a computer file, it becomes part of what are known in Microsoft Windows as the most recently used (MRU) documents. As such, when you click the Office Button, the right side of the menu shows a list of MRUs.

The number of files that the right column can display can be decreased as low as 1 or increase as high as 9. To change this number, access the Options dialog box by clicking the Office Button and clicking Access Options. In the left frame, click Advanced. In the right frame and in the Display section, change the value of the Show This Number Of Recent Documents.

Database Properties

Whether you work alone or in a group, communication and documentation are important. Your database project has its own properties that you can use to find out some details about your file, to enter some notes about the project, or to give directives to other people who have access to the database. This can be done using a dialog box called the Database Properties. The Database properties allow you to provide additional information about your database. To view the Database properties, click Database Properties on the File menu. You can set these properties by entering information in the Summary or Custom tabs in the DatabaseName Properties dialog box or in a Microsoft Access database (.mdb), by using Visual Basic.

The Database properties appear in the DatabaseName Properties dialog box as shown in Table 7.1.

Size of a Database

A database is primarily a computer file, just like those created with other applications. As such, it occupies an amount of space in the computer memory. In some circumstances, you should know how much space a database is using. This can be important when you need to back it up or when it is time to

Table 7.1: Database properties

Tab	*Description*
General	This is the same information that is displayed when you right-click the name of a file in Windows Explorer and then click Properties on the shortcut menu. The only difference is that when these properties are viewed in Microsoft Access, the Attributes settings are read-only.
Summary	This information is similar to the summary information you can provide in other Microsoft Office applications. Summary information allows the user to better identify a database both from within Microsoft Access and from other programs such as the Windows Find Files program. In Microsoft Access databases (.mdb), the information you enter on this tab is added to the SummaryInfo Document object in the Documents collection for Microsoft Access databases. The Hyperlink Base setting on the Summary tab is used to create the base hyperlink path that is appended to the beginning of relative Hyperlink-Address property settings.
Statistics	This information includes the date and time the active database was created, and the last date and time it was modified, accessed, and printed.
Contents	This information includes the names of the objects contained in your database.
Custom	In Microsoft Access databases (.mdb), the custom properties you enter become properties of the UserDefined Document object in the Documents collection.

distribute it. Also, when adding and deleting objects from your database, its file can grow or shrink without your direct intervention.

Like any other computer file, to know the size of a database, you can right-click it in Windows Explorer or My Computer and click Properties. If you are already using the database, to check its size, you can click the Office Button, position the mouse on Manage and click Database Properties. In the Properties dialog box, click General and check the Size label.

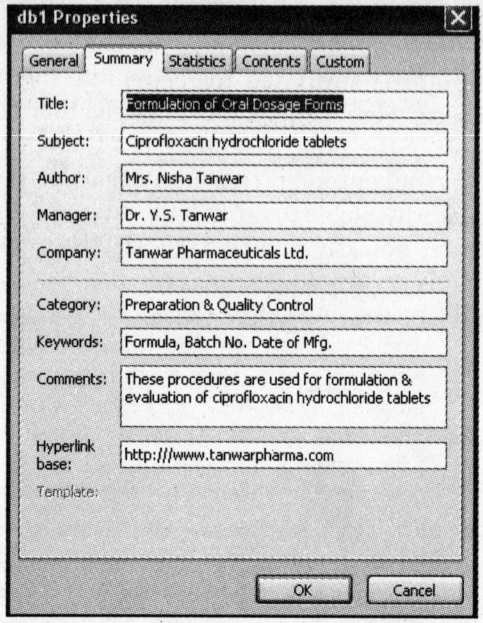

Compacting and Repairing a Database

As mentioned already, once you have created a database file, it occupies a certain amount of memory space that can grow or shrink without your direct intervention:

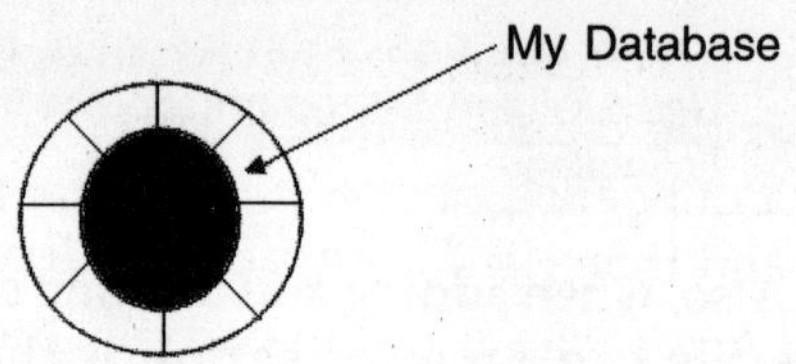

When you add an object to the database, the database's file grows as needed. When you remove an object, the memory

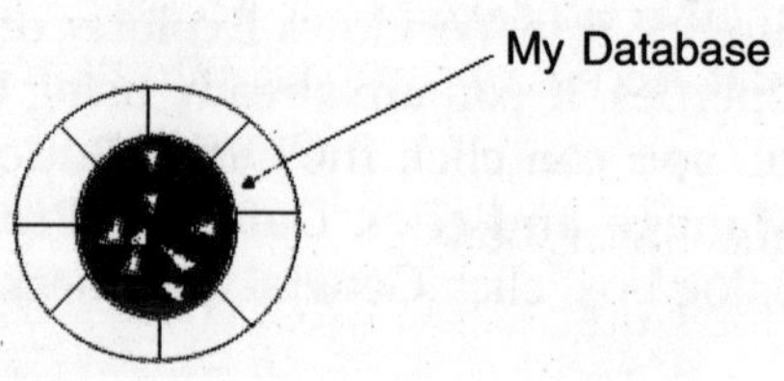

space it was occupying is left empty. This also applies when you keep removing objects:

The computer is supposed to recuperate the space those previous objects were using. Unfortunately, that is not always the case. Most of the time, that space is left empty but cannot be accessed by the computer. This means that the memory space cannot be made available to other applications. To recover this memory space, you can compact the database. When this is done, the file is shrunk to occupy only the necessary amount of space and free the unused sections:

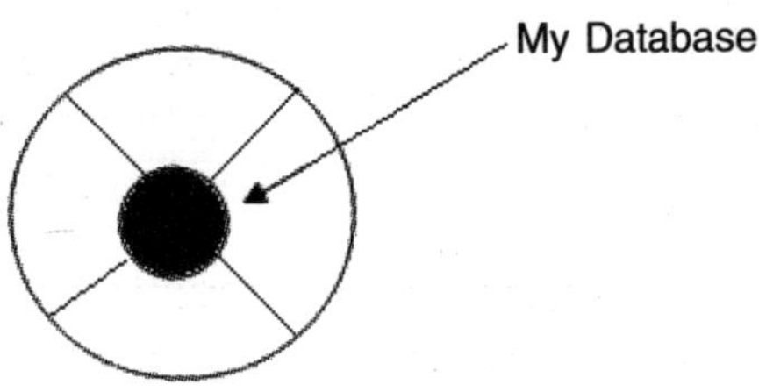

To ensure optimal performance, compact your Microsoft Access databases and Microsoft Access projects on a regular basis. Compacting and repairing have been improved, and they are now integrated into a single process that is safer and more effective.

To compact a database, you have two options:

1. To compact a database, you have two options. To compact and repair the database that is currently opened, and to compact it only once, on the Tools menu, point to Database Utilities, and then click Compact and Repair Database.
2. Microsoft Access can also automatically compact a Microsoft Access database or Microsoft Access project every time you close it.
    - Open the Access database or Access project that you want Microsoft Access to compact automatically.
    - On the Tools menu, click Options.
    - Click the General tab.
    - Select the Compact On Close check box.

TABLES

A table is a collection of data about a specific topic, such as students or contacts. Using a separate table for each topic means that you store that data only once, which makes your database more efficient, and reduces data-entry errors. Tables organize data into columns (called fields) and rows (called records).

Each field in Students Record table contains the same type of information for every student, such as I.D. No. This is an example of a COLUMN

I.D. No	Student Name	Date of Birth	Address	City
1111	Amita Sharma	16 March 1984	5, BN Road	Udaipur
1112	Neha Singh	15 Sept. 1982	21, Avenue Qt.	Delhi
1113	Roop Kumar	05 July 1980	09, Maal Road	Shimla
1114	Om Trivedi	11 Sept. 1986	123 N, Union	Mumbai
1115	Raj Kumar	14 April 1982	1, St. Village	Bangalore
1116	Mona Lal	05 Jan.1980	74, Vaishali Qt.	Jaipur
1117	Ram Kumar	25 May 1985	25, Vasant Kj.	Indore
1118	Mohan Meena	22 June 1982	12 Gandhi Park	Assam

Each record in a Students Record table contains all information about one student such as name, birthday, address, city. This is an example of ROW.

Create a table from scratch in design view:

1. If you have not already done so, switch to the Database Window You can press F11 to switch to the Database window from any other window.

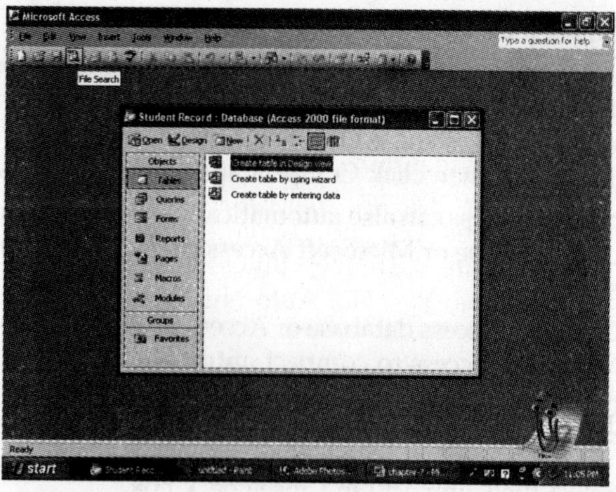

2. Double-Click on "Create table in Design view".

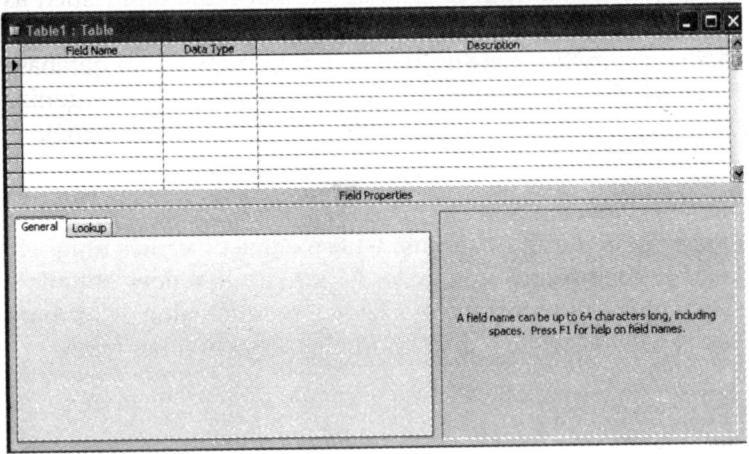

3. Define each of the fields in your table:
   a. Under the Field Name column, enter the categories of your table.
   b. Under Data Type column, enter the type you want for you categories.
      - The attribute of a variable or field that determines what kind of data it can hold. For example, in a Microsoft Access database, the Text and Memo field data types allow the field to store either text or numbers, but the Number data type will allow the field to store numbers only. Number data type fields store numerical data that will be used in mathematical calculations. Use the Currency data type to display or calculate currency values. Other data types are Date/Time, Yes/No, Auto Number, and OLE object (Picture).
   c. Under the Description column, enter the text that describes what you field is (This field is optional).

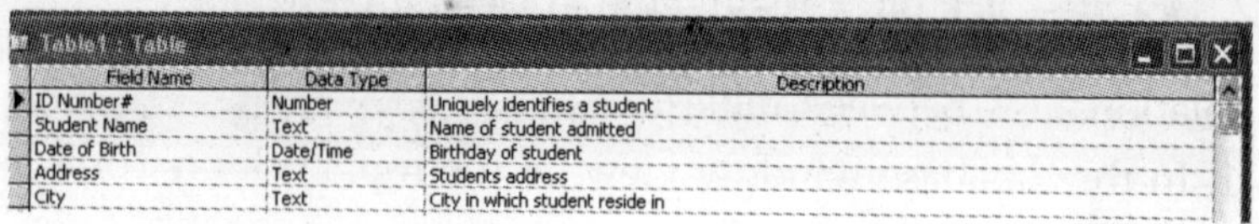

Field Name	Data Type	Description
ID Number#	Number	Uniquely identifies a student
Student Name	Text	Name of student admitted
Date of Birth	Date/Time	Birthday of student
Address	Text	Students address
City	Text	City in which student reside in

Primary Key

One or more fields (columns) whose value or values uniquely identify each record in a table. A primary key does not allow Null values and must always have a unique value. A primary key is used to relate a table to foreign keys in other tables.

RELATIONSHIPS

After you have set up multiple tables in your Microsoft Access database, you need a way of telling Access how to bring that information back together again. The first step in this process is to define relationships between your tables. After you have done that, you can create queries, forms, and reports to display information from several tables at once.

A relationship works by matching data in key fields—usually a field with the same name in both tables. In most cases, these matching fields are the primary key from one table, which provides a unique identifier for each record, and a foreign key in the other table. For example, teachers can be associated with the students they are responsible for by creating a relationship between the teacher's table and the student's table using the TeacherID fields.

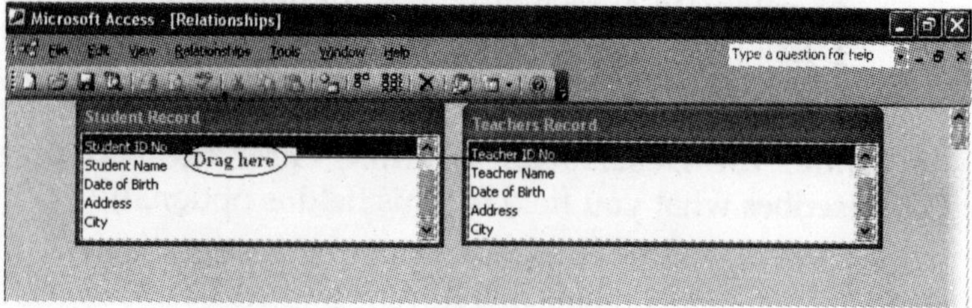

Having met the criteria above, follow these steps for creating relationships between tables.

1. In the database window view, at the top, click on Tools → Relationships.
2. Select the Tables you want to link together, by clicking on them and selecting the Add Button.
3. Drag the primary key of the Parent table (Teacher in this case), and drop it into the same field in the Child table (Student in this case).
4. Select Enforce Referential Integrity:
   a. When the Cascade Update Related Fields check box is set, changing a primary key value in the primary table automatically updates the matching value in all related records.
   b. When the Cascade Delete Related Records check box is set, deleting a record in the primary table deletes any related records in the related table.
5. Click Create and Save the Relationship.

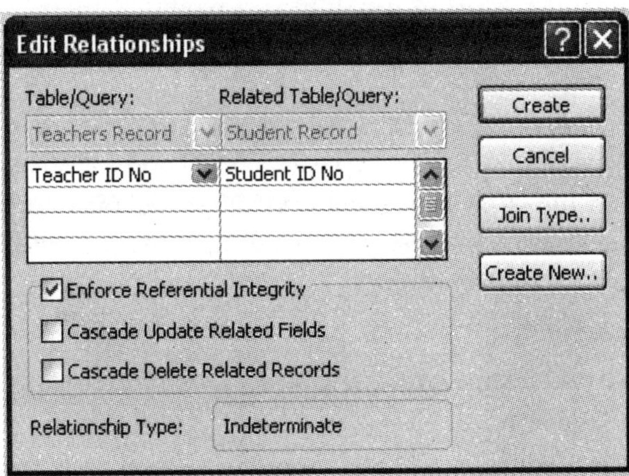

FORM

A form is nothing more than a graphical representation of a table. You can add, update, delete records in your table by using a form. Although a form can be named different from a table, they both still manipulate the same information and the same exact data. Hence, if you change a record in a form, it will be changed in the table also.

A form is very good to use when you have numerous fields in a table. This way you can see all the fields in one screen, whereas if you were in the table view (datasheet) you would have to keep scrolling to get the field you desire.

It is a very good idea to create a form using the wizard, unless you are an advanced user and know what you are doing. Microsoft Access does a very good job of creating a form using the wizard. The following steps are needed to create a basic form:

1. Switch to the Database Window. You can do this by pressing F11 on the keyboard.
2. Click on the Forms button under Objects on the left side of screen.
3. Double click on Create Form Using Wizard.
4. On the next screen select the fields you want to view on your form. Most of the time you would select all of them.
5. Click Next.
6. Select the layout you wish.
7. Click Next.
8. Select the style you desire...HINT: if you plan on printing your form, I suggest you use a light background to save on printer toner and ink.
9. Click Next.
10. Give you form a name, and select Open the Form and enter information.
11. Select Finish.
12. You should see your form. To adjust the design of your form, simply hit the design button (same as with the tables), and adjust your form accordingly.

REPORT

A report is an effective way to present your data in a printed format. Because you have control over the size and appearance of everything on a report, you can display the information the way you want to see it.

As with the Form, it is a very good idea to create a report using the wizard, unless you are an advanced user. Microsoft Access does a very good job using the wizard to create reports:

1. Switch to the Database Window. You can do this by pressing F11 on the keyboard.
2. Click on the Reports button under Objects on the left side of screen.
3. Double click on Create Report Using Wizard.
4. On the next screen select the fields you want to view on your form. Most of the time you would select all of them.
5. Click Next.
6. Select if you would like to group your files. Keep repeating this step for as many groupings as you would like.
7. Click Next.
8. Select the layout and the paper orientation you desire.
9. Click Next.
10. Select the style you desire...HINT: if you plan on printing your report, you can use a light background to save on printer toner and ink
11. Click Next.
12. Give you report a name, and select Preview the Report.
13. Select Finish.
14. You should see your report. To adjust the design of your report, simply hit the design button (same as with the tables), and adjust your report accordingly.

QUERY

You use queries to view, change, and analyze data in different ways. You can also use them as the source of records for forms, reports, and data access pages. The power of queries lies in being able to bring together or perform an action on data from more than one table or query. Each query has property settings that you can change to alter the way the query behaves and how the query results look.

An action query is a query that makes changes to many records in just one operation. There are four types of action queries: delete, update, append, and make-table (Table 7.2).

Table 7.2: Types of action query

Type	*Meaning*	*Example*
Delete query	Deletes a group of records from one or more tables. With delete queries, you always delete entire records, not just selected fields within records.	You could use a delete query to remove products that are discontinued or for which there are no orders.
Update query	Makes global changes to a group of records in one or more tables. With an update query, you can change data in existing tables.	You can raise prices by 10 percent for all dairy products, or you can raise salaries by 5 percent for the people within a certain job category.
Append query	Adds a group of records from one or more tables to the end of one or more tables.	Suppose that you acquire some new customers and a database containing a table of information on those customers. To avoid typing all this information in, you would like to append it to your customers table.
Make-table query	Creates a new table from all or part of the data in one or more tables.	You might want to create a table that contains several fields from your Employees table, and then export that table to a database used by your personnel department.

Open a query in design view:

1. In the Database window, click Queries under Objects.
2. Click the query you want to open, and then click Design on the Database window toolbar.
3. If a form, report, or data access page is based on a query, you can open the query to modify its design directly from the form, report, or data access page.

Create a query for you:

Microsoft Access can often create a query for you so you do not have to design one from scratch:

1. To create a query to use as the basis of a form, report, or data access page, try the form, report, or data access page wizards. They create the form, report or data access page, and if it is based on more than one table, they also create its underlying SQL statement. If you want, you can save the SQL statement as a query.
2. To easily create queries that you want to run independently or base multiple forms, reports, and data access pages on, try one of the query wizards. Query wizards do all the basic work for you after you provide answers to a series of questions. Even if you have created many queries, you may want to use a wizard to quickly design the query. Then you can switch to Design view to customize it.
3. To create queries from filters you created using Filter By Form, Filter By Selection, or Filter For Input, save the filter as a query.

CREATING MAIL MERGE LABELS USING A WIZARD

Microsoft Access lets you create Mailing Labels for your database that you have. To do this do the following:

1. Switch to the Database Window. You can do this by pressing F11 on the keyboard.
2. Click on the Reports button under Objects on the left side of screen.
3. Click on New.

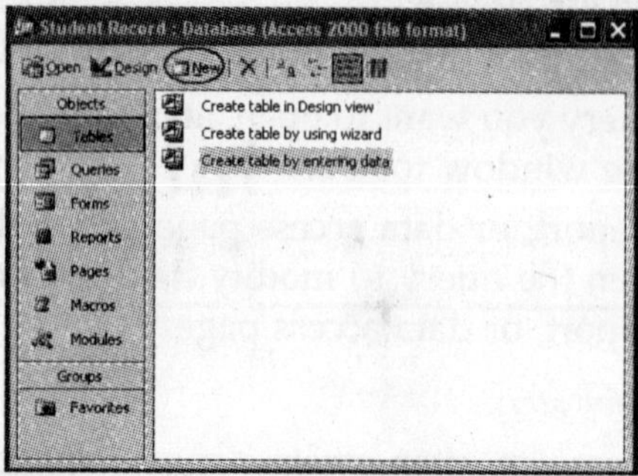

4. Select Label Wizard and the table you would like to get your information from.

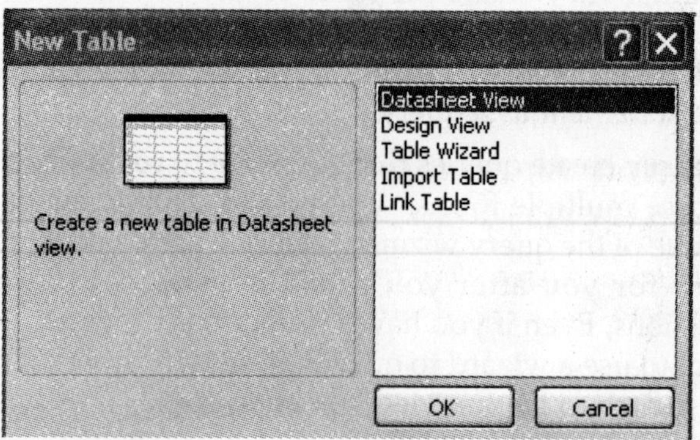

5. Click OK.
6. Select the layout of your labels.
7. Click Next.
8. Select the font size and color you want on each label.
9. Click Next.
10. Select how you want your label to look.
11. Click Next.
12. Select how you want your labels sorted.
13. Give your label report a name and preview it.

Introduction to Internet

NETWORKING

One way to categorize the different types of computer network designs is by their scope or scale. For historical reasons, the networking industry refers to nearly every type of design as some kind of area network. Common examples of area network types are:

- LAN (Local Area Network).
- WLAN (Wireless Local Area Network).
- WAN (Wide Area Network).
- MAN (Metropolitan Area Network).
- SAN (Storage Area Network, System Area Network, Server Area Network, or sometimes Small Area Network).
- CAN (Campus Area Network, Controller Area Network, or sometimes Cluster Area Network).
- PAN (Personal Area Network).
- DAN (Desk Area Network).

LAN and WAN were the original categories of area networks, while the others have gradually emerged over many years of technology evolution.

1. ***Local area network:*** LAN supplies networking capability to a group of computers in close proximity to each other such as in an office building, a school, or a home. A LAN is useful for sharing resources like files, printers, games or other applications. A LAN in turn often connects to other LANs, and to the Internet or other WAN. Most local area networks are built with relatively inexpensive hardware such as Ethernet cables, network adapters and hubs. Wireless LAN and other

more advanced LAN hardware options also exist. Specialized operating system software may be used to configure a local area network. For example, most flavors of Microsoft Windows provide a software package called Internet Connection Sharing (ICS) that supports controlled access to LAN resources. The term LAN partly refers to a multiplayer gaming event where participants bring their own computers and build a temporary LAN.

2. ***Wide area network:*** As the term implies, a WAN spans a large physical distance. The Internet is the largest WAN, spanning the Earth. A WAN is a geographically dispersed collection of LANs. A network device called a router connects LANs to a WAN. In IP networking, the router maintains both a LAN address and a WAN address. A WAN differs from a LAN in several important ways. Most WANs (like the Internet) are not owned by any one organization but rather exist under collective or distributed ownership and management. WANs tend to use technology like ATM, Frame Relay and X.25 for connectivity over the longer distances.

3. ***Other types of area networks:*** While LAN and WAN are by far the most popular network types mentioned, you may also commonly see references to these others:

- *Wireless local area network:* A LAN based on WiFi wireless network technology.
- *Metropolitan area network:* A network spanning a physical area larger than a LAN but smaller than a WAN, such as a city. A MAN is typically owned and operated by a single entity such as a government body or large corporation.
- *Campus area network:* A network spanning multiple LANs but smaller than a MAN, such as on a university or local business campus.
- *Storage area network:* Connects servers to data storage devices through a technology like Fibre Channel.
- *System area network:* Links high-performance computers with high-speed connections in a cluster configuration. Also known as Cluster Area Network.

LAN, WAN and Home Networking: Residences typically employ one LAN and connect to the Internet WAN via an Internet Service Provider (ISP) using a broadband modem. The ISP provides a WAN IP address to the modem, and all of the computers on the home network use LAN (so-called private) IP addresses. All computers on the home LAN can communicate directly with each other but must go through a central gateway, typically a broadband router, to reach the ISP.

WHAT IS INTERNET?

The Internet is a computer network made up of thousands of networks worldwide. No one knows exactly how many computers are connected to the Internet. It is certain, however, that these number in the millions and are growing.

No one is in charge of the Internet. There are organizations which develop technical aspects of this network and set standards for creating applications on it, but no governing body is in control. The Internet backbone, through which Internet traffic flows, is owned by private companies.

All computers on the Internet communicate with one another using the Transmission Control Protocol / Internet Protocol suite, abbreviated to TCP / IP. Computers on the Internet use a client / server architecture. This means that the remote server machine provides files and services to the user's local client machine. Software can be installed on a client computer to take advantage of the latest access technology.

An Internet user has access to a wide variety of services: electronic mail, file transfer, vast information resources, interest group membership, interactive collaboration, multimedia displays, real-time broadcasting, breaking news, shopping opportunities and much more.

The Internet consists primarily of a variety of access protocols. Many of these protocols feature programs that allow users to search for and retrieve material made available by the protocol.

HISTORY OF INTERNET

The Internet was the result of some visionary thinking by people in the early 1960s who saw great potential value in allowing computers to share information on research and development in scientific and military fields. J.C.R. Licklider of MIT, first proposed a global network of computers in 1962, and moved over to the Defense Advanced Research Projects Agency (DARPA) in late 1962 to head the work to develop it. Leonard Kleinrock of MIT and later UCLA developed the theory of packet switching, which was to form the basis of Internet connections. Lawrence Roberts of MIT connected a Massachusetts computer with a California computer in 1965 over dial-up telephone lines. It showed the feasibility of wide area networking, but also showed that the telephone line's circuit switching was inadequate. Kleinrock's packet switching theory was confirmed. Roberts moved over to DARPA in 1966 and developed his plan for ARPANET. These visionaries and many more left unnamed here are the real founders of the Internet.

The Internet, then known as ARPANET, was brought online in 1969 under a contract let by the renamed Advanced Research Projects Agency (ARPA), which initially connected four major computers at universities in the southwestern US (UCLA, Stanford Research Institute, UCSB, and the University of Utah).

The Internet was designed in part to provide a communications network that would work even if some of the sites were destroyed by nuclear attack. If the most direct route was not available, routers would direct traffic around the network via alternate routes.

The early Internet was used by computer experts, engineers, scientists and librarians. There was nothing friendly about it. There were no home or office personal computers in those days, and anyone who used it, whether a computer professional or an engineer or scientist or librarian, had to learn to use a very complex system. e-mail was adapted for ARPANET by Ray Tomlinson of BBN in 1972. He picked the @ symbol from the available symbols on his teletype to link the username and address.

As the commands for e-mail, FTP, and telnet were standardized, it became a lot easier for non-technical people to learn to use the nets. It was not easy by today's standards by any means, but it did open up use of the Internet to many more people in universities in particular. Other departments besides the libraries, computer, physics, and engineering departments found ways to make good use of the nets—to communicate with colleagues around the world and to share files and resources.

Since the Internet was initially funded by the government, it was originally limited to research, education, and government uses. Commercial uses were prohibited unless they directly served the goals of research and education. This policy continued until the early 90's, when independent commercial networks began to grow. It then became possible to route traffic across the country from one commercial site to another without passing through the government funded NSFNet Internet backbone.

Delphi was the first national commercial online service to offer Internet access to its subscribers. It opened up an e-mail connection in July 1992 and full Internet service in November 1992. Microsoft's full-scale entry into the browser, server, and Internet Service Provider market completed the major shift over to a commercially based Internet.

ADVANTAGES OF INTERNET

1. ***Communication:*** The foremost target of Internet has always been the communication and Internet has excelled beyond the expectations. Still innovations are going on to make it faster, more reliable. By the advent of computer's Internet, our earth has reduced and has attained the form of a global village. Now we can communicate in a fraction of second with a person who is sitting in the other part of the world. Today for better communication, we can avail the facilities of e-mail; we can chat for hours with our loved ones. There are plenty messenger services in offering. With the help of such services, it has become very easy to establish a kind of global friendship where you can share your thoughts, can explore other cultures of different ethnicity.

2. ***Information:*** Information is probably the biggest advantage Internet is offering. The Internet is a virtual treasure trove of information. Any kind of information on any topic under the sun is available on the Internet. The search engines like Google, Yahoo is at your service on the Internet. You can almost find any type of data on almost any kind of subject that you are looking for. There is a huge amount of information available on the Internet for just about every subject known to man, ranging from government law and services, trade fairs and conferences, market information, new ideas and technical support, the list is endless. Students and children are among the top users who surf the Internet for research. Today, it is almost required that students should use the Internet for research for the purpose of gathering resources. Teachers have started giving assignments that require research on the Internet. Almost every coming day, researches on medical issues become much easier to locate. Numerous websites available on the net are offering loads of information for people to research diseases and talk to doctors online at sites such as America's Doctor.

3. ***Entertainment:*** Entertainment is another popular reason why many people prefer to surf the Internet. In fact, medium of Internet has become quite successful in trapping multifaceted entertainment factor. Downloading games, visiting chat rooms or just surfing the web are some of the uses people have discovered. There are numerous games that may be downloaded from the Internet for free. The industry of online gaming has tasted dramatic and phenomenal attention by game lovers. Chat rooms are popular because users can meet new and interesting people. In fact, the Internet has been successfully used by people to find lifelong partners. When people surf the web, there are numerous things that can be found. Music, hobbies, news and more can be found and shared on the Internet.

4. ***Services:*** Many services are now provided on the Internet such as online banking, job seeking, purchasing tickets for your favorite movies, guidance services on array of topics engulfing the every aspect of life, and hotel reservations. Often these services are not available off-line and can cost you more.

5. ***e-Commerce:*** e-Commerce is the concept used for any type of commercial manufacturing or business deals that involves the transfer of information across the globe via Internet. It has become a phenomenon associated with any kind of shopping, almost anything. You name it and E-commerce with its giant tentacles engulfing every single product and service will make you available at your doorsteps. It has got a real amazing and wide range of products from household needs, technology to entertainment.

DISADVANTAGES OF INTERNET

1. ***Theft of personal information:*** If you use the Internet, you may be facing grave danger as your personal information such as name, address, credit card number, etc. can be accessed by other culprits to make your problems worse.

2. ***Spamming:*** Spamming refers to sending unwanted e-mails in bulk, which provide no purpose and needlessly obstruct the entire system. Such illegal activities can be very frustrating for you, and so instead of just ignoring it, you should make an effort to try and stop these activities so that using the Internet can become that much safer.

3. ***Virus threat:*** Virus is nothing but a program, which disrupts the normal functioning of your computer systems. Computers attached to Internet are more prone to virus attacks and they can end up into crashing your whole hard disk.

4. ***Pornography:*** This is perhaps the biggest threat related to your children's healthy mental life. A very serious issue concerning the Internet. There are thousands of pornographic sites on the Internet that can be easily found and can be a detrimental factor to letting children use the Internet. Though, Internet can also create havoc, destruction and its misuse can be very fatal, the advantages of it outweigh its disadvantages.

USES OF INTERNET

1. ***e-Mail:*** The concept of sending electronic text messages between parties in a way analogous to mailing letters or memos predates the creation of the Internet. Even today it can be

important to distinguish between Internet and internal e-mail systems. Internet e-mail may travel and be stored unencrypted on many other networks and machines out of both the sender's and the recipient's control. During this time it is quite possible for the content to be read and even tampered with by third parties, if anyone considers it important enough. Purely internal or intranet mail systems, where the information never leaves the corporate or organization's network, are much more secure, although in any organization there will be IT and other personnel whose job may involve monitoring, and occasionally accessing, the e-mail of other employees not addressed to them.

2. ***Chat and instant messaging:*** Chat programs allow users on the Internet to communicate with each other by typing in real time. They are sometimes included as a feature of a website, where users can log into the "chat room" to exchange comments and information about the topics addressed on the site. Chat may take other, more wide-ranging forms. For example, America Online is well known for sponsoring a number of topical chat rooms. Internet Relay Chat (IRC) is a service through which participants can communicate to each other on hundreds of channels. These channels are usually based on specific topics. While many topics are frivolous, substantive conversations are also taking place. To access IRC, you must use an IRC software program.

Instant messaging offers real-time communication and allows easy collaboration, which might be considered more akin to genuine conversation than e-mail's "letter" format. In contrast to e-mail, the parties know whether the peer is available. Most systems allow the user to set an online status or away message so peers are notified when the user is available, busy, or away from the computer. On the other hand, people are not forced to reply immediately to incoming messages. For this reason, some people consider communication via instant messaging to be less intrusive than communication via phone.

3. ***Internet fax:*** Internet fax uses the Internet to receive and send faxes. Internet fax achieves a dramatic reduction in communication costs, especially when long faxes are frequently

exchanged with overseas or distant offices. Since there is no telephone connection charge when sending a fax over the Internet, the cost of sending faxes is covered entirely by the fixed line Internet connection fee. The recipient machine must also be compatible with Internet fax.

4. ***The World Wide Web:*** Through keyword-driven Internet research using search engines, like Yahoo! and Google, millions of people worldwide have easy, instant access to a vast and diverse amount of online information. Compared to encyclopedias and traditional libraries, the World Wide Web has enabled a sudden and extreme decentralization of information and data. It is also easier, using the web, than ever before for individuals and organisations to publish ideas and information to an extremely large audience.

Collections of personal web pages published by large service providers remain popular, and have become increasingly sophisticated. Whereas operations such as Angelfire and GeoCities have existed since the early days of the web, newer offerings from, for example, Facebook and MySpace currently have large followings. These operations often brand themselves as social network services rather than simply as web page hosts. Advertising on popular web pages can be lucrative, and e-commerce or the sale of products and services directly via the web continues to grow.

5. ***Remote access:*** The Internet allows computer users to connect to other computers and information stores easily, wherever they may be across the world. They may do this with or without the use of security, authentication and encryption technologies, depending on the requirements. This is encouraging new ways of working from home, collaboration and information sharing in many industries.

6. ***Collaboration:*** The low cost and nearly instantaneous sharing of ideas, knowledge, and skills has made collaborative work dramatically easier. Not only can a group cheaply communicate and test, but the wide reach of the Internet allows such groups to easily form in the first place, even among niche interests. An example of this is the free software movement in software development which produced GNU and Linux from

scratch and has taken over development of Mozilla and OpenOffice.org (formerly known as Netscape Communicator and StarOffice).

7. ***File sharing:*** A computer file can be e-mailed to customers, colleagues and friends as an attachment. It can be uploaded to a website or FTP server for easy download by others. It can be put into a "shared location" or onto a file server for instant use by colleagues. The load of bulk downloads to many users can be eased by the use of "mirror" servers or peer-to-peer networks.

8. ***Voice telephony:*** Voice over Internet Protocol (VoIP) is a protocol optimized for the transmission of voice through the Internet or other packet switched networks. VoIP is often used abstractly to refer to the actual transmission of voice (rather than the protocol implementing it). Thus VoIP is maturing into a viable alternative to traditional telephones. Interoperability between different providers has improved and the ability to call or receive a call from a traditional telephone is available. Simple inexpensive VoIP modems are now available that eliminate the need for a PC.

9. ***Streaming media:*** An Internet-connected device, such as a computer or something more specific, can be used to access online media in much the same way as was previously possible only with a television or radio receiver. Webcams can be seen as an even lower-budget extension of this phenomenon. Video chat rooms, video conferencing and remote controllable webcams are also popular.

HOW DOES INTERNET WORK?

The Internet is a worldwide network that adheres to specific methods of data transfer in order to establish a standardized communication highway. Anyone with access can send and receive information over the Internet by using Internet-enabled software, which understands the online protocols or language of the Internet.

The backbone of the Internet consists of a powerful set of telephone lines including T3 lines, capable of transferring data at a very fast rate of about 45 megabytes per second. The lines link metropolitan cities and include national access points or feeds. If you imagine a geographic map, there are equivalent major highways, explaining why the Internet is often referred to as the Information Superhighway.

The backbone of the Internet is operated and maintained by various companies and organizations working cooperatively without centralized ownership. Redundancy is built into the backbone of the Internet so that if one or more major lines go down, traffic can be rerouted, much like a traffic detour when a highway is temporarily under construction. While this might slow Internet traffic, it will not 'break' the Internet.

While T3 lines provide the backbone for the Internet, smaller tributaries provide local support by establishing dedicated lines that link into the Internet's backbone at national access points. Revisiting the map analogy, these can be equated with boulevards and major streets that lead to freeways. These secondary lines are leased and maintained by various Internet Service Provider (ISP) co-ops using routers to direct traffic.

Every computer connected to the Internet is assigned a unique Internet Protocol (IP) address. When you point-and-click on a link, your browser sends out a request that is addressed to the website that houses the content you want. Routers along the way read the data packet's address and relay it along the best route available.

When the data packet arrives at the website, the server reads the request and sends the requested page back to your computer via a return address in the data packet: this is your computer's IP address. The data packet is routed back to you (in actuality, several data packets) and your browser interprets the content and displays the page for you.

THE WORLD WIDE WEB

The World Wide Web is a set of programs, standards and protocols that allows the multimedia and hypertext files to be created, displasyed and linked on the Internet. The World Wide Web is a system of interlinked, hypertext documents accessed via the Internet. With a web browser, a user views web pages that may contain text, images, videos, and other multimedia and navigates between them using hyperlinks. The World Wide Web was created in 1989 by Sir Tim Berners-Lee, working at CERN in Geneva, Switzerland. Since then, Berners-Lee has played an active role in guiding the development of web standards (such as the markup languages in which Web pages are composed), and in recent years has advocated his vision of a semantic web. The World Wide Web is often abbreviated as the web or WWW.

The World Wide Web is a system of Internet servers that supports hypertext to access several Internet protocols on a single interface. Almost every protocol type available on the Internet is accessible on the web. This includes e-mail, FTP, Telnet, and Usenet News. In addition to these, the World Wide Web has its own protocol: HyperText Transfer Protocol or HTTP.

The World Wide Web provides a single interface for accessing all these protocols. This creates a convenient and user-friendly environment. It is not necessary to be conversant in these protocols within separate, command-level environments, as was typical in the early days of the Internet. The web gathers together these protocols into a single system. Because of this feature, and because of the web's ability to work with multimedia and advanced programming languages, the web is the most popular component of the Internet.

The operation of the web relies primarily on hypertext as its means of information retrieval. HyperText is a document containing words that connect to other documents. These words are called links and are selectable by the user. A single hypertext document can contain links to many documents. In the context of the web, words or graphics may serve as links to other documents, images, video, and sound. Links may or may not follow a logical path, as each connection is programmed by the creator of the source document. Overall, the web contains a complex virtual web of connections among a vast number of documents, graphics, videos, and sounds.

Producing hypertext for the web is accomplished by creating documents with a language called HyperText Markup

Language, or HTML. With HTML, tags are placed within the text to accomplish document formatting, visual features such as font size, italics and bold, and the creation of hypertext links. Graphics and multimedia may also be incorporated into an HTML document.

HTML is an evolving language, with new tags being added as each upgrade of the language is developed and released. For example, visual formatting features are now often separated from the HTML document and placed into Cascading Style Sheets (CSS). This has several advantages, including the fact that an external style sheet can centrally control the formatting of multiple documents. The World Wide Web Consortium (W3C), led by web founder Tim Berners-Lee, coordinates the efforts of standardizing HTML. The W3C now calls the language XHTML and considers it to be an application of the XML language standard.

The World Wide Web consists of files, called pages or home pages, containing links to documents and resources throughout the Internet. The web provides a vast array of experiences including multimedia presentations, real-time collaboration, interactive pages, radio and television broadcasts, and the automatic "push" of information to a client computer or to an RSS reader. Programming languages such as Java, JavaScript, Visual Basic, Cold Fusion and XML extend the capabilities of the web. Much information on the web is served dynamically from content stored in databases. The web is, therefore, not a fixed entity, but one that is in a constant state of development and flux.

Access to web pages may be accomplished by:

1. Entering an Internet address and retrieving a page directly.
2. Browsing through pages and selecting links to move from one page to another.
3. Searching through subject directories linked to organized collections of web pages.
4. Entering a search statement at a search engine to retrieve pages on the topic of your choice.

Viewing a web page on the World Wide Web normally begins either by typing the URL of the page into a web browser, or by following a hyperlink to that page or resource. The web browser then initiates a series of communication messages, behind the scenes, in order to fetch and display it.

First, the server-name portion of the URL is resolved into an IP address using the global, distributed Internet database known as the domain name system, or DNS. This IP address is necessary to contact and send data packets to the web server.

The browser then requests the resource by sending an HTTP request to the web server at that particular address. In the case of a typical web page, the HTML text of the page is requested first and parsed immediately by the web browser, which will then make additional requests for images and any other files that form a part of the page. Statistics measuring a website's popularity are usually based on the number of 'page views' or associated server 'hits', or file requests, which take place.

Having received the required files from the web server, the browser then renders the page onto the screen as specified by its HTML, CSS, and other web languages. Any images and other resources are incorporated to produce the on-screen web page that the user sees.

Most web pages will themselves contain hyperlinks to other related pages and perhaps to downloads, source documents, definitions and other web resources. Such a collection of useful, related resources, interconnected via hypertext links, is what was dubbed a "web" of information.

HYPERTEXT MARKUP LANGUAGE

HTML (Hypertext Markup Language) is the predominant markup language for web pages. It provides a means to describe the structure of text-based information in a document by denoting certain text as headings, paragraphs, lists, and so on and to supplement that text with interactive forms, embedded images, and other objects. HTML is written in the form of labels (known as tags or elements), surrounded by angle brackets. HTML can also describe, to some degree, the appearance and semantics of a document, and can include embedded scripting language code which can affect the behavior of web browsers and other HTML processors. HTML is a language to specify the structure of documents for retrieval across the Internet using browser programs of the World Wide Web.

- HTML stands for Hyper Text Markup Language.
- An HTML file is a text file containing small markup tags.
- The markup tags tell the web browser how to display the page.
- An HTML file must have an htm or html file extension.
- An HTML file can be created using a simple text editor.

File extension	.html, .htm
MIME type:	text/html
Type code:	TEXT
Uniform Type Identifier:	public.html
Developed by:	World Wide Web Consortium
Type of format:	Markup language
Extended from:	SGML
Extended to:	XHTML
Standard(s):	W3C HTML 4.01
	W3C HTML 3.2

If you are running windows, start Notepad or if you are on a Mac, start SimpleText. In OSX start TextEdit and change the following preferences: Open the "Format" menu and select "Plain text" instead of "Rich text". Then open the "Preferences" window under the "Text Edit" menu and select "Ignore rich text commands in HTML files". Your HTML code will probably not work if you do not change the preferences above.

Type in the following text:

```
<html>
<head>
<title> Title of page </title>
```

```
</head>
<body>
This is my first homepage. <b> This text is bold </b>
</body>
</html>
```

Save the file as "mypage.htm". Start your Internet browser. Select "Open" (or "Open Page") in the File menu of your browser. A dialog box will appear. Select "Browse" (or "Choose File") and locate the HTML file you just created - "mypage.htm" - select it and click "Open". Now you should see an address in the dialog box, for example "C:\MyDocuments\mypage.htm". Click OK, and the browser will display the page.

HTML Elements

- Each HTML element has an element name (body, h1, p, br).
- The start tag is the name surrounded by angle brackets: <h1>.
- The end tag is a slash and the name surrounded by angle brackets </h1> .
- The element content occurs between the start tag and the end tag.
- Some HTML elements have no content.
- Some HTML elements have no end tag.

Remember the HTML example from the previous page:

```
<html>
<head>
<title> Title of page </title>
</head>
<body>
This is my first homepage. <b> This text is bold </b>
</body>
</html>
```

This is an HTML element:

<b> This text is bold </b>

The HTML element starts with a start tag: <b>

The content of the HTML element is: This text is bold

The HTML element ends with an end tag: </b>. The purpose of the <b> tag is to define an HTML element that should be displayed as bold.

This is also an HTML element:

<body>

This is my first homepage. <b>This text is bold</b>

</body>

This HTML element starts with the start tag <body>, and ends with the end tag </body>. The purpose of the <body> tag is to define the HTML element that contains the body of the HTML document.

Basic HTML Tags

The most important tags in HTML are tags that define headings, paragraphs and line breaks.

- HTML tags are used to mark-up HTML elements.
- HTML tags are surrounded by the two characters < and >.
- The surrounding characters are called angle brackets.
- HTML tags normally come in pairs like <b> and </b>.
- The first tag in a pair is the start tag, the second tag is the end tag.
- The text between the start and end tags is the element content.
- HTML tags are not case sensitive, <b> means the same as <B>.

a. ***Headings:*** Headings are defined with the <h1> to <h6> tags. <h1> defines the largest heading. <h6> defines the smallest heading.

<h1> This is a heading </h1>

<h2> This is a heading </h2>

<h3> This is a heading </h3>

<h4> This is a heading </h4>

<h5> This is a heading </h5>

<h6> This is a heading </h6>

HTML automatically adds an extra blank line before and after a heading.

b. ***Paragraphs:*** Paragraphs are defined with the <p> tag.

<p> This is a paragraph </p>

<p> This is another paragraph </p>

HTML automatically adds an extra blank line before and after a paragraph.

c. ***Line breaks:*** The <br> tag is used when you want to break a line, but do not want to start a new paragraph. The <br> tag forces a line break wherever you place it.

<p> This <br> is a para <br> graph with line breaks </p>

HTML Standard Attributes

HTML tags can have attributes. The special attributes for each tag are listed under each tag description. The attributes listed here are the core and language attributes that are standard for all tags (with a few exceptions):

a. ***Core attributes:*** Not valid in base, head, html, meta, param, script, style, and title elements. These are given in Table 8.1.

Table 8.1: Core attributes

Attribute	*Value*	*Description*
class	class_rule or style_rule	The class of the element
id	id_name	A unique id for the element
style	style_definition	An inline style definition
title	tooltip_text	A text to display in a tool tip

b. ***Language attributes:*** Not valid in base, br, frame, frameset, hr, iframe, param, and script elements. These are given in Table 8.2.

Table 8.2: Language attributes

Attribute	*Value*	*Description*
dir	ltr | rtl	Sets the text direction
lang	language_code	Sets the language code

c. ***Keyboard attributes:*** These are described in Table 8.3.

Table 8.3: Keyboard attributes

Attribute	*Value*	*Description*
accesskey	character	Sets a keyboard shortcut to access an element
tabindex	number	Sets the tab order of an element

HTML Text Formatting

HTML defines a lot of elements for formatting output, like bold or italic text (Tables 8.4 to 8.6).

Table 8.4: Text formatting tags

Tag	*Description*
<b>	Defines bold text
<big>	Defines big text
<em>	Defines emphasized text
<i>	Defines italic text
<small>	Defines small text
<strong>	Defines strong text
<sub>	Defines subscripted text
<sup>	Defines superscripted text
<ins>	Defines inserted text
<del>	Defines deleted text
<s>	Deprecated. Use <del> instead
<strike>	Deprecated. Use <del> instead
<u>	Deprecated. Use styles instead

Table 8.5: Computer output tags

Tag	*Description*
<code>	Defines computer code text
<kbd>	Defines keyboard text
<samp>	Defines sample computer code
<tt>	Defines teletype text
<var>	Defines a variable
<pre>	Defines preformatted text
<listing>	Deprecated. Use <pre> instead
<plaintext>	Deprecated. Use <pre> instead
<xmp>	Deprecated. Use <pre> instead

Table 8.6: Citations, quotations and definition tags

Tag	*Description*
<abbr>	Defines an abbreviation
<acronym>	Defines an acronym
<address>	Defines an address element
<bdo>	Defines the text direction
<blockquote>	Defines a long quotation
<q>	Defines a short quotation
<cite>	Defines a citation
<dfn>	Defines a definition term

HTML Character Entities

Some characters like the < character, have a special meaning in HTML, and therefore, cannot be used in the text. To display a less than sign (<) in HTML, we have to use a character entity. Some characters have a special meaning in HTML, like the less than sign (<) that defines the start of an HTML tag. If we want the browser to actually display these characters we must insert character entities in the HTML source. A character entity has three parts: an ampersand (and), an entity name or a # and an entity number, and finally a semicolon (;) as shown in Table 8.7.

Table 8.7: Commonly used character entities

Result	*Description*	*Entity name*	*Entity number*
	non-breaking space		and#160;
<	less than	<	and#60;
>	greater than	>	and#62;
and	ampersand	&	and#38;
"	quotation mark	"	and#34;
'	apostrophe	' (does not work in IE)	and#39;
¢	cent	¢	and#162;
£	pound	£	and#163;
¥	yen	¥	and#165;
•	euro	€	and#8364;
§	section	§	and#167;
©	oopyright	©	and#169;
®	registered trademark	®	and#174;
×	multiplication	×	and#215;
÷	division	÷	and#247;

To display a less than sign in an HTML document we must write: < or and#60; The advantage of using a name instead of a number is that a name is easier to remember. The disadvantage is that not all browsers support the newest entity names, while the support for entity numbers is very good in almost all browsers. The most common character entity in HTML is the non-breaking space.

HTML Links

a. *Anchor tag and Href attribute:* HTML uses the <a> (anchor) tag to create a link to another document. An anchor can point to any resource on the web: an HTML page, an image, a sound file, a movie, etc.

The syntax of creating an anchor:

<a href="url"> Text to be displayed </a>

The <a> tag is used to create an anchor to link from, the href attribute is used to address the document to link to, and the words between the open and close of the anchor tag will be displayed as a hyperlink.

For example, this anchor defines a link to W3Schools:

<a href="http://www.w3schools.com/">Visit W3Schools!</a>

Named anchors are often used to create "table of contents" at the beginning of a large document. Each chapter within the document is given a named anchor, and links to each of these anchors are put at the top of the document.

b. ***Target attribute:*** With the target attribute, you can define where the linked document will be opened. The line below will open the document in a new browser window:
<a href="http://www.w3schools.com/"
target="_blank">Visit W3Schools!</a>

c. ***Anchor tag and name attribute:*** The name attribute is used to create a named anchor. When using named anchors we can create links that can jump directly into a specific section on a page, instead of letting the user scroll around to find what he/she is looking for. Below is the syntax of a named anchor:
<a name="label">Text to be displayed</a>

The name attribute is used to create a named anchor. The name of the anchor can be any text you care to use. The line below defines a named anchor:

<a name="tips">Useful Tips Section</a>

To link directly to the "tips" section, add a # sign and the name of the anchor to the end of a URL, like this:

<a href="http://www.w3schools.com/html_links.asp#tips">
Jump to the Useful Tips Section</a>

HTML Frames

With frames, you can display more than one web page in the same browser window.

With frames, you can display more than one HTML document in the same browser window. Each HTML document is called a frame, and each frame is independent of the others.

The disadvantages of using frames are:

- The web developer must keep track of more HTML documents.
- It is difficult to print the entire page.

a. The frameset tag:

- The <frameset> tag defines how to divide the window into frames
- Each frameset defines a set of rows or columns
- The values of the rows/columns indicate the amount of screen area each row/column will occupy.

b. ***The frame tag:*** The <frame> tag defines what HTML document to put into each frame. In the example below we have a frameset with two columns. The first column is set to 25% of the width of the browser window. The second column is set to 75% of the width of the browser window. The HTML document "frame_a.htm" is put into the first column, and the HTML document "frame_b.htm" is put into the second column:

```
<frameset cols="25%,75%">
 <frame src="frame_a.htm">
 <frame src="frame_b.htm">
</frameset>
```

HTML Tables

Tables are defined with the <table> tag. A table is divided into rows (with the <tr> tag), and each row is divided into data cells (with the <td> tag). The letters td stand for "table data," which is the content of a data cell. A data cell can contain text, images, lists, paragraphs, forms, horizontal rules, tables, etc (Table 8.8).

```
<table border="1">
<tr>
<td>row 1, cell 1</td>
<td>row 1, cell 2</td>
</tr>
```

```
<tr>
<td>row 2, cell 1</td>
<td>row 2, cell 2</td>
</tr>
</table>
```

a. ***Tables and border attribute:*** To display a table with borders, you will have to use the border attribute.

```
<table border="1">
<tr>
<td>Row 1, cell 1</td>
<td>Row 1, cell 2</td>
</tr>
</table>
```

b. ***Headings in a table:*** Headings in a table are defined with the <th> tag.

```
<table border="1">
<tr>
<th>Heading</th>
<th>Another heading</th>
</tr>
<tr>
<td>row 1, cell 1</td>
<td>row 1, cell 2</td>
</tr>
<tr>
<td>row 2, cell 1</td>
<td>row 2, cell 2</td>
</tr>
</table>
```

c. ***Empty cells in a table:*** Table cells with no content are not displayed very well in most browsers.

```
<table border="1">
<tr>
<td>row 1, cell 1</td>
<td>row 1, cell 2</td>
</tr>
<tr>
<td>row 2, cell 1</td>
<td></td>
</tr>
</table>
```

The borders around the empty table cell are missing. To avoid this, add a non-breaking space to empty data cells, to make the borders visible:

```
<table border="1">
<tr>
<td>row 1, cell 1</td>
<td>row 1, cell 2</td>
</tr>
<tr>
<td>row 2, cell 1</td>
<td> </td>
</tr>
</table>
```

HTML Lists

HTML supports ordered, unordered and definition lists.

a. ***Unordered lists:*** An unordered list is a list of items. The list items are marked with bullets (typically small black circles). An unordered list starts with the <ul> tag. Each list item starts with the <li> tag.

```
<ul>
<li>Coffee</li>
<li>Milk</li>
</ul>
```

Table 8.8: Table tags

Tag	*Description*
<table>	Defines a table
<th>	Defines a table header
<tr>	Defines a table row
<td>	Defines a table cell
<caption>	Defines a table caption
<colgroup>	Defines groups of table columns
<col>	Defines the attribute values for one or more columns in a table
<thead>	Defines a table head
<tbody>	Defines a table body
<tfoot>	Defines a table footer

b. ***Ordered lists:*** An ordered list is also a list of items. The list items are marked with numbers. An ordered list starts with the <ol> tag. Each list item starts with the <li> tag.

```
<ol>
<li>Coffee</li>
<li>Milk</li>
</ol>
```

c. ***Definition lists:*** A definition list is not a list of items. This is a list of terms and explanation of the terms. A definition list starts with the <dl> tag. Each definition-list term starts with the <dt> tag. Each definition-list definition starts with the <dd> tag.

```
<dl>
<dt>Coffee</dt>
<dd>Black hot drink</dd>
<dt>Milk</dt>
<dd>White cold drink</dd>
</dl>
```

HTML Forms and Input

HTML forms are used to select different kinds of user input.

a. ***Forms:*** A form is an area that can contain form elements. Form elements are elements that allow the user to enter information (like text fields, textarea fields, drop-down menus, radio buttons, checkboxes, etc.) in a form. A form is defined with the <form> tag.

```
<form>
<input>
<input>
</form>
```

b. ***Input:*** The most used form tag is the <input> tag. The type of input is specified with the type attribute. The most commonly used input types are explained below.

i. *Text fields:* Text fields are used when you want the user to type letters, numbers, etc. in a form.

```
<form>
First name:
<input type="text" name="firstname">
<br>
Last name:
<input type="text" name="lastname">
</form>
```

How it looks in a browser:

First name:

Last name:

ii. *Radio buttons:* Radio buttons are used when you want the user to select one of a limited number of choices.

```
<form>
<input type="radio" name="sex" value="male"> Male
<br>
<input type="radio" name="sex" value="female"> Female
</form>
```

How it looks in a browser:

Male

Female

iii. *Checkboxes:* Checkboxes are used when you want the user to select one or more options of a limited number of choices.

```
<form>
I have a bike:
<input type="checkbox" name="vehicle" value="Bike">
<br>
I have a car:
<input type="checkbox" name="vehicle" value="Car">
<br>
I have an airplane:
<input type="checkbox" name="vehicle" value="Airplane">
</form>
```

How it looks in a browser:

I have a bike:

I have a car:

I have an airplane:

iv. Form's action attribute and submit button: When the user clicks on the "Submit" button, the content of the form is sent to another file. The form's action attribute defines the name of the file to send the content to. The file defined in the action attribute usually does something with the received input.

```
<form name="input" action="html_form_action.asp"
method="get">
Username:
<input type="text" name="user">
<input type="submit" value="Submit">
</form>
```

How it looks in a browser:

Username:

HTML Images

With HTML you can display images in a document.

a. ***Image tag and src attribute:*** In HTML, images are defined with the <img> tag. The <img> tag is empty, which means that it contains attributes only and it has no closing tag. To display an image on a page, you need to use the src attribute. Src stands for "source". The value of the src attribute is the URL of the image you want to display on your page.

The syntax of defining an image:

<img src="url">

The URL points to the location where the image is stored. An image named "boat.gif" located in the directory "images" on "www.w3schools.com" has the URL: http://www.w3schools.com/images/boat.gif. The browser puts the image where the image tag occurs in the document. If you put an image tag between two paragraphs, the browser shows the first paragraph, then the image, and then the second paragraph.

b. ***Alt attribute:*** The alt attribute is used to define an "alternate text" for an image. The value of the alt attribute is an author-defined text:

<img src="boat.gif" alt="Big Boat">

The "alt" attribute tells the reader what he or she is missing on a page if the browser cannot load images. The browser will then display the alternate text instead of the image. It is a good practice to include the "alt" attribute for each image on a page, to improve the display and usefulness of your document for people who have text-only browsers.

HTML Backgrounds

The <body> tag has two attributes where you can specify backgrounds. The background can be a color or an image.

a. ***Bgcolor:*** The bgcolor attribute specifies a background-color for an HTML page. The value of this attribute can be a hexadecimal number, an RGB value, or a color name:

<body bgcolor="#000000">

<body bgcolor="rgb(0,0,0)">

<body bgcolor="black">

The lines above all set the background-color to black.

b. ***Background:*** The background attribute specifies a background-image for an HTML page. The value of this attribute is the URL of the image you want to use. If the image is smaller than the browser window, the image will repeat itself until it fills the entire browser window.

<body background="clouds.gif">

<body background="http://www.w3schools.com/clouds.gif">

HTML Colors

Colors are displayed combining red, green, and blue light sources.

a. ***Color values:*** HTML colors can be defined as a hexadecimal notation for the combination of red, green, and blue color values (RGB). The lowest value that can be given to one light source is 0 (hex #00) and the highest value is 255 (hex #FF).

   The combination of red, green and blue values from 0 to 255 gives a total of more than 16 million different colors to play with (256 × 256 × 256). Most modern monitors are capable of displaying at least 16384 different colors.

b. ***W3C standard color names:*** W3C has listed 16 color names that will validate with an HTML validator. The color names are: aqua, black, blue, fuchsia, gray, green, lime, maroon, navy, olive, purple, red, silver, teal, white and yellow.

c. ***Cross-browser color names:*** A collection of nearly 150 color names are supported by all major browsers.

d. ***Cross-browser color values:*** Some years ago, when most computers only supported 256 different colors, a list of 216 web safe colors was suggested as a web standard. The reason for this was that the Microsoft and Mac operating system used 40 different "reserved" fixed system colors (about 20 each).

We are not sure how important this is now, since most computers today have the ability to display millions of different colors, but the choice is left to you. The 216 cross-browser color palette was created to ensure that all computers would display the colors correctly when running a 256 color palette:

HTML Links

When you click on a link in an HTML document like this: Last Page, an underlying <a> tag points to a place (an address) on the web with an href attribute value like this: <a href="lastpage.htm">Last Page</a>.

a. ***Uniform resource locators:*** A uniform resource locator (URL) is used to address a document (or other data) on the World Wide Web. A full web address like this: http://www.w3schools.com/html/lastpage.htm follows these syntax rules:

scheme://host.domain:port/path/filename

- The scheme is defining the type of Internet service. The most common type is http.
- The domain is defining the Internet domain name like w3schools.com.
- The host is defining the domain host. If omitted, the default host for http is www.
- The port is defining the port number at the host. The port number is normally omitted. The default port number for http is 80.
- The path is defining a path (a sub directory) at the server. If the path is omitted, the resource (the document) must be located at the root directory of the website.
- The filename is defining the name of a document. The default filename might be default.asp, or index.html or something else depending on the settings of the web server.

Some examples of the most common schemes are given in Table 8.9.

Table 8.9: Examples of schemes

Schemes	*Access*
file	a file on your local PC
ftp	a file on an FTP server
http	a file on a World Wide Web server
gopher	a file on a Gopher server
news	a Usenet newsgroup
telnet	a Telnet connection
WAIS	a file on a WAIS server

b. ***Accessing a newsgroup:*** The following HTML code:

<a href="news:alt.html">HTML Newsgroup</a>

creates a link to a newsgroup like this HTML newsgroup

c. ***Downloading with FTP:*** The following HTML code:

<a href="ftp://www.w3schools.com/ftp/winzip.exe">Download WinZip</a>

creates a link to download a file like this: Download WinZip.

d. ***Link to your mail system:*** The following HTML code:

<a href="mailto:someone@w3schools.com">someone@w3schools.com</a>

creates a link to your own mail system like this: someone@w3schools.com

WEBSITES

A website is a collection of web pages, images, videos or other digital assets that is hosted on one or more web servers, usually accessible via the Internet. A web page is a document, typically written in (X)HTML, that is almost always accessible via HTTP, a protocol that transfers information from the web server to display in the user's web browser.

The pages of a website can usually be accessed from a common root URL called the homepage, and usually reside on the same physical server. The URLs of the pages organize them into a hierarchy, although the hyperlinks between them control how the reader perceives the overall structure and how the traffic flows between the different parts of the site.

Some websites require a subscription to access some or all of their content. Examples of subscription sites include many business sites, parts of many news sites, academic journal sites, gaming sites, message boards, web-based e-mail services, social networking websites, and sites providing real-time stock market data. Because they require authentication to view the content they are technically an Intranet site.

A website is hosted on a computer system known as a web server, also called an HTTP server, and these terms can also refer to the software that runs on these systems and that retrieves and delivers the web pages in response to requests from the website users. Apache is the most commonly used web server software (according to Netcraft statistics) and Microsoft's Internet Information Server (IIS) is also commonly used.

Website Styles

1. ***Static website:*** A static website is one that has web pages stored on the server in the same form as the user will view them. It is primarily coded in HTML (Hyper-text Markup Language).

A static website is also called a Classic website, a 5-page website or a Brochure website because it simply presents pre-defined information to the user. It may include information about a company and its products and services via text, photos, flash animation, audio/video and interactive menus and navigation.

2. ***Dynamic website:*** A dynamic website is one that does not have web pages stored on the server in the same form as the user will view them. Instead, the web page content changes automatically and/or frequently based on certain criteria. It generally collates information on the hop each time a page is requested.

A website can be dynamic in one of two ways. The first is that the web page code is constructed dynamically, piece by piece. The second is that the web page content displayed varies based on certain criteria. The criteria may be pre-defined rules or may be based on variable user input.

A dynamic website is also called a Web Application, a Data-driven website or an OCRAFT (Online Customer Request and Fulfillment Tools) website because it presents variable information that is tailored to a particular user. It may accept a user's input and respond to the request. For example, a user can enter text into a login form or keyword search, which prompts the website to fulfill the request and return a unique result. In addition, the user may be able to perform tasks that may alter the website itself, such as post a comment or update a user profile. Examples of task-based websites include, online banking, shopping, e-learning, and social networking. Furthermore, the website may be able to make instant decisions on the fly in various situations, such as online quiz scoring or credit card processing.

Types of Websites

There are many varieties of websites, each specializing in a particular type of content or use, and they may be arbitrarily classified in any number of ways. A few such classifications might include:

- ***Affiliate:*** Enabled portal that renders not only its custom CMS but also syndicated content from other content providers for an agreed fee. There are usually three relationship tiers: Affiliate agencies (e.g. Commission Junction), Advertisers (e.g. Ebay) and Consumer (e.g. Yahoo).
- ***Archive site:*** Used to preserve valuable electronic content threatened with extinction. Two examples are: Internet Archive, which since 1996 has preserved billions of old (and new) web pages; and Google Groups, which in early 2005 was archiving over 845,000,000 messages posted to Usenet news/discussion groups.
- ***Blog (or web log) site:*** Sites generally used to post online diaries which may include discussion forums (e.g. blogger, Xanga).

- ***Content site:*** Sites whose business is the creation and distribution of original content (e.g. Slate, About.com).
- ***Corporate website:*** Used to provide background information about a business, organization, or service.
- ***Commerce site (or e-commerce site):*** For purchasing goods, such as Amazon.com, CSN Stores, and Overstock.com.
- ***Community site:*** A site where persons with similar interests communicate with each other, usually by chat or message boards, such as MySpace.
- ***City site:*** A site that shows information about a certain city or town and events that take place in that town. Usually created by the city council or other "movers and shakers".
- ***Database site:*** A site whose main use is the search and display of a specific database's content such as the Internet Movie Database or the Political Graveyard.
- ***Dating site:*** A website where single people could find dates by using social networking like technologies.
- ***Development site:*** A site whose purpose is to provide information and resources related to software development, web design and the like.
- ***Directory site:*** A site that contains varied contents which are divided into categories and subcategories, such as Yahoo! directory, Google directory and Open Directory Project.
- ***Download site:*** Strictly used for downloading electronic content, such as software, game demos or computer wallpaper.
- ***Employment site:*** Allows employers to post job requirements for a position or positions and prospective employees to fill an application.
- ***Fan site:*** A website created and maintained by fans of and for a particular celebrity, as opposed to a website created, maintained, and controlled by a celebrity through their own paid webmaster. May also be known as a Shrine in the case of certain subjects, such as anime, and manga characters.
- ***Game site:*** A site that is itself a game or "playground" where many people come to play (e.g. MSN games and Pogo.com).

- Geodomain refers to domain names that are the same as those of geographic entities, such as cities and countries. For example, Richmond.com is the geodomain for Richmond, Virginia.
- ***Gripe site:*** A site devoted to the critique of a person, place, corporation, government, or institution.
- ***Humor site:*** Satirizes, parodies or otherwise exists solely to amuse.
- ***Information site:*** Contains content that is intended to inform visitors, but not necessarily for commercial purposes, such as: RateMyProfessors.com, Free Internet Lexicon and Encyclopedia. Most government, educational and non-profit institutions have an informational site.
- ***Java applet site:*** Contains software to run over the web as a web application.
- ***Mirror (computing) site:*** A complete reproduction of a website.
- ***News site:*** Similar to an information site, but dedicated to dispensing news and commentary.
- ***Personal homepage:*** Run by an individual or a small group (such as a family) that contains information or any content that the individual wishes to include. These are usually uploaded using a web hosting service such as Geocities.
- ***Political site:*** A site on which people may voice political views.
- ***Rating site:*** A site on which people can praise or disparage what is featured.
- ***Review site:*** A site on which people can post reviews for products or services.
- ***School site:*** A site on which teachers, students, or administrators can post information about current events at or involving their school. U.S. websites generally use k12 in the URL such as kearney.k12.mo.us.
- ***Video sharing:*** A site that enables user to upload videos, such as YouTube and Google Video.

- ***Search engine site:*** A site that provides general information and is intended as a gateway or lookup for other sites. A pure example is Google, and the most widely known extended type is Yahoo!.
- ***Warez:*** A site designed to host and let users download copyrighted materials illegally.
- ***Web portal:*** A site that provides a starting point or a gateway to other resources on the Internet or an intranet.
- ***Wiki site:*** A site which users collaboratively edit (such as Wikipedia and Wikihow).

WEB SERVER

It is a computer program that is responsible for accepting HTTP requests from web clients, which are known as web browsers, and serving them HTTP responses along with optional data contents, which usually are web pages such as HTML documents and linked objects (images, etc.).

The basic common features of web programs include:

1. ***HTTP:*** Every web server program operates by accepting HTTP requests from the client, and providing an HTTP response to the client. The HTTP response usually consists of an HTML document, but can also be a raw file, an image, or some other type of document (defined by MIME-types). If some error is found in client request or while trying to serve it, a web server has to send an error response which may include some custom HTML or text messages to better explain the problem to end users.
2. ***Logging:*** Usually web servers have also the capability of logging some detailed information, about client requests and server responses, to log files; this allows the webmaster to collect statistics by running log analyzers on log files.
3. ***Authentication:*** Optional authorization request (request of user name and password) before allowing access to some or all kinds of resources.
4. ***Content:*** Handling of static content (file content recorded in server's file systems) and dynamic content by supporting

one or more related interfaces (SSI, CGI, SCGI, FastCGI, JSP, PHP, ASP, ASP.NET, Server API such as NSAPI, ISAPI, etc.).

5. ***HTTPS support (by SSL or TLS):*** To allow secure (encrypted) connections to the server on the standard port 443 instead of usual port 80.
6. ***Content compression:*** By gzip encoding to reduce the size of the responses to lower bandwidth usage, etc.
7. ***Virtual hosting:*** To serve many websites using one IP address.
8. ***Large file support:*** To be able to serve files whose size is greater than 2 GB on 32 bit OS.
9. ***Bandwidth throttling:*** To limit the speed of responses in order to not saturate the network and to be able to serve more clients.

WEB SEARCH ENGINES (Table 8.10)

It is a program that searches documents for specified keywords and returns a list of the documents where the keywords were found. Search engines are the key to finding specific information on the vast expanse of the World Wide Web. Without sophisticated search engines, it would be virtually impossible to locate anything on the web without knowing a specific URL.

There are basically three types of search engines: (i) those that are powered by robots (called crawlers; ants or spiders), (ii) those that are powered by human submissions; and (iii) those that are a hybrid of the two.

- Crawler-based search engines are those that use automated software agents (called crawlers) that visit a website, read the information on the actual site, read the site's meta tags and also follows the links that the site connects to performing indexing on all linked websites as well. The crawler returns all that information back to a central depository, where the data is indexed. The crawler will periodically return to the sites to check for any information that has changed. The frequency with which this happens is determined by the administrators of the search engine.

- Human-powered search engines rely on humans to submit information that is subsequently indexed and catalogued. Only information that is submitted is put into the index.

A search engine works with the help of the following three elements:

1. ***Spiders or webcrawlers or bots or agents:*** The search engine uses software called spider or webcrawler or bot or agent, which comb the Internet looking for documents and their web addresses. The spiders or webcrawalers perform the methodical searches needed to find information. The bots or spiders are given direction by the search engine and they crawl from one server to another, compiling the huge lists of URLs given by search engine.
2. ***Indexing software and database:*** The lists of documents and web addresses collected by bots are sent to the indexing software. The indexing software extracts information from the document and web addresses, prepares on index of it and stores in a database. The kind of information indexed depends upon the particular search engine.

Table 8.10: Some popular search engines

Search engine	*URL*
AltaVista	http://www.altavista.com/
AOL Search	http://search.aol.com/
Complete Planet	http://www.completeplanet.com/
ICQ Search	http://search.icq.com/
Google	http://www.google.com/
Lycos	http://www-english.lycos.com/
MSN Search	http://search.msn.com/
Netscape Search	http://search.netscape.com/
Search the net	http://www.searchthe.net/
Virtual search engines	http://www.virtualfreesites.com/search.html
Web Search	http://www.web-search.com/
Webcrawler	http://www.webcrawler.com/
Yahoo!	http://www.yahoo.com/

3. ***Search algorithm:*** When you perform a search by entering keywords, the search engine software searches using a particular search method called search algorithm and then it displays the matching documents or web addresses.

Typically, a search engine works by sending out a spider to fetch as many documents as possible. Another program, called an indexer, then reads these documents and creates an index based on the words contained in each document. Each search engine uses a proprietary algorithm to create its indices such that, ideally, only meaningful results are returned for each query.

ELECTRONIC MAIL

Electronic mail, or e-mail, allows computer users locally and worldwide to exchange messages. Each user of e-mail has a mailbox address to which messages are sent. Messages sent through e-mail can arrive within a matter of seconds.

A powerful aspect of e-mail is the option to send electronic files to a person's e-mail address. Non-ASCII files, known as binary files, may be attached to e-mail messages. These files are referred to as MIME attachments. MIME stands for Multimedia Internet Mail Extension, and was developed to help e-mail software, handle a variety of file types. For example, a document created in Microsoft Word can be attached to an e-mail message and retrieved by the recipient with the appropriate e-mail program. Many e-mail programs offer the ability to read files written in HTML, which is itself a MIME type.

1. ***e-Mail systems:*** They are store-and-deliver software systems, which transport messages from one computer user to another. e-Mail systems range in scope and size from a local area network e-mail system which shuffles messages to users within an agency or office; to a wide area network e-mail system which carries messages to various users in various physical locations; to Internet e-mail which allows users with an Internet address to send and receive messages from other Internet users around the world.

2. ***e-Mail messages:*** They are text documents, which are created, stored, and delivered, in an electronic format. As such, e-mail messages are similar to other forms of communicated messages, such as correspondence, memoranda, and circular letters. e-Mail messages also contain features commonly associated with traditional record systems, including calendars, directories, distribution lists, and attachments such as word processing documents, spreadsheets, or images that are incorporated into an e-mail message.

3. ***e-Mail addresses:*** Each Internet domain has an associated e-mail server that manages all e-mail addresses at that domain. Each e-mail address is expressed in the form "name@domain" and is unique at that domain, as in for example rohit@twenty.net.

4. ***e-Mail client protocols:*** Your e-mail client application communicates with an e-mail server over the Internet to login, get mail status, and send and receive e-mail. The most common client connection protocols are:

- Post Office Protocol 3:
- Internet Message Application Protocol.
- Messaging Application Programming Interface.

5. ***e-Mail servers:*** e-Mail servers exchange e-mail with the Simple Mail Transfer Protocol (SMTP). Each Internet domain has a corresponding e-mail server. When you send e-mail, your client application first sends it to your e-mail server, which then contacts the addressee's e-mail server and carries out a conversation over the Internet according to the rules defined by SMTP. Your e-mail server asks the other e-mail server if the user name is valid, and, if it is, transfers the e-mail, where the receiving e-mail server stores it until the addressee logs on and downloads it. By far the most common SMTP server in use is the venerable sendmail system, first distributed for free with the Unix operating system.

6. ***e-Mail composition:*** The text of an e-mail is entered in the main body of the message. Remember that you can copy text from a document or another e-mail and paste it into a new e-mail, so you do not have to retype text. Many e-mail programs

will also let you paste pictures and documents directly into your message.

7. ***Sending e-Mail:*** You can send an e-mail in five basic actions:

   1. Press <ctrl>-n to create a new e-mail,
   2. Type the message,
   3. Enter the subject,
   4. Enter the addressee's e-mail address,
   5. Send.

8. ***Reading e-Mail:*** It is usually most convenient to sort your e-mail by the date received. You might also configure your client to automatically check for new e-mail. When you check your mail, your e-mail program connects to your e-mail provider's e-mail server over the Internet, often with the POP3 protocol, and downloads incoming mail and stores it in your e-mail application's Inbox. If your Inbox is not currently open, you can open it so you can see any new mail.

9. ***Replying to e-Mail:*** e-Mail replies are usually informal, and often brief. You can reply to an e-mail by selecting <ctrl>-r or the "reply" menu item. This action will do two useful things:

   a. Automatically transfer the person's e-mail address into the "To:" field.

   b. Automatically put a copy of the original e-mail in the reply e-mail, with a reply character such as ">" in front of each line (unless your client is configured not to do so).

10. ***Forwarding e-Mail:*** You can forward an e-mail to someone else, and forward all of your e-mail from one of your addresses to another. The forward function can usually be found under a menu item like "Message/Forward", or by right-clicking on an e-mail and then selecting "Forward" from the resulting pop-up menu. Many e-mail providers let you configure a setting to forward your messages direct from the mail server, so that your e-mail is forwarded as soon as it is received. You can also configure some e-mail program filters to automatically forward certain e-mail as soon immediately after they are downloaded.

11. ***Saving e-Mail:*** You can easily manage your e-mail volume if you set up a separate mailbox for each person you correspond

with. Your e-mail program should automatically save all outgoing e-mail in your Out mailbox. Do not bother trying to manage your sent mail–you can always sort the Out mailbox by the "To" field to organize it into sections ordered by the name of the people you sent to. You can also sort the Outbox by "Date" and scan the messages sent by hour, day, and week. Never take mail out of the Outbox and file it somewhere else unless you have a very good reason for doing so.

12. ***Sending e-Mail attachments:*** In most applications, you can attach any file on your computer to an e-mail with an "Attach" button, menu item, or by right-clicking on the e-mail, which brings up a standard file open window. Select the file you want to attach, double-click it or select the OK button, and you should see either a document icon or a header line indicating the file attached. Multiple attachments result in multiple icons (often at the end of the e-mail) or multiple header lines. The attached file(s) will then be transmitted to the recipient with the e-mail.

13. ***Filtering e-Mail:*** You can configure most e-mail applications to automatically filter incoming e-mail based on selected keywords in the message and take various useful actions. On most applications you can find this function under a menu item named "Filters", and on Microsoft Outlook under "Inbox assistant".

14. ***Deleting e-Mail:*** You can delete any e-mail that you really do not want, usually by selecting it and pressing the Del key.

e-COMMERCE

What is e-Commerce?

Electronic commerce (e-commerce) is the use of electronic communication to do business. It may be used to carry out business-to-business or business-to-consumer transactions. The real benefit of e-commerce is not that it makes old processes work better, but rather it provides a means to break with tradition and create new ways of doing business. For example, using the Internet will allow some businesses to remain small while building a larger turnover by reducing the cost of doing business.

Electronic Commerce (EC) is the paperless exchange of business information using Electronic Data Interchange (EDI) and related technologies. If you are familiar with Electronic Mail (e-Mail), computer bulletin boards, facsimile machines (faxes), Electronic Funds Transfer (EFT), you can very well understand what is e-commerce. These are all forms of EC. All EC systems replace all or key parts of paper-based work flow with faster, cheaper, more efficient, and more reliable communications between machines.

e-Commerce is a term for any type of business, or commercial transaction, that involves the transfer of information across the Internet. It covers a range of different types of businesses, from consumer-based retail sites, through auction or music sites, to business exchanges trading goods and services between corporations. It is currently one of the most important aspects of the Internet to emerge.

e-Commerce includes electronic trading, electronic messaging, electronic data interchange (EDI), electronic mail (e-mail), electronic catalogues, Internet, intranet and extranet services. The department has developed fact sheets that provide incisive information on how some leading Queensland small businesses have seized the opportunity and benefited from embracing the challenges and rewards of e-commerce.

e-Commerce is online commerce verses real-world commerce. e-Commerce includes retail shopping, banking, stocks and bonds trading, auctions, real estate transactions, airline booking, movie rentals-nearly anything you can imagine in the real world. Even personal services such as hair and nail salons can benefit from e-commerce by providing a website for the sale of related health and beauty products, normally available to local customers exclusively.

e-Commerce allows consumers to electronically exchange goods and services with no barriers of time or distance. Electronic commerce has expanded rapidly over the past five years and is predicted to continue at this rate, or even accelerate. In the near future the boundaries between "conventional" and "electronic" commerce will become increasingly blurred as more and more businesses move sections of their operations onto the Internet.

e-Commerce is referred to as a profitable business area by experts. A lot of businessmen get into e-commerce because it gives them a wider scope for conducting business with anyone and everyone around the globe.

The Internet is now a valuable communication tool, which offers small business a great opportunity to market itself internationally and reach a global client base. It is estimated that 81% of small businesses in Australia are connected to the Internet.

The best e-commerce solution is dependent on the type of data trading partners need to exchange to run their businesses effectively. It is important to focus on the business process rather than the technical issues such as hardware and software. Different e-commerce tools are suited to different business objectives and different trading partners.

According to experienced organizations, the introduction of e-commerce can potentially:

- Lower transaction costs
- Reduce inventory holdings
- Provide a competitive business advantage
- Expand one's market
- Increase speed to market
- Streamline supply chain management.

e-Commerce can provide the following benefits over non-electronic communication:

- ***Reduced costs:*** Reduced labour, reduced paper work, reduced errors in keying in data, etc.
- ***Reduced time:*** Shorter lead times, faster delivery of product.
- ***Flexibility with efficiency:*** The ability to handle complex situations, product ranges and customer profiles without the situation becoming unmanageable.
- ***Enhanced long-term trading partner relationships:*** Improved communication between trading partners leads to enhanced long-term relationships.

- ***Lock in customers***: The closer you are to your customer and the more you work with them to change from normal business practices to best practice e-commerce the harder it is for a competitor to upset your customer relationship.
- ***New markets:*** The Internet has the potential to expand your business into wider geographical locations. However, it is necessary to develop the appropriate production capacity and distribution channels to support market demands generated by promoting your business to a larger marketplace.

History of e-Commerce

One of the most popular activities on the web is shopping. It has much allure in it—you can shop at your leisure, anytime, and in your pajamas. Literally anyone can have their pages built to display their specific goods and services.

History of e-commerce dates back to the invention of the very old notion of "sell and buy", electricity, cables, computers, modems, and the Internet. e-Commerce became possible in 1991 when the Internet was opened to commercial use. Since that date thousands of businesses have taken up residence at websites.

At first, the term e-commerce meant the process of execution of commercial transactions electronically with the help of the leading technologies such as Electronic Data Interchange (EDI) and Electronic Funds Transfer (EFT) which gave an opportunity for users to exchange business information and do electronic transactions. The ability to use these technologies appeared in the late 1970s and allowed business companies and organizations to send commercial documentation electronically.

Although the Internet began to advance in popularity among the general public in 1994, it took approximately four years to develop the security protocols (for example, HTTP) and DSL, which allowed rapid access and a persistent connection to the Internet. In 2000 a great number of business companies in the United States and Western Europe represented their services in the World Wide Web. At this time the meaning of the word e-commerce was changed. People began to define the term e-commerce as the process of purchasing of available goods and services over the Internet using secure connections and electronic payment services. Although the dot-com collapse in 2000 led to unfortunate results and many of e-commerce companies disappeared, the "brick and mortar" retailers recognized the advantages of electronic commerce and began to add such capabilities to their websites (e.g. after the online grocery store Webvan came to ruin, two supermarket chains, Albertsons and Safeway, began to use e-commerce to enable their customers to buy groceries online). By the end of 2001, the largest form of e-commerce, Business-to-Business (B2B) model, had around $700 billion in transactions.

According to all available data, e-commerce sales in USA continued to grow in the next few years and, by the end of 2007, e-commerce sales accounted for 3.4 percent of total sales (Fig. 8.1).

e-Commerce has a great deal of advantages over "brick and mortar" stores and mail order catalogs. Consumers can easily search through a large database of products and services. They can see actual prices, build an order over several days and e-mail it as a "wish list" hoping that someone will pay for their selected goods. Customers can compare prices with a click of the mouse and buy the selected product at best prices.

Online vendors, in their turn, also get distinct advantages. The web and its search engines provide a way to be found by customers without expensive advertising campaign. Even small online shops can reach global markets. Web technology also allows to track customer preferences and to deliver individually-tailored marketing.

History of e-commerce is unthinkable without Amazon and EBay, which were among the first Internet companies to allow electronic transactions. Thanks to their founders we now have a handsome e-commerce sector and enjoy the buying and selling advantages of the Internet. Currently there are 5 largest and most famous worldwide Internet retailers: Amazon, Dell, Staples, Office Depot and Hewlett Packard. According to

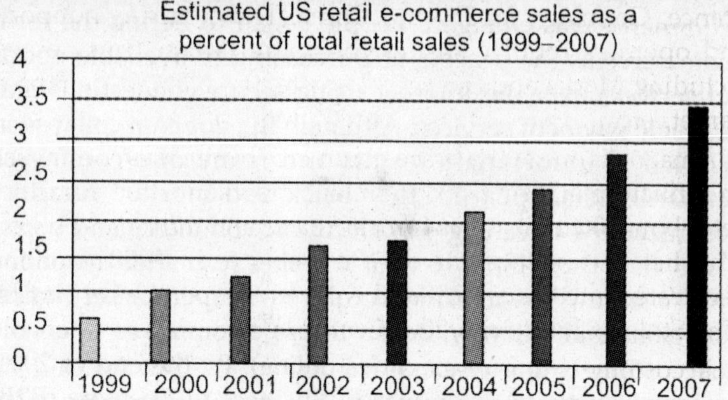

Fig. 8.1: US retail e-commerce sales from 1999–2007

statistics, the most popular categories of products sold in the World Wide Web are music, books, computers, office supplies and other consumer electronics.

Amazon.com, Inc. is one of the most famous e-commerce companies and is located in Seattle, Washington (USA). It was founded in 1994 by Jeff Bezos and was one of the first American e-commerce companies to sell products over the Internet. After the dot-com collapse Amazon lost its position as a successful business model, however, in 2003 the company made its first annual profit, which was the first step to the further development.

At the outset Amazon.com was considered as an online bookstore, but in time it extended a variety of goods by adding electronics, software, DVDs, video games, music CDs, MP3s, apparel, footwear, health products, etc. The original name of the company was Cadabra.com, but shortly after it became popular in the Internet Bezos decided to rename his business "Amazon" after the world's most voluminous river. In 1999 Jeff Bezos was entitled as the Person of the Year by Time Magazine in recognition of the company's success. Although the company's main headquarters is located in the USA, WA, Amazon has set up separate websites in other economically developed countries such as the United Kingdom, Canada,

France, Germany, Japan, and China. The company supports and operates retail websites for many famous businesses, including Marks and Spencer, Lacoste, the NBA, Bebe Stores, Target, etc.

Amazon is one of the first e-commerce businesses to establish an affiliate marketing program, and nowadays the company gets about 40% of its sales from affiliates and third party sellers who list and sell goods on the website. In 2008 Amazon penetrated into the cinema and is currently sponsoring the film "The Stolen Child" with 20th Century Fox.

According to the research conducted in 2008, the domain Amazon.com attracted about 615 million customers every year. The most popular feature of the website is the review system, i.e. the ability for visitors to submit their reviews and rate any product on a rating scale from one to five stars. Amazon.com is also well-known for its clear and user-friendly advanced search facility which enables visitors to search for keywords in the full text of many books in the database.

One more company which has contributed much to the process of e-commerce development is Dell Inc., an American company located in Texas, which stands third in computer sales within the industry behind Hewlett-Packard and Acer.

Launched in 1994 as a static page, Dell.com has made rapid strides, and by the end of 1997 was the first company to record a million dollars in online sales. The company's unique strategy of selling goods over the World Wide Web with no retail outlets and no middlemen has been admired by a lot of customers and imitated by a great number of e-commerce businesses. The key factor of Dell's success is that Dell.com enables customers to choose and to control, i.e. visitors can browse the site and assemble PCs piece by piece choosing each single component based on their budget and requirements. According to statistics, approximately half of the company's profit comes from the website.

In 2007, Fortune magazine ranked Dell as the 34th largest company in the Fortune 500 list and 8th on its annual Top 20 list of the most successful and admired companies in the USA in recognition of the company's business model.

e-Commerce Advantages

e-Commerce does have unique advantages for business hours. Imagine a shop, a showroom or an office that is open 24 hours a day, 7 days a week. You have no staff to pay, no rates or rent, you do not even have to sweep the floor. This is not a dream, just a few of the business advantages of using e-commerce. A website can bring your prospect from the point of advertising and information directly to the point of sale, seamlessly, without involving any other medium.

1. ***New marketing time opportunities:*** People are often at their best when sat relaxed in the evening using their computer, surfing the net for pleasure and keen to interact with interesting business websites. This is a good time, emotionally speaking, to make a sale. Much better than the next morning when they get up to go to work and find a pile of bills sitting on their doormat (along with your competitors junk mail!). Let us suppose your client finds an advert you have placed in a magazine or local paper. He/she notices the website address, connects to the Internet... you may take an order without even being there-24 hours a day. One of the advantages of using e-commerce to do business is that it gives you access to your client base at times you have never been able to dream of before. It also means that time zones are not a problem.

2. ***Business advantages of using e-Commerce:*** e-Commerce is conducted solely on computers, which are by default very good at generating data and recording statistics. This makes market research, measuring statistics and identifying valuable patterns very easy. Try the metrics calculator to get started with a scientific approach to doing business. e-Commerce needs e-business to make it work. E-business is the process of doing market research, getting qualified traffic, converting hits to business advantages and using information to generate new e-commerce from existing clients. Without e-business, e-commerce is like owning a car on an island with no roads.

3. ***Electronic bill presentment and payment services:*** Services that enable customers to leverage the Internet for bill presentment and payments in order to reduce cost with bill and statement delivery and payment processing.

4. ***Catalog flexibility and online fast updating:*** Direct "link" capabilities to content information and visual displays already existing on other client website. You can update your E-catalog anytime, whether it is adding new products, or adjusting prices, without the expense and time of a traditional print catalog. Extensive search capabilities by item, corporate name, division name, location, manufacturer, partner, price or any other specified need.

5. ***Shrinks the competition gap:*** Reduce marketing / advertising expenses, compete on equal footing with much bigger companies; easily compete on quality, price, and availability.

6. ***Unlimited market place and business access which extend customer base:*** The Internet gives customers the opportunity to browse and shop at their convenience and at their place. They can access your services from home, office, or on the road, 24 hours a day, 7 days a week. The Internet allows you to reach people around the world, offering your products to a global customer base.

7. ***24 hour store reduced sale cycle:*** Reduce unnecessary phone calls and mailings.

8. ***Lower cost of doing business:*** Reduce inventory, employees, purchasing costs, order processing costs associated with faxing, phone calls, and data entry, and even eliminate physical stores. Reduce transaction costs.

9. ***Eliminate middlemen:*** Sell directly to your customers.

10. ***Easier business administration:*** With right software, store inventory levels, shipping and receiving logs, and other business administration tasks can be automatically stored, categorized and updated in real-time, and accessed on demand.

11. ***Frees your staff:*** Reduce customer service and sales support.

12. ***Customers will love it:*** Gives customers control of sales process. Builds loyalty.

13. ***More efficient business relationships:*** Better way to deal with dealers and suppliers.

14. ***Workflow automation:*** Shipping, real-time inventory accounting system, which adjusts stock levels and site, location availability instantaneously. Secured, automated registration verification, account entry and transaction authorization features Automated RFP and RTQ features for vendor bid development and selection. Banking and accounting features customized for pre-approved third party direct sales, vendor, consignment or internal transfer transactions.

15. ***Secure payment systems:*** Recent advancements in payment technologies allow encrypted, secure payment online.

16. ***e-Commerce website development and design overview:*** The e-commerce solutions cover all the basic and advanced features with respect to e-commerce applications, from the easy to surf front end to the user-friendly content management at the back end. Our shopping cart solutions is search engine friendly, easy to manage and provides a high level experience for your customers. Our e-commerce solution is more than just a website—it converts site users into buyers thus improving the ROI.

The advantages of e-commerce are basically increased sales and decreased costs through the use of electronical media, especially the web. The advantages of e-commerce will be divided into the benefits it provides to organizations, consumers, and society.

i. ***Advantages to organizations:*** Due to the global reach of the Internet, businesses organizations are able to send messages worldwide, exploring new markets and opportunities. This breaks down geographic limitations, and reaches narrow markets that traditional businesses have difficulties accessing. Through the Internet, business now offers a wide range of choices and higher levels of customer information and details for individuals to search and compare. Some build-to-order companies such as Dell Computer Corp can even provide a competitive advantage by inexpensive customization of products and services.

In terms of cost reduction, e-commerce helps organizations decrease costs in creating, processing, distributing, storing and retrieving information. For example, the communication and advertising costs could be lower by sending e-mails and using online advertising channels, than by using television commercials or the print media. In terms of online ordering and online auction organizations, the costs could be lower than running an actual shop with the associated manpower.

Extended trading hours is another benefit, the 24 hours a day. 7 days a week in 365 days allows business always free to open on the Internet without overtime and extra cost. Other advantages include the up-to-date company material, current inventories, improved customers service, better customers communication, increased operating and trading flexibility.

ii. ***Advantages to consumers:*** For customers, the advantages occur in the buying process, product research, evaluation and execution. e-Commerce provides customers with a platform to search product information through global markets with a wider range of choices, which makes comparison and evaluation easier and more efficient. With the ubiquity in accessing the Internet, consumers are able to search for shops or perform other transactions anytime in almost location. Cheaper goods and services is one of the benefits for consumers who purchase online. Furthermore, delivery time and costs can be saved by buyers when they purchase digital goods and services. Examples are e-books, music and audio clips, software, games, and distance education delivered via the Internet.

iii. ***Advantages to society:*** By telecommuting, individuals can nowadays work and do their purchasing at home rather than by traveling around. This will result in less traffic and air pollution. For people in Third World countries, many services and products are now available which were unavailable in the past; opportunities and higher education services are more achievable for students. Non-profit organizations, including government services, also benefit from e-commerce by the online payment system which supports the payment of tax refunds and pensions quickly and securely. Public services such as health care, education, and public social service also benefit from e-commerce. For example, rural doctors and nurses can access professional information and the latest health care technologies. Overall, e-commerce makes products and services more easily available without geographic limitations.

e-Commerce Disadvantages and Constraints

Some disadvantages and constraints of e-commerce include the following:

1. ***Time for delivery of physical products:*** It is possible to visit a local music store and walk out with a compact disc, or a book store and leave with a book. e-Commerce is often used to buy goods that are not available locally from businesses all over the world, meaning that physical goods need to be delivered, which takes time and costs money. In some cases there are ways around this, for example, with electronic files of the music or books being accessed across the Internet, but then these are not physical goods.

2. ***Physical product, supplier and delivery uncertainty:*** When you walk out of a shop with an item, it is yours. You have it; you know what it is, where it is and how it looks. In some respects e-commerce purchases are made on trust. This is because, firstly, not having had physical access to the product, a purchase is made on an expectation of what that product is and its condition. Secondly, because supplying businesses can be conducted across the world, it can be uncertain whether or not they are legitimate businesses and are not just going to take your money. It is pretty hard to knock on their door to complain or seek legal recourse! Thirdly, even if the item is sent, it is easy to start wondering whether or not it will ever arrive.

3. ***Perishable goods:*** Forget about ordering a single gelato ice cream from a shop in Rome! Though specialized or refrigerated transport can be used, goods bought and sold via the Internet tend to be durable and non-perishable: they need to survive the trip from the supplier to the purchasing business or consumer. This shifts the bias for perishable and/or non-durable goods back towards traditional supply chain arrangements, or towards relatively more local e-commerce-based purchases, sales and distribution. In contrast, durable

goods can be traded from almost anyone to almost anyone else, sparking competition for lower prices. In some cases this leads to disintermediation in which intermediary people and businesses are bypassed by consumers and by other businesses that are seeking to purchase more directly from manufacturers.

4. ***Limited and selected sensory information:*** The Internet is an effective conduit for visual and auditory information: seeing pictures, hearing sounds and reading text. However, it does not allow full scope for our senses: we can see pictures of the flowers, but not smell their fragrance; we can see pictures of a hammer, but not feel its weight or balance. Further, when we pick up and inspect something, we choose what we look at and how we look at it. This is not the case on the Internet. If we were looking at buying a car on the Internet, we would see the pictures the seller had chosen for us to see but not the things we might look for if we were able to see it in person. And, taking into account our other senses, we can not test the car to hear the sound of the engine as it changes gears or sense the smell and feel of the leather seats. There are many ways in which the Internet does not convey the richness of experiences of the world. This lack of sensory information means that people are often much more comfortable buying via the Internet generic goods-things that they have seen or experienced before and about which there is little ambiguity, rather than unique or complex things.

5. ***Returning goods:*** Returning goods online can be an area of difficulty. The uncertainties surrounding the initial payment and delivery of goods can be exacerbated in this process. Will the goods get back to their source? Who pays for the return postage? Will the refund be paid? Will I be left with nothing? How long will it take? Contrast this with the offline experience of returning goods to a shop.

6. ***Privacy, security, payment, identity, contract:*** Many issues arise—privacy of information, security of that information and payment details, whether or not payment details (e.g. credit card details) will be misused, identity theft, contract, and, whether we have one or not, what laws and legal jurisdiction apply.

7. ***Defined services and the unexpected:*** e-Commerce is an effective means for managing the transaction of known and established services, that is, things that are everyday. It is not suitable for dealing with the new or unexpected. For example, a transport company used to dealing with simple packages being asked if it can transport a hippopotamus, or a customer asking for a book order to be wrapped in blue and white polka dot paper with a bow. Such requests need human intervention to investigate and resolve.

8. ***Personal service:*** Although some human interaction can be facilitated via the web, e-commerce cannot provide the richness of interaction provided by personal service. For most businesses, e-commerce methods provide the equivalent of an information-rich counter attendant rather than a salesperson. This also means that feedback about how people react to product and service offerings also tends to be more granular or perhaps lost using e-commerce approaches. If your only feedback is that people are (or are not) buying your products or services online, this is inadequate for evaluating how to change or improve your e-commerce strategies and / or product and service offerings. Successful business use of e-commerce typically involves strategies for gaining and applying customer feedback. This helps businesses to understand, anticipate and meet changing online customer needs and preferences, which is critical because of the comparatively rapid rate of ongoing Internet-based change.

9. ***Size and number of transactions:*** e-Commerce is most often conducted using credit card facilities for payments, and as a result very small and very large transactions tend not to be conducted online. The size of transactions is also impacted by the economics of transporting physical goods. For example, any benefits or conveniences of buying a box of pens online from a US-based business tend to be eclipsed by the cost of having to pay for them to be delivered to you in India. The delivery costs also mean that buying individual items from a range of different overseas businesses is significantly more expensive than buying all of the goods from one overseas business because the goods can be packaged and shipped together.

Types of e-Commerce

There are a number of different types of e-commerce:

1. ***B2B-business to business:*** Business-to-business e-commerce has been in use for quite a few years and is more commonly known as EDI (electronic data interchange). In the past EDI was conducted on a direct link of some form between the two businesses whereas today the most popular connection is the Internet. The two businesses pass information electronically to each other. B2B e-commerce currently makes up about 94% of all e-commerce transactions.

Business-to-business electronic commerce, also known as e-business, is experiencing an explosive growth rate on the Internet. Companies of all sizes and types are now mutually buying and selling products and services on the Internet. B2B also offers unique benefits such as less human intervention, less overhead expenses, fewer inadvertent errors, more efficiency, more advertising exposure, new markets and new physical territories equate to an intelligent method of mutual business. It is a win-win situation for both buyer and seller.

Currently there are 2 main issues to deal with when conducting a B2B e-commerce:

- ***Supply chain management:*** In the 80's, concepts like Lean Manufacturing, Design for Manufacturability, Just-in-Time, and Stockless Production emerged. If properly managed, the operating costs of such systems can be substantially reduced. Reduction in costs can be in the form of reduced inventory cost, obsolescence, transportation and other logistics costs, overhead and direct labor costs. All have pointed out potential savings in costs that could amount to billions when companies can engage in supply chain integration efforts.
- ***Electronic procurement system:*** Using Internet technologies to handle product distribution to the buyer and from supplier while at the same time removing the complexity of multi-level paper and processing which are labour intensive. This allows the business to run more efficiently and allows purchasing professionals to have more time to focus on complex acquisitions and supplier negotiation. Besides

reducing cost and hassle, it must be designed expressly for casual use by untrained employees and it must also provide extensive management controls, reporting, and integration with existing systems.

2. ***B2C-business to consumer:*** Business to consumer e-commerce is relatively new. This is where the consumer accesses the system of the supplier. It is still a two-way function but is usually done solely through the Internet.

B2C is basically a concept of online marketing and distributing of products and services over the Internet. It is a natural progression for many retailers or marketers who sell directly to the consumer. The general idea is, if you could reach more customers, service them better, make more sales while spending less to do it, that would the formula of success for implementing a B2C e-commerce infrastructure. For the consumer, it is relatively easy to appreciate the importance of e-commerce. Why waste time fighting the very real crowds in supermarkets, when, from the comfort of home, one can shop online at any time in virtual Internet shopping malls, and have the goods delivered home directly.

3. ***C2B-consumer to business:*** Consumer to business is a growing arena where the consumer requests a specific service from the business.

Example: Harry is planning a holiday in Darwin. He requires a flight in the first week of December and is only willing to pay $250. Harry places a submission within a web-based C2B facility. Dodgy Brothers Airways accesses the facility and sees Harry's submission. Due to it being a slow period, the airline offers Harry a return fare for $250.

4. ***B2E-business to employee:*** Business to employee e-commerce is growing in use. This form of e-commerce is more commonly known as an 'Intranet'. An intranet is a website developed to provide employees of an organization with information. The intranet is usually accessed through the organization's network, though it can and is often extended to an entrant who uses the Internet but restricts uses by sign on and password.

5. ***C2C-consumer to consumer:*** These sites are usually some form of an auction site. The consumer lists items for sale with a commercial auction site. Other consumers access the site and place bids on the items. The site then provides a connection between the seller and buyer to complete the transaction. The site provider usually charges a transaction cost. In reality this site should be called C2B2C.

e-Commerce Development

e-Commerce is referred to as a profitable business area by experts. A lot of businessmen get into e-commerce because it gives them a wider scope for conducting business with anyone and everyone around the globe. If you are running an e-commerce business what are the tools and ways to see it go into development stage? Let us take a look.

1. ***e-Commerce product support development:*** You could be selling a lot of products on your e-commerce website. How can you ensure product support development for your clients? Install a product tracking software in your e-commerce site. You could ask your e-commerce solution providers for the software if you do not have it. A lot of e-commerce businesses like to have this product tracking software, as it will let them check to see when it was bought and when is it scheduled for delivery. Your customers could be keen to know about the time taken for delivery so if you let them log on to your site and check with their product code or id they will be glad to check the status of their product. At the same time they will like to shop in your store again as you are providing convenient service for them.

2. ***e-Commerce customer service development:*** In any business the client is to be pleased. If the customers think that they can get service elsewhere you may lose them to your competitors. So how can you look into the development of customer service for your e-commerce business site? Experts say that it is the best to make the clients feel happy about using your e-commerce business. Let us say that a customer has bought something from you through your e-commerce store. How can

you make that customer know that you appreciate him using your service? Send a thank you e-card or e-mail. This can help to create a more positive outlook to your business and your customers will like to return again because of your friendly and warm customer service. This is a good way to get customer service development for the e-commerce business.

3. ***e-Commerce marketing development:*** Marketing is a very essential factor to determine if your e-commerce business can grow and be a success. Without marketing you cannot see your e-commerce business reach into development. So what tools can you use for marketing and promoting your e-commerce business? One simple and cheap tool which all e-commerce businessmen think of when it comes to marketing their e-commerce business is the e-mail. You can use the e-mail as a marketing tool to keep in touch with your customers and alert them of any new promotions you have in your e-commerce store. Apart from e-mail you can also use electronic newsletters as another tool to keep your customers updated on any sales and these newsletters can remind them to visit your e-commerce site again. You can also use banner advertisements to promote and create more awareness of your online e-commerce business.

Essential Internet Tools for e-Commerce

1. ***Develop your website:*** Contact an Internet Service Provider (ISP) who will register a domain name for your business (for example: www.mynewbusiness.com.in). A listing of all Internet Service Providers may be obtained from the Internet Industry Association. The website must:

- Serve as a commercial site to generate sales of a range of products and services.
- Build company awareness, i.e. serve as an advertising and marketing tool for your business.
- Serve as a channel of communication between your business, existing customers and potential customer.
- Serve as a conduit for customer service and basic market research.

- Use a database application for easy and immediate update.
- Incorporate catalogue facilities within the database.
- Include a search engine.
- Make it easy for visitors to find what they are looking for in a very short period of time.
- Navigation controls should be clearly labeled or be otherwise recognizable.
- Provide information to visitors or customers about how to contact the business.
- Attracting visitors to the website, sustaining visitor attention, and encouraging repeated visits, by making the site interesting enough so that visitors stay, explore and return.
- The website must not only present content and information. It must also be relevant, engaging and encourage interaction with your business.
- Convincing visitors to follow the site's links to obtain information.
- Offering easily accessible facts about the business.
- Offering easily accessible information about products and services, and how to use and/or acquire them.
- Converting visitors into customers.
- Providing visitors with a meaningful, two-way communication link with the business.
- Creating an impression consistent with the business's desired image.
- Reinforcing positive images that the visitor might already have about the business.
- Integrating the opportunity for enhancing the image of the business with the provision of information.
- Design of consistency across pages in terms of layout/page composition, design features, theme and color.
- Registration of the website with search engines and directories; as well as the inclusion of as many relevant metatags as possible.

- Interaction with the ISP hosting the website and obtaining web usage statistics.

2. ***Produce appropriate electronic information for your website:*** Customers around the world will view your website, so it is important to produce appropriate business and product information. Usually the saying "less is more" can also be applied to websites. You may offer downloadable product samples, information and other interactive online discussion services, but significant publications and products should be offered as a follow-up service.

3. ***Provide online ordering facilities:*** Many websites act simply as a corporate brochure for a company. However, effective websites for Queensland exporters should provide online ordering facilities. In this fashion overseas visitors to your site can directly place orders for your products and services.

4. ***Provide online payment facilities:*** As well as offering online ordering facilities, your website should also offer online payment facilities. Not only will this mean that the company receives payment before the order is filled, it will be a boon to the business cash flow, as you are no longer waiting for payment.

5. ***Promote your web address:*** It is all very well to have an effective website with terrific corporate information, as well as online ordering and payment facilities, but if no one knows the address this website will be a useless marketing tool. Promoting the web address for your business will become essential:

- Ensure the address is included in all appropriate search engines.
- Hyperlink your site to other web addresses, e.g. many industry associations provide links from their website to their members.
- Print your web address on all stationery, advertisements, brochures, packaging, orders, invoices and anywhere else you promote your business.

Issues to consider when designing an effective business website include:

i. ***Speed:*** Slow sites will deter online users. Heavy graphics or wrong servers for site hosting can cause performance problems; however, as more and more Internet users gain access to broadband this problem will decrease.

ii. ***Navigation:*** More and more web pages are beginning to look the same as they start to adopt similar navigation tools to help the user move around the site. While this may not seem very creative it does set a standard to frequent online shoppers.

iii. ***Content:*** More often than not, less is best. The follow-up material that you can post or e-mail to your customers will bring them back to your site.

iv. ***Interactivity:*** Ask your customers for their input. Also offer facilities to enable your customers to order goods, check their account balances, view inventory, check order status and update their contact information.

v. ***Suppliers:*** Offer the facilities to enable your suppliers to retrieve purchase orders and send invoices to your website.

e-Commerce Today

e-Commerce allows consumers to electronically exchange goods and services with no barriers of time or distance. Electronic commerce has expanded rapidly over the past five years and is predicted to continue at this rate, or even accelerate. In the near future the boundaries between "conventional" and "electronic" commerce will become increasingly blurred as more and more businesses move sections of their operations onto the Internet.

e-Commerce today is a remarkable experience. It has transformed traditional shopping beyond recognition. It is so much better than any other way of shopping that it has already attracted a great many of e-commerce-lovers.

If some years ago e-commerce was a buzzword, now it has become the order of the day. People seem to shop literally everywhere—at their workplaces during lunch times, in rush hour when there is nothing else to do but switch on their laptops and start surfing.

e-Commerce today gained so much popularity because its underlying technologies are evolving at giant steps. We are even offered to "feel" the product with a 3D mouse to better understand its shape, size and texture. Why go somewhere out when all you have to do is make an order, choose the shipping method, put up your feet and wait till the order is delivered right to your door-step?

e-Commerce today offers so much luxury that even conventional stores have already signaled the alarm. Although, everyone agrees that it is a long way for an e-commerce to replace "brick-and-mortar" stores, it has every chance to happen in the future. e-Commerce which we are witnessing today brings in so much adventure into our lives that it is enjoyed by the whole online community. e-Commerce today reflects what we created at the very dawn of online electronic commerce. It is made by us and meant for us.

Future of e-Commerce

Experts predict a promising and glorious future of e-commerce in the 21st century. In the foreseeable future e-commerce will further confirm itself a major tool of sale. Successful e-commerce will become a notion absolutely inseparable from the web, because e-shopping is becoming more and more popular and natural. At the same time severe rivalry in the sphere of e-commerce services will intensify their development. Thus prevailing future trends of e-commerce will be the growth of Internet sales and evolution.

Each year number of e-commerce deals grows enormously. Sales volumes of online stores are more than comparable with those of "brick-and-mortar" ones. And the tendency will continue, because a lot of people are "imprisoned" by work and household duties, while Internet saves a lot of time and gives opportunity to choose goods at the best prices. Present-day Internet sales boom is the foundation for magnificent e-commerce future.

The "quantity to quality" tendency of e-commerce is also becoming more and more obvious, as the Internet has excluded geographical factor from the sale. So it does not matter anymore whether your store is situated in New York or London or in a small town. To survive, merchants will have to adapt rapidly to the new conditions. To attract more customers e-store-owners will have not only to increase the number of available services, but to pay more attention to such elements like attractive design, user-friendliness, appealing goods presentation, they will have to opportunely employ modern technologies for their businesses to become parts of e-commerce future.

Of course, those, who acquire e-stores earlier, get better chance for future success and prosperity, though an e-commerce site itself does not guarantee you anything. Only an appropriate e-commerce solution in combination with thorough e-marketing and advertising can buy you business insurance.

PUBMED

PubMed is a service of the U.S. National Library of Medicine that includes over 18 million citations from MEDLINE and other life science journals for biomedical articles back to the 1950s. PubMed includes links to full text articles and other related resources.

PubMed is a free search engine for accessing the MEDLINE database of citations and abstracts of biomedical research articles. The core subject is medicine, and PubMed covers fields related to medicine, such as nursing and other allied health disciplines. It also provides very full coverage of the related biomedical sciences, such as biochemistry and cell biology. It is offered by the United States National Library of Medicine at the National Institutes of Health as part of the Entrez information retrieval system. As with other indexes, the inclusion of an article or journal in PubMed is not endorsement. In 2007 MEDLINE contained over 17,000,000 records from more than 5,000 journals published in the United States and more than 80 other countries primarily from 1950 onwards. In addition to MEDLINE, PubMed also offers access to:

- OLDMEDLINE for pre-1966 citations. This has recently been enhanced, and records for 1951+, even those parts in the printed indexes, are now included within the main portion.
- Citations to all articles, even those that are out-of-scope (e.g. covering plate tectonics or astrophysics) from certain MEDLINE journals, primarily the most important general science and chemistry journals, from which the life sciences articles are indexed for MEDLINE.
- In-process citations which provide a record for an article before it is indexed with MeSH and added to MEDLINE or converted to out-of-scope status.
- Citations that precede the date that a journal was selected for MEDLINE indexing (when supplied electronically by the publisher).
- Some life science journals that submit full text to PubMed Central and may not have been recommended for inclusion in MEDLINE although they have undergone a review by NLM, and some physics journals that were part of a prototype PubMed in the early to mid-1990s.

Many PubMed citations contain links to full text articles which are freely available, often in the PubMed Central digital library. In late 2007, the Consolidated Appropriations Act of 2007 (H.R. 2764) was signed into law and included a provision requiring the NIH to modify its policies and require inclusion into PubMed Central complete electronic copies of their peer-reviewed research and findings from its funded research. This is the first time the US government has required an agency to provide open access to research and is an evolution from the 2005 policy, in which the NIH asked researchers to voluntarily add their research to PubMed Central. With an effective date of April 7, 2008, the Department of Health and Human Services has given notice: "The Director of the National Institutes of Health shall require that all investigators funded by the NIH submit or have submitted for them to the National Library of Medicine's PubMed Central an electronic version of their final, peer-reviewed manuscripts upon acceptance for publication, to be made publicly available no later than 12 months after the official date of publication: Provided, that the NIH shall implement the public access policy in a manner consistent with copyright law."

PubMed is one of a number of search engines through which it is possible to search the MEDLINE database; the National Library of Medicine also leases the MEDLINE information to a number of private vendors such as Ovid and SilverPlatter—as well as many other vendors. PubMed has been available free on the Internet since the mid-1990s.

Information about the journals indexed in PubMed is found in its journals database, searchable by subject or journal title, title abbreviation, the NLM ID (NLM's unique journal identifier), the ISO abbreviation, and both the print and electronic International Standard Serial Numbers (pISSN and eISSN). The database includes all journals in all Entrez databases. As of 20 October 2008, PubMed has 16,880,015 citations going back to the year 1865.

PubMed Central

PubMed Central (PMC) is the U.S. National Institutes of Health (NIH) free digital archive of biomedical and life sciences journal literature. All the articles in PMC are free (sometimes on a delayed basis). PMC's utilities include an OAI service that provides XML of the full-text of some articles, functions for scripting PMC searches and linking to specific PMC articles from your site. The PMC journal list comprises journals that deposit material in PMC on a routine basis and generally make all their published articles available here. PMC also has the author manuscripts of articles published by NIH-funded researchers in various non-PMC journals.

PubMed Features

- Sophisticated search capabilities, including spell checker and special tools for searching clinical topics.
- Assistance in finding search terms using the MeSH database, a guide to MEDLINE's controlled vocabulary.

- Ability to store and automatically receive e-mail updates for saved searches using PubMed's My NCBI.
- Links to full-text articles and to information about library holdings.
- Links to other NLM search systems, such as ClinicalTrials.gov®, MedlinePlus®, NIH Clinical Alerts and Advisories, NLM Gateway® and PubMed.

PubMed Content

- MEDLINE®, NLM's database of millions of references to articles published in biomedical journals.
- OLDMEDLINE®, journal article citations from 1949 through 1965.
- In-process citations that have not yet been analyzed and indexed for MEDLINE.
- Publisher supplied citations that may not receive full indexing for MEDLINE because they are not biomedical in nature.
- Links to Entrez molecular biology databases.

PubMed Services

1. ***Journal database:***
   - Search by topic, journal title or abbreviation, ISSN, or browse by subject terms.
   - Limit searches to PubMed journals and/or currently indexed.
   - Lists of all Entrez journals and those with links to full-text websites are available.
2. ***MeSH database:*** MeSH is the U.S. National Library of Medicine's controlled vocabulary used for indexing articles for MEDLINE/PubMed. MeSH terminology provides a consistent way to retrieve information that may use different terminology for the same concepts.
   - Use the MeSH database to find Medical Subject Heading Terms and build a search strategy.

3. ***Single citation matcher:*** Use this tool to find PubMed citations. You may omit any field.
   - Journal may be the full title or the title abbreviation.
   - For first and last author searching, use smith jc format.

Journal:

Date: yyyy/mm/d (month and day are optional)

Volume: Issue: First page:

Author name (see help)

Only as first author Only as last author

Title words:

4. ***Batch citation matcher:*** To retrieve PubMed or PMC UIs for fewer than 100 citations enter each citation string on a separate line using the following input format:

journal_title | year | volume | first_page | author_name | your_key |

To retrieve more than 100 citations use the e-mail function instead of the text box below:

- Enter your e-mail address. Citations will be sent via e-mail if an address is provided.

Select database: PubMed

Email: File: Browse

Go

- Create a file using the citation input format and save it locally, then enter the filename or browse to choose it from your system directory.
- e-Mail requests may take a few minutes to process and be sent to your e-mail address.

5. ***Clinical queries:*** Results of searches on these pages are limited to specific clinical research areas. For comprehensive searches, use PubMed directly (Table 8.11).

i. ***Search by clinical study category:*** This search finds citations that correspond to a specific clinical study category. The search may be either broad and sensitive or narrow and specific. The search filters are based on the work of Haynes RB et al.

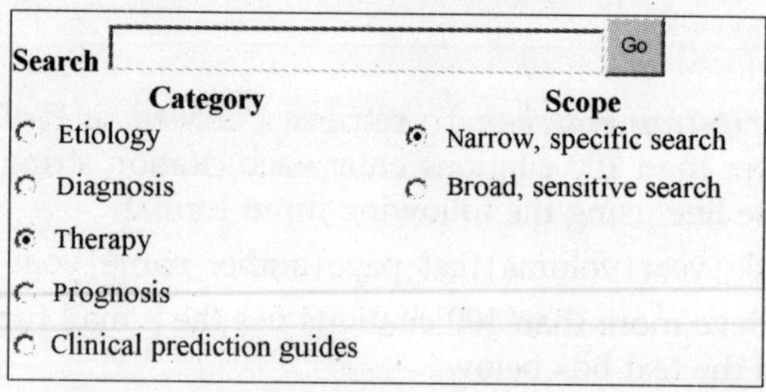

ii. ***Find systematic reviews:*** For your topic(s) of interest, this search finds citations for systematic reviews, meta-analyses,

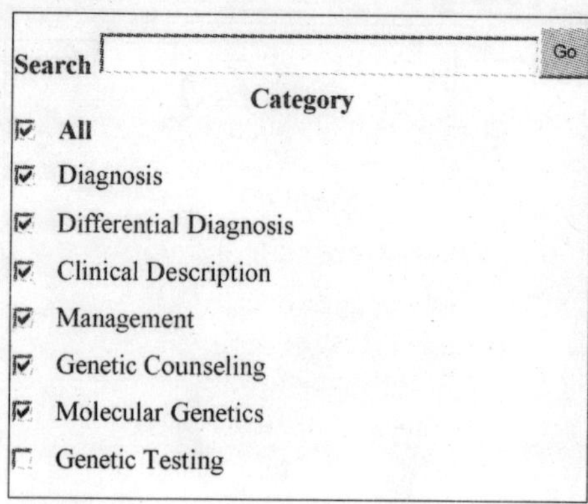

reviews of clinical trials, evidence-based medicine, consensus development conferences and guidelines.

iii. ***Medical genetics searches:*** This search finds citations and abstracts related to various topics in medical genetics.

6. ***Special queries:*** It is directory of topic-related PubMed queries.

Table 8.11: Queries targeted for clinicians and health services researchers

Clinical queries	A search interface to find citations in the areas of: • *Clinical study categories:* Find citations corresponding to a specific clinical study category. • *Systematic reviews:* Find citations for systematic reviews, meta-analyses, reviews of clinical trials, evidence-based medicine, consensus development conferences, and guidelines. • *Medical genetics:* Find citations related to various topics in medical genetics.
Health services research (HSR) queries	A search interface to find PubMed citations relating to health care quality or to health care costs
Cancer topic searches	A search interface to retrieve PubMed citations on more than 100 major cancer topics
Healthy people 2010	A search interface providing searches for published literature related to the Healthy People 2010 focus areas of the HP2010 Information Access Project.
	Subjects
AIDS	Limits search to the PubMed AIDS subset
Bioethics	Bioethics Information Resource page providing a PubMed search function using the PubMed Bioethics subset, and links to additional bioethics-related resources.

Contd...

Contd...

Cancer	Limits search to the PubMed Cancer subset
Complementary medicine	Limits search to the PubMed Complementary Medicine subset
Health disparities	PubMed search and links to other health disparities information resources
Health literacy	PubMed search and links to other health literacy information resources
History of medicine	Limits search to the PubMed History of Medicine subset
Space life sciences	Limits search to the PubMed Space Life Sciences subset
Smallpox	Comprehensive PubMed search and links to other smallpox information resources
Toxicology	Limits search to the PubMed Toxicology subset
Veterinary medicine/ animal health	PubMed search and links to other veterinary information resources
Additional Search Queries/Interfaces	
ALTBIB	Provides a PubMed interface to search animal alternatives for biomedical research and testing
CAM on PubMed	Provides information on searching for complementary and alternative medicine citations in PubMed
Medlineplus health topics	Provides several search mechanisms for searching for health topics of interest to the general public in PubMed
National institutes of health funding support	Provides a search in PubMed for citations designated as funded by NIH Institutes.
Retracted publication	Provides a search in PubMed for all citations designated as a retracted publication
TOXNET	Provides a series of toxicological databases, several of which include a PubMed search option/function

Contd...

Contd...

	Journal Collections
Core clinical journals	Limits search to the PubMed Core clinical journal subset
Dental journals	Limits search to the PubMed Dental journal subset
Nursing journals	Limits search to the PubMed Nursing journals subset

7. ***My NCBI:*** PubMed's My NCBI feature stores search strategies, provides automatic e-mail updates, and stores search results as collections. You must register for My NCBI by creating a User Name and Password. Click on My NCBI on the blue sidebar to sign on. My NCBI includes additional features for filtering search results. The tool icon to the right of the features tabs links to a page where up to five search filters may be selected.
8. ***Saving search results:*** To save search results, select file from the Send to pull down menu. You can use the Clipboard to collect citations from multiple searches. To save citations for citation management software, change the display format to MEDLINE before downloading or e-mailing.

How to Search PubMed?

For comprehensive, optimal searching in PubMed, it is necessary to have a thorough understanding of its core component, MEDLINE, and especially of the MeSH (Medical Subject Headings) controlled vocabulary used to index MEDLINE articles.

1. ***Telegram-style search:*** However, simple telegram-style search formulations can also be used, and they generally produce acceptable results. PubMed automatically links textwords to relevant MeSH terms. Aspects of the question can then be added successively, in a Google-like fashion, until a number of 'hits' judged manageable is achieved. No knowledge of actual MeSH terms, Boolean operators, English or American

spelling, 'nesting', or record-fields is required. PubMed's intelligent search algorithm does (or implies) this in the background.

2. ***Clinical queries/systematic reviews:*** A special feature of PubMed is the 'Clinical Queries' and 'Systematic Reviews' option which can be used to identify more relevant (robust) studies by automatically applying 'quality filters' to be applied to each search.

3. ***Related articles:*** After a quick search, references which are judged particularly relevant can be marked and 'related articles' can be identified. If relevant, several studies can be selected and 'related articles' to all of them can be generated. The 'related articles' are then listed on order or 'relatedness' (not chronological order). To create the list of 'Related Articles' PubMed compares words from the Title and Abstract of each citation, as well as the MeSH headings assigned, using a powerful word-weighted algorithm.

4. ***Mapping to MeSH (headings) and subheadings:*** A strong feature of PubMed is its ability to automatically link to Medical Subject Headings (MeSH) and Subheadings. Examples would be: 'bad breath' links to (and includes in the search) 'Halitosis', 'Writers cramp' to 'focal dystonia', 'breast cancer' to 'breast neoplasms'. Where appropriate, these MeSH terms are automatically 'expanded'. Terms like 'nursing' are automatically linked to 'Nursing [Mesh]' or 'Nursing [Subheading]'. This important feature makes PubMed searches automatically more sensitive and avoids false-negative (missed) hits by compensating for the diversity of medical terminology.

5. ***Searching with tags and boolean operators:***

   i. ***Tags:*** Search-field tags can be used for searching PubMed, some of the most common being:

   - [au] -- author -- e.g. Miller RA [au] or miller ra [au] (not case sensitive)
   - [dp] -- date published -- e.g. 1998 [dp] or 1998/11/06 (YYYY/MM/DD, where MM/DD are optional)
   - [ip] -- issue, part or supplement -- e.g. 4 [ip] (for issue four of a volume)

- [la] -- language -- e.g. eng [la] (to only find articles in English)
- [pg] -- first page number of the article -- e.g. 673 [pg] (for an article starting on page 673)
- [pmid] -- PubMed ID -- e.g. 15094092 [pmid] (to find the PubMed article with ID 15094092)
- [pt] -- publication type -- e.g. review [pt] (to only see review articles)
- [ta] -- journal title -- e.g. rejuvenation res [ta] (all articles in the journal Rejuvenation Research)
- [ti] -- title words -- e.g. endothelial [ti] (all articles with "endothelial" in the title)
- [vi] -- volume -- e.g. 101 [vol] (for volume number 101)

It should be noted that using field qualifiers automatically disables PubMed's 'mapping' function.

ii. ***Boolean operators:*** There are three Boolean operators: AND (intersection); OR (union); NOT (exclusion). NOT should be used with care as it may generate 'false-negative' results.

For example: cdd tanwar ys 2007

will yield a single reference, and is the equivalent of

cdd AND tanwar ys AND 2007

whereas

cdd OR tanwar ys OR 2007

will yield hundreds of thousands of articles, including all articles published in 2007, all articles in CDD (Current Drug Delivery) and all articles by Y.S. Tanwar.

All Boolean operators are processed in a left-to-right sequence. The order in which PubMed processes a search statement can be changed by enclosing concepts in parentheses. The terms inside the parentheses are processed first as a unit and then incorporated into the overall strategy.

PubMed Search Results: After clicking on the Go button, PubMed displays a list of results in summary format. To retrieve more information about the search results, use the menu next to Display to pick Abstract, Citation, or MEDLINE format.

PATENT DATABASES

Intellectual property refers to creations of the mind: inventions, literary and artistic works, and symbols, names, images, and designs used in commerce. Intellectual property is divided into two categories: Industrial property, which includes inventions (patents), trademarks, industrial designs, and geographic indications of source; and copyright, which includes literary works such as novels, poems and plays, films, musical works, and artistic works such as drawings, paintings, photographs and sculptures, and architectural designs. Rights related to copyright include those of performing artists in their performances, producers of phonograms in their recordings, and those of broadcasters in their radio and television programs.

Patents-Key Databases

1. ***Britain patents status enquiry:*** The British Patent Office's patent register giving published numbers for filing, ownership details and if still in force. Enter a British patent application number (check digit not required) or a published patent number (British, or a granted EP designating GB) in the format GB2300000, EP0500000 and so on. Note that changed ownership is often not recorded.

2. ***DEPATISnet:*** Database hosted by German Patent Office offering links to Adobe copies of German patents and many foreign patents. Often supplements what is on Esp@cenet®.

3. ***Esp@cenet:*** Esp@cenet, pronounced espacenet, is a free patent search service developed by the European Patent Office (EPO). It provides access to our patents database and those of over 20 European patent offices, the EPO and the World Intellectual Property Office. This is the European Patent Office gateway. If it is temporarily unavailable the British Intellectual Property Office or Irish sites may work.

Esp@cenet defaults to the worldwide database, which contains more than 60 million patents from around the world. However, you can choose a more specific database to focus your search on patents covering a particular country, for example, GB - esp@cenet for patents covering the United Kingdom (UK).

The 'worldwide' format enables searching across a vast amount of data (back to 1895 by name, title or abstract for Britain, for example). Different formats can be chosen: brief results list, detailed results list, abstract plus drawing, 'mosaic' of drawings, etc. by choosing among the formats. PDFs of the complete specifications are often available. Machine translations from German or French into English are available from the 'Description' formats. Later citations of the document being looked at are also available. A useful tutorial can be found at 'Get Assistance' in the Advanced search option.

Some European B and A4 (top up search reports after PCT publications) are also included. Those specifications suffixed U or Y should have these added to the end of the number or they will not be retrieved. There is a Global Patent Data Coverage tool where clicking on the country provides details of its coverage. British 'B' specifications are not yet available. Title or abstract words can be truncated by *, or by ? for zero or one character.

4. ***Epoline®:*** Status register of European patent specifications (only to end of opposition period). Click on Register Plus to search for a known application or published number (or go downwards on arrow to pick other options). Use in format EP1300000, etc. In results, click on All Documents on left hand side to see citations to copies of correspondence (click on title to open that copy). There are also subscriber features. Links to the Esp@cenet database for the actual specifications and also to the EPO Board of Appeal decisions.

5. ***European patent database:*** European patent server is the official site for publication of European Patent Office A and B specifications (omits those published only as WO (PCT) documents). The entire specification forms a single document. New publications go up every Wednesday at 14.00 hours Central European time. You can search by publication/ application number, IPC (to 4 digit level, e.g. A61K), publication date and kind of publication (A1, B8, etc.). All the documents

published in a given week can be identified by checking the box for "all kind codes" and selecting the week and year from drop down menus. A subset can then be found by checking the box for the document kind code.

6. ***Patent abstracts of Japan:*** English abstracts plus drawing of Japanese patent applications from 1976 includes legal status data. Machine translations are available at this site (but only from 1993/94). After the search is entered, click on "index indication" for list of hits. Click on the wanted hit. When the abstract appears, click on "Detail" at top to begin translating. The Japanese document is available as "Japanese". There is a delay in placing material on the database of months.

When searching for specific patent numbers the search box defaults to filing numbers. For A (kokai) publications click on "publication number". A more up-to-date source for machine translations where the document number is known is the Patent and Utility Model Gazette.

7. ***Patent scope:*** Contains images of specifications (including revised, amended, etc.), often in different formats, and often priority, etc. documents, and has searchable text for Latin character languages from the beginning. May include priority documents and some data on entering national phases. It is updated about noon each Thursday.

8. ***US patent full-text and full-page image databases:*** From 1976 searchable front page data of US patents (but with revised US classification) plus text of claims and description. Revised versions of patents following litigation, and correction slips, are not included. Images of patents from 1790 are available and can be searched for by patent number or current US classification. Published applications from 15 March 2001 are available as a separate database in the same way as grants. The 'assignees' are often not given.

9. ***Australian patent information:*** More than 30 million patent documents have been published worldwide with almost a million new disclosures added each year. Each patent document has a unique identifying number and includes a detailed description of an invention, usually with drawings, and information about the inventor and applicant.

Abstracts of published Australian patent applications from 1975 onwards are available at AU Published Patent Data Searching. They can also be viewed at any of their state offices and are available on subscription on CD-ROM.

10. ***Canadian patent database:*** The Canadian Intellectual Property Office (CIPO), a Special Operating Agency (SOA) associated with Industry Canada, is responsible for the administration and processing of the greater part of intellectual property in Canada. CIPO's areas of activity include:

- Patents cover new inventions (process, machine, manufacture, composition of matter), or any new and useful improvement of an existing invention;
- Trade marks are words, symbols or designs (or a combination of these), used to distinguish the wares or services of one person or organization from those of others in the marketplace;
- Copyrights provide protection for artistic, dramatic, musical or literary works (including computer programs), and three other subject-matter known as: performance, sound recording and communication signal;
- Industrial designs are the visual features of shape, configuration, pattern or ornament (or any combination of these features), applied to a finished article of manufacture;
- Integrated circuit topographies refer to the three-dimensional configurations of electronic circuits embodied in integrated circuit products or layout designs.

This database lets you access over 75 years of patent descriptions and images. You can search, retrieve and study more than 1,900,000 patent documents.

11. ***Indian patent database:*** Patent applications filed in India as published in the issues of the Gazette of India (Part III, Section 2) from January 1995 onwards.

- *Ekaswa-A database:* Patent applications filed in India as published in the issues of the Gazette of India (Part III, Section 2) from January 1995 to December 2004.

- *Ekaswa-B database:* Patent applications notified for opposition in the Gazette of India (Part III, Section 2) published from January 1995 to December 2004.
- *Ekaswa-C database:* Patent applications published in official Journal of Patent office published from January 2005 onwards.

12. ***Fullerene patent database:*** This database is brought to you by the laboratory of Prof. M. S. Dresselhaus, at M.I.T. Currently, only U.S. Patents are available here. The patents are listed in chronological order. Clicking on a patent number will bring up the abstract of that patent (courtesy the CNIDR/ USPTO U.S. Patent Bibliographic Database). Note that you will need a Table capable browser (such as Netscape Navigator) in order to properly display the abstracts. For some patents, the full text is available, accessible by clicking on the patent's title.

Internet Sites for Patent Search (Table 8.12)

1. ***National informatic center (NIC):*** http://pk2id.delhi.nic.in/

Provides free online access to INPADOC-EPIDOS database to the registered users. Registration is open to all and is free of cost. The INPADOC-EPIDOS database is produced by the European Patent Office (EPO). It is possible to conduct bibliographic searches through this site. The bibliographic data includes publication number and date, priority number(s) and date(s), application number and date, International Patent Classification Code (IPC), name of inventor, applicant's name, title of the invention and other details. About 70% of the titles are in English, remaining 30% in 13 other languages.

This database is claimed to be the largest database on patents, dealing with patent applications filed or granted in 65 countries. The data includes patent applications filed through the Patent Cooperation Treaty (PCT), patents published by African Intellectual Property Organisation (ARIPO), European Patent Office (EPO), Organisation Africaine de Propriéeté Intellectuelle (OAPI) and the countries of Argentina, Austria, Australia,

Belgium, Brazil, Bulgaria, Canada, Czech Republic, China, Croatia, Cuba, Cyprus, Denmark, Egypt, Finland, France, Germany, Greece, Hong Kong, Hungary, India, Ireland, Israel, Italy, Japan, Kenya, Latvia, Lithuania, Luxembourg, Malawi, Malaysia, Malta, Mexico, Moldova, Singapore, Mongolia, Monaco, New Zealand, Netherlands, Norway, Philippines, Poland, Portugal, Rep. of Korea, Romania, Russia, Spain, Sweden, Slovenia, Slovakia, South Africa, Switzerland, Turkey, United Kingdom, U.S.S.R, U.S.A., Vietnam, Yugoslavia, Zambia and Zimbabwe.

The database is being updated weekly, subject to availability of data from the member countries. Nearly 30,000 new records are added every week. Data for almost all countries are complete since 1973. Data prior to 1973 are also available in respect of some countries.

2. ***European patent office-Europe's network of patent databases:*** http://ep.espacenet.com/

This site is hosted by European Patent Office, which provides the free access to all European patent applications filed and granted by EPO. The site also provides access to EPO's collection of patent databases named Globlepat of about 60 countries, more than 30 million patents and also to Japanese abstracts. In addition to this the site also guides to the databases of the National Patent Offices sites of espacenet of the members of EPO, where one can search on patent database of national patent offices of the members of EPO. Abstracts and claims of patents except a few countries are also available on the site free of cost; all European patents and patent for some other countries; full text documents along with images (150 million pages) are also available on site for free access.

3. ***US patent and trademark office:*** http://www.uspto.gov/

Patent searches on patents issued by USPTO since 1976. This site provides facilities to conduct key word searches on abstracts and full texts. Searches based on specified fields are also possible. The site provides wide range information on the activities at USPTO.

Table 8.12: URL for patent databases of different countries

Country/Organization	*URL*
Australia	http://www.ipaustralia.gov.au/patents/search_index.htm (Patents)
Benelux	http://register.boip.int/bmbonline/intro/select.do?language=en (Trademarks)
Canada	http://patents1.ic.gc.ca/intro-e.html (Patents)
	http://strategis.ic.gc.ca/cipo/trademarks/search/tmSearch.do (Marks)
Chile	http://www.dpi.cl/dpi_web/Frm_Login_default2.htm (Patents and Trademarks)
China	http://www.sipo.gov.cn/sipo_English/zljs/ (Patents)
Czech Republic	http://isdvapl.upv.cz/pls/portal30/pt.ptfrm (Patents)
	http://isdvapl.upv.cz/pls/portal30/oz.ozfrm (Trademarks)
European Patent Office	http://www.espacenet.com/ (Patents)
Finland	http://www.prh.fi/en/patentit/tietokannat/patinfo.html (Patents)
France	http://www.inpi.fr/front/show_rub.php?rub_id=8 (Patents)
Germany	http://www.dpma.de/suche/suche.html (Patents)
Hungary	http://www.hpo.hu/English/adatbazis/ (Patents)
India	http://www.pfc.org.in/db/db.htm (Patents)
Ireland	http://www.patentsoffice.ie/eregister/Query/PTQuery.asp (Patents)
Japan	http://www.jpo.go.jp/quick_e/index_search.htm (Patents and Trademarks)
Latin America	http://invenes.oepm.es/ (Patents)
LUSOPAT (Portal of	http://www.portal-lusofonia.org/

Contd...

Contd...

Portuguese language IP collections)	
New Zealand	http://www.iponz.govt.nz/search/cad/dbssiten.main (Patents and Trademarks)
OHIM (Office for Harmonization in the Internal Market - Trademarks and Designs)	http://oami.europa.eu/en/default.htm
Republic of Korea	http://www.kipo.go.kr/kpo2/user.tdf?a=user.english.html.HtmlApp&c=50100&catmenu=ek50100 (Patents)
Romania	http://193.230.133.4/cgi-bin/invsearch (Patents)
Russian Federation	http://www.fips.ru/ensite/ (Patents and Trademarks)
Singapore	http://www.epatents.gov.sg/PE/ (Patents)
Slovakia	http://www.indprop.gov.sk/eskipo.php?lang=en&idd=2&idd2=
Slovenia	http://www2.uil-sipo.si/dse.htm
Spain	http://invenes.oepm.es/ (Patents)
Switzerland	http://www.swissreg.ch/ (Patents and Trademarks)
Thailand	http://www1.ipic.moc.go.th/dipdcd/owa/p5query1.main?LANG=1 (Patents)
United Kingdom	hhttp://www.ipo.gov.uk/patent.htm (Patents)
United States of America	http://www.uspto.gov/patft/index.html (Patents)
	http://tess2.uspto.gov/bin/gate.exe?f=login&p_lang=english&p_d=trmk (Trademarks)

4. ***Department of intellectual property, Thailand:*** http://www.ipic.moc.go.th/search5.html

   Patents granted in Thailand can be searched in Thai and English language.

5. ***World intellectual property Organization (WIPO)-PCT database:*** http://pctgazette.wipo.int/

   Search patents filed through PCT route since January 1998.

6. ***http://www.library.ubc.ca/patscan/:*** This site provides free access to more than 1.4 million patent documents issued by Canadian Patent Office (CIPO) since 1920. Database is available in English and French. Search can be done in any field individually or simultaneously.

9 Antivirus Software

INTRODUCTION

A computer virus is a computer program that can copy itself and infect a computer without the permission or knowledge of the owner. The term "virus" is also commonly but erroneously used to refer to other types of malware, adware, and spyware programs that do not have the reproductive ability. A true virus can only spread from one computer to another (in some form of executable code) when its host is taken to the target computer; for instance because a user sent it over a network or the Internet, or carried it on a removable medium such as a floppy disk, CD, DVD, or USB drive. Viruses can increase their chances of spreading to other computers by infecting files on a network file system or a file system that is accessed by another computer.

The term "computer virus" is sometimes used as a catch-all phrase to include all types of malware. Malware includes computer viruses, worms, Trojan horses, most rootkits, spyware, dishonest adware, crimeware, and other malicious and unwanted software, including true viruses. Viruses are sometimes confused with computer worms and Trojan horses, which are technically different. A worm can exploit security vulnerabilities to spread itself to other computers without needing to be transferred as part of a host, and a Trojan horse is a program that appears harmless but has a hidden agenda. Worms and Trojans, like viruses, may cause harm to a computer system's hosted data, functional performance, or networking throughput, when they are executed. Some viruses and other malware have symptoms noticeable to the computer user, but many are surreptitious.

Most personal computers are now connected to the Internet and to local area networks, facilitating the spread of malicious code. Today's viruses may also take advantage of network services such as the World Wide Web, e-mail, Instant Messaging, and file sharing systems to spread.

WHAT IS MALWARE?

The word malware comes from the words 'malicious' and 'software'. Malware (malicious software) is software designed to infiltrate or damage a computer system without the owner's informed consent. The expression is a general term used by computer professionals to mean a variety of forms of hostile, intrusive, or annoying software or program code. Types of malware include:

- Computer viruses
- Computer worms
- Trojan horses
- Logic bombs
- Spyware
- Adware
- Spam
- Popups

Various factors make a system more vulnerable to malware:

- ***Homogeneity:*** For example, when all computers in a network run the same OS, if you can exploit that OS, you can break into any computer running it.
- ***Defects:*** Malware leveraging defects in the OS design.
- ***Unconfirmed code:*** Code from a floppy disk, CD-ROM or USB device may be executed without the user's agreement.
- ***Over-privileged users:*** Some systems allow all users to modify their internal structures.
- ***Over-privileged code:*** Most popular systems allow code executed by a user to access all rights of that user.

As malware attacks become more frequent, attention has begun to shift from viruses and spyware protection to malware protection, and programs have been developed to specifically combat them.

COMPUTER VIRUSES

What is Computer Virus?

A virus is a malicious computer program which can replicate itself. It is created to change what your computer does. Viruses can be contracted without your permission and you might not know anything about the infection until you run a virus scan. Computer viruses have become much more widespread throughout subsequent years. Thanks to networks and the Internet the spread of viruses was made easier.

- ***First virus:*** The first virus, which was released in the wild and affected normal computers, was created in 1982. There were previous viruses created before this time but these were never released from the labs where they were written. This first virus attacked Apple Dos 3.3 and was spread by disks. This virus was written by Rich Skrenta.
- ***First PC virus:*** The first virus to attack PCs was called ©Brain and it was released in 1986. This was a boot sector virus written by brothers from Pakistan. Apparently the reason for this computer virus was to prevent people pirating their software.

Some signs that may indicate that your computer is infected include:

- Your computer functions slower than normal.
- Your computer responds slowly and freezes often.
- Your computer restarts itself often.
- You see uncommon error messages, distorted menus, and dialog boxes.
- You notice applications on your computer fail to work correctly.
- You fail to print correctly.

The History of the Computer Virus

When we think about computer viruses and their creation, the way they work, where they come from and the problems they create, we believe that it is a recent phenomenon that has threatened the PC world to a great extent today. But the actual truth is that computer viruses have been around for longer than most people might think.

The first computer virus popularly known as the 'brain virus' was created in 1986 by two Pakistani brothers, Amjad and Basit Farooq Alvi. This virus, which spread via floppy disks, was known only to infect boot records and not computer hard drives like most viruses today. The virus also known as the Lahore, Pakistani, Pakistani Brain, Brain-A and UIUC would occupy unused space on the floppy disk so that it could not be used and would hide from detection. It would also disguise itself by displaying the uninfected boot sector on the disk.

In 1987, the Lehigh virus was discovered at Lehigh University in the United States. The Lehigh virus was the first memory resident file infector that attacked executable files and took control when a file was opened. The Jerusalem virus also appeared around this time at Hebrew University in Israel. Like the Lehigh virus, the Jerusalem virus was also a memory resident file infector. It contained bugs to re-infect programs that were already infected.

In March 1988, the first antivirus was designed to detect and remove the brain virus.

The antivirus also immunized floppy disks to get rid of the Brian infection. At the same time, the Cascade virus appeared in Germany. The Cascade virus was the first encrypted virus, which was coded and could not be changed or removed.

Thus, during the late 1980's and the early 1990's, viruses on the loose which infected files, disks, etc. on the computer and caused a great deal of damage received a lot of media attention.

In 1991, Symantec released the Norton Antivirus software. Antivirus products from IBM, McAfee, Digital Dispatch and Iris also became available. A few years ago, in 2000, the ILOVEYOU virus wreaked havoc around the world. The virus that was created in the Philippines was sent through e-mail and spread around the world in one day infecting 10 percent of computers connected to the Internet and causing $5.5 billion dollars in damage. Hence, viruses are still common and still create chaos even today. It is hard to determine the reasons for all these actions and why virus writers create computer viruses. Some do it for their personal gain, for research projects, pranks, vandalism, etc. while others want to help make improvements in programs.

Types of Computer Viruses

There are different types of computer viruses, and each type has its own separate features and factors that make them different from one another. Among the different types of computer viruses the most familiar ones are computer virus types and Internet types of virus. Viruses can now affect every computer platform including Mac OS, Windows and Linux. Linux viruses are becoming a major problem for anyone using the operating system.

The list of viruses is quiet long and complex. So, we simplified the list by mentioning a few broad categories of viruses that can put your computer and all your personal data on it, in danger (Table 9.1). These computer viruses include:

1. ***Boot sector viruses:*** A boot sector virus infects diskettes and hard drives. All disks and hard drives contain smaller sections called sectors. The first sector is called the boot. The boot carries the Mater Boot Record (MBR). MBR functions to read and load the operating system. So, if a virus infects the boot or MBR of a disk, such as a floppy disk, your hard drive can become infected, if you re-boot your computer while the infected disk is in the drive. Once your hard drive is infected all diskettes that you use in your computer will be infected. Boot sector viruses often spread to other computers by the use of shared infected disks and pirated software applications. The best way to disinfect your computer of the boot sector virus is by using antivirus software.

2. ***Program viruses:*** A program virus becomes active when the program file (usually with extensions .BIN, .COM, .EXE, .OVL, .DRV) carrying the virus is opened. Once active, the virus will make copies of itself and will infect other programs on the computer.

3. ***Multipartite viruses:*** A multipartite virus is a hybrid of a boot sector and program viruses. It infects program files and when the infected program is active it will affect the boot record. So the next time you start up your computer it will infect your local drive and other programs on your computer.

The multipartite virus combines the characteristics of more than one type which gives it the ability to infect boot system sectors as well as program files. It often infects the section on a hard drive that contains data which instructs the machine on how to boot up. Whenever the computer starts, the virus is automatically distributed throughout the system. This enables it to spread and infect program files, causing a user to unknowingly invoke the virus, resulting in more destructive payloads being delivered into the system. Ghostball, the first multipartite virus, was discovered by a member of the Icelandic company, FRISK Software International Corporation. Later variants include the Emperor, Tequila and Anthrax.

4. ***Stealth viruses:*** A stealth virus can disguise itself by using certain tactics to prevent being detected by antivirus software. These tactics include altering its file size, concealing itself in memory, and so on. This type of virus is nothing new, in fact, the first computer virus, dubbed Brain, was a stealth virus. A good antivirus should be able to detect a stealth virus lurking on your hard drive by checking the areas, the virus infected and evidence in memory.

A stealth virus is one that conceals the changes it makes. This is done by taking control of system functions that interpret files or system sectors. When other applications request data from portions of the system modified by the virus, the infection reports back the accurate, unchanged data, instead of the malicious code. In order for this to occur, the virus must be actively present in the memory.

An example of a stealth infection is Brain, the very fist DOS virus. Brain is a system infector that begins by monitoring physical disks. It then redirects all attempts to read an infected sector to sections on the disk where the original, uninfected boot sector is located. Other viruses to follow this trend were

Frodo and the Number of the Beast, two viruses classified as file infectors.

Virus coders mainly use the stealth approach to elude virus scanners. Those that have not been designed to do so, because the malicious code is fairly new or the user's antivirus software is not up to date, are often described as stealth viruses as well. The stealth technique is a contributing factor to why most antivirus programs function best when the system is booted from a clean CD or floppy disk. By doing this, the infection is not able to seize control of the system and the changes it makes can be exposed and immediately dealt with.

In general, a stealth virus will hide itself in system memory every time a program scanner is run. It employs various techniques to hide any changes so that when the scanner looks for altered sections, the virus redirects it to any area that contains the clean, uninfected data. A more advanced antivirus program can detect a stealth virus by searching for evidence of changes within system sectors along with areas that are more susceptible to attack, regardless of how it is booted.

5. ***Polymorphic viruses:*** A polymorphic virus acts like a chameleon, changing its virus signature (also known as binary pattern) every time it multiples and infects a new file. By changing binary patterns, a polymorphic virus becomes hard to detect by an antivirus program.

The polymorphic virus is one of the more complex computer threats. During the process of infection, it creates slightly modified, fully functional copies of itself. This is primarily done to elude the detection of a virus scanner as some are not able to identify different instances of an infection. One method it commonly uses to bypass a scanner involves self-encryption performed with a variable key. In order to create an effective polymorphic virus, a coder chooses from a number of different encryption schemes that require different methods of decryption, only one of which will remain plainly visible to all instances of the infection. A virus scanner based on a string-driven detection would have to find many different strings, one for each probable decryption scheme. This is the best technique for reliably identifying this type of virus.

More advanced forms of the polymorphic virus alter the instruction sequences of their variants by interspersing decryption instructions with other instructions designed to fail the process of encryption. It may also interchange mutually independent instructions to load inaccurate arbitrary values such as moving "0" to "A" or replacing "A" with "B". A basic virus scanner would have no way to effectively identify all variants of the infection. Even a more advanced program has to thoroughly research this type of virus and make special configurations to their scanner in order to detect it.

6. ***Macro viruses:*** A macro virus is programmed as a macro embedded in a document. Many applications, such as Microsoft Word and Excel, support macro languages. Once a macro virus gets on to your computer, every document you produce will become infected. This type of virus is relatively new and may slip by your antivirus software if you do not have the most recent version installed on your computer.

A macro virus is a computer infection written in macro language, which is commonly built into word processing applications. In general, macros is a series of commands and executions that help automate specific tasks. Regardless of how they are created, they must be executed by a system able to interpret stored commands. Some macro systems are actually self-contained utilities while others are built into more advanced applications that allow users to easily repeat a sequence of commands or enable a programmer to customize the application to suite the user's needs.

A macro virus may be distributed via e-mail, floppy disk, network sharing, a modem and compromised sites on the Internet. Since most macros automatically start when a documented is opened and closed, a macro virus seeks to replace the original with its malicious code. From there, the infection tags the replacement code with the same name and functions when the command is executed which happens when a user accesses the file.

Once opened, the macro virus begins to embed itself within other documents and templates. It also makes preparations to infect any files that will eventually be created. Depending on what resources it is able to access, a macro virus can damage other areas of the operating system. This occurs as the infected documents are shared amongst other users and devices.

One of the most popular variations of this infection is the Melissa virus, first detected in 1999. It spread via e-mail attachment and infected any recipient who opened it. This virus manipulated the victim's address book and distributed itself to numerous e-mail contacts, enabling it to replicate at an alarming rate.

A macro virus has the ability to infect nearly any system running word processing software. This is because it seeks to corrupt that application opposed to the operating system. The virus has been known to attack computers running Mac OS X, Windows and other platforms that are compatible with Microsoft Word.

7. ***e-Mail viruses:*** E-mail viruses are different types of viruses, which use e-mail messages to transport, and can automatically send itself to hundreds, and thousands of people depending on whose e-mail address they victimize. There are certain basic rules that you can follow which will help you to avoid e-mail viruses. Some of them include never open any attachment unless you know the sender and you were expecting it. If you happen to receive a particular e-mail message with an attachment from someone you do not know you should delete it immediately and never open it. Always use antivirus software and remember to constantly check for updates. Always let someone know when you will be sending them an attachment in an e-mail so that they can be expecting it; and always use spam filters to block unwanted and unrecognizable mail.

8. ***Companion viruses:*** Companion viruses can be considered file infector viruses like resident or direct action types. They are known as companion viruses because once they get into the system they "accompany" the other files that already exist. In other words, in order to carry out their infection routines, companion viruses can wait in memory until a program is run (resident viruses) or act immediately by making copies of themselves (direct action viruses).

Companion viruses take advantage of MS-DOS. This virus creates a new file with typically the .COM extensions, but sometimes the .EXD extension as well. When a user manually types in a program they desire without adding .EXE or any other specific extension, DOS will make the assumption that the user wants the file with the extension that comes first in alphabetical order, and thus running the virus. The companion virus is rare among Windows XP computers as this particular operating system does not use the MS-DOS.

9. ***FAT virus:*** FAT12, the oldest version of the File Allocation Table, uses a 12-bit binary system. This type of system is no longer used to format a hard drive as the maximum volume size was quite limited. If a computer running Windows 95 or higher displays the File Allocation Table as FAT12, it is likely that the hard drive is terribly corrupted and may be infected with a virus.

A FAT virus can be rather dangerous as it infects a vital part of the computer's operational process. It has the ability to prevent access to certain sections on the hard drive where important files are located. As the virus spreads its infection, these files or even entire directories can be overwritten and permanently lost.

A common threat to the File Allocation Table is the link virus. Instead of inserting a malicious code directly into infected files, it distributes itself by manipulating the method in which files are accessed by the FAT file system. Once an infected file is executed, a link virus typically slithers into resident memory and writes a hidden file to the disk. Subsequently, it alters the FAT in a way that cross-links other files to a sector of the disk that contains the viral code. As a result, the operating system jumps to the original code and launches it whenever an infected file is run, granting complete control to the virus.

10. ***File infectors:*** This type of virus infects programs or executable files (files with an .EXE or .COM extension). When one of these programs is run, directly or indirectly, the virus is activated, producing the damaging effects it is programmed to carry out. The majority of existing viruses belong to this

category, and can be classified depending on the actions that they carry out.

The following is a list of extensions for files which may be infected by a virus:

Extensions

386, ACE, ACM, ACV, ARC, ARJ, ASD, ASP, AVB, AX, BAT, ,BMP, BIN, BOO, BTM, CAB, CLA, CLASS, CDR, CHM, CMD, CNV, COM, CPL, CPT, CSC, CSS, DAT, DLL, DOC, DOT DRV, DVB, DWG, EML, EXE, FON, GIF, GMS, GVB, HLP, HTA, HTM, HTML, HTA, HTT, INF, INI, JS, JSE, JPG, LNK, MDB, MHT, MHTM, MHTML, MPD, MPP, MPT, MSG, MSI, MSO, NWS, OBD, OBJ, OBT, OBZ, OCX, OFT, PCI, PIF, PL, PPT, PWZ, POT, PRC, QPW, RAR, SCR, SBF, SH, SHB, SHS, SHTML, SHW, SMM, SYS, TAR.GZ, TD0, TGZ, TLB, TSK, TSP, TXT, VBE, VBS, VBX, VOM, VWP, VXE, VXD, WBK, WBT, WIZ, WAV, WPC, WPD, WML, WSH, WSC, XML, XLS, XLT, ZIP

COMPUTER WORMS

What is Computer Worm?

A computer worm is a self-replicating computer program. It uses a network to send copies of itself to other nodes (computers on the network) and it may do so without any user intervention. Unlike a virus, it does not need to attach itself to an existing program. Worms almost always cause at least some harm to the network, if only by consuming bandwidth, whereas viruses almost always corrupt or devour files on a targeted computer.

A computer worm is a program which copies itself across a network. A computer worm differs from a computer virus in that a computer worm can run itself. A virus needs a host program to run, and the virus code runs as part of the host program. A computer worm can spread without a host program, although some modern computer worms also use files to hide inside. The typical computer virus must be activated by way of user intervention. This may include double-clicking on a website link or opening the attachment of an e-mail message. A worm bypasses user intervention by

Table 9.1: Characteristics of viruses

Type of virus	*Characteristics*	*Examples*
Boot viruses	These viruses infect floppy disk boot records or master boot records in hard disks. They replace the boot record program (which is responsible for loading the operating system in memory) copying it elsewhere on the disk or overwriting it. Boot viruses load into memory if the computer tries to read the disk while it is booting.	Form, Disk Killer, Michelangelo and Stone virus
Program viruses	These infect executable program files, such as those with extensions like .BIN, .COM, .EXE, .OVL, .DRV (driver) and .SYS (device driver). These programs are loaded in memory during execution, taking the virus with them. The virus becomes active in memory, making copies of itself and infecting files on disk.	Sunday, Cascade
Multipartite viruses	A hybrid of Boot and Program viruses. They infect program files and when the infected program is executed, these viruses infect the boot record. When you boot the computer next time the virus from the boot record loads in memory and then starts infecting other program files on disk.	Invader, Flip and Tequila
Stealth viruses	These viruses use certain techniques to avoid detection. They may either redirect the disk head to read another sector instead	Frodo, Joshi, Whale

Contd...

Contd...

	of the one in which they reside or they may alter the reading of the infected file's size shown in the directory listing. For instance, the Whale virus adds 9216 bytes to an infected file; then the virus subtracts the same number of bytes (9216) from the size given in the directory.	
Polymorphic viruses	A virus that can encrypt its code in different ways so that it appears differently in each infection. These viruses are more difficult to detect.	Involuntary, Stimulate, Cascade, Phoenix, Evil, Proud, Virus 101
Macro viruses	It is a new type of computer virus that infects the macros within a document or template. When you open a word processing or spreadsheet document, the macro virus is activated and it infects the Normal template (Normal.dot)—a general purpose file that stores default document formatting settings. Every document you open refers to the Normal template, and hence gets infected with the macro virus. Since this virus attaches itself to documents, the infection can spread if such documents are opened on other computers.	DMV, Nuclear, Word Concept, Melissa. A

Contd...

Contd...

FAT viruses	This type of virus attack can be especially dangerous, by preventing access to certain sections of the disk where important files are stored. Damage caused can result in information losses from individual files or even entire directories.	FAT12 virus
Companion viruses	They can wait in memory until a program is run or act immediately by making copies of themselves.	Stator, Asimov.1539, and Terrax.1069
Network viruses	These viruses rapidly spread through LAN and sometimes throughout the Internet. Generally, network viruses multiply through shared resources, i.e. shared drives and folders. When the virus infects a computer, it searches through the network to attack its new potential prey. When the virus finishes infecting that computer, it moves on to the next and the cycle repeats itself	Nimda and SQL Slammer

releasing a document containing the infected macro and distributing itself from computer to computer. A computer virus is generally the more harmful of the two, although worms have been known to cripple entire networks due to multiple.

Well-known examples of computer worm include:

- The original computer worm was (perhaps accidentally) unleashed on the Internet by Robert Tappan Morris in 1988. The Internet worm unix sendmail, Finger, and rsh/rexec to spread itself across the Internet.
- The SQL Slammer worm of 2003 used vulnerability in Microsoft SQL Server 2000 to spread itself across the Internet. The Blaster worm, also of 2003, used vulnerability in Microsoft DCOM RPC to spread itself.
- The Melissa worm of 1999, the Sobig worms of 2003 and the Mydoom worm of 2004 all spread through e-mail. These worms shared some features of a Trojan horse, in that they spread by enticing a user to open an infected e-mail attachment.
- Mydoom also attempted to spread itself through the peer-to-peer file sharing application KaZaA. The Mydoom worms attempted a Denial of Service (DoS) attack against SCO and Microsoft.

The History of Computer Worms

A worm is a program that makes copies of itself and can spread outside your operating system; it can copy itself from one computer to another by using e-mail or another transport mechanism. Worms can damage computer data and security in much the same ways as viruses, but are different from viruses in that they copy themselves from system to system.

Malware with self-replicating capability has been an issue in the world of computing for several years, dating back to the first self-replicating code created by Ken Thompson in 1984. Over the past few years, both worms and viruses have become major problems, mainly due to widespread use of the Internet. This wide open platform enables these infections to spread rapidly with no geographic restrictions. Worms in particular are becoming more sophisticated as malicious coders have learned from their mistakes and successes as well.

Early infections: Self-replicating applications date back to the early days of the Unix operating system. Ken Thompson's code was essentially a compiler modification that manipulated login procedures and the compiler itself. The conventional virus became a common plague in the era of the Apple II system. This infection moved rather slowly, yet provided the means of distributing some of the most known viruses, such as Chernobyl and Michelangelo.

The first Internet infection that required no human intervention to propagate was the Morris Worm, discovered in 1988 and released by Robert Morris. It spread very quickly, infecting a number of vulnerable computers in a matter of hours. The Morris worm infected various machines and also used multiple exploits including buffer overflows, debugging routines in mail components, password sniffing, and other streams of execution to improve its ability to attack other computers.

Modern worms: Active computer worms have returned to prominence in recent times. The first one to cause an eruption was Code Red. This infection proved how quickly a simple self-replicating program could spread via the Internet's current infrastructure. Code Red exploited a buffer flow condition in the Microsoft IIS (Internet Information Server). It was able to propagate quickly because of the "always on" nature of IIS and many versions of the Windows operating system. Code Red was also equipped with scanning capabilities that improved its throughput and gave it the ability to elude numerous IP address security features.

Examples of Computer Worms

1. ***Sober X worm:*** Sober X is known as the most damaging worm of 2005. This is a rapidly spreading infection worked by distributing messages that looked like official e-mail from the FBI and CIA. The contents of the message include a statement

claiming that the government recently discovered that you were viewing illegal sites on the Internet, singling out your computer by its IP address. The message is usually written in English or German. You are then instructed to open an attached file which includes official questions that need to be answered. If the attachment is opened, the computer becomes instantly infected. Sober X has the ability to disable system security settings and a firewall. It can also send mass mailings of similar e-mails to other users found in your address book. Sober X often blocks access to sites hosting malware solutions, such as those by McAfee and Symantec. Unlike the average computer worm, this one can create backdoors and leave a user exposed to various exploits. Exploits like Sober X and others are commonly attempted by numerous malicious programmers. These infections may come disguised as love letters, software, explicit videos and photographs, free screensavers or even Microsoft security patches and program updates.

2. ***Slapper worm:*** The Slapper worm was first discovered in September 2002 on Friday the 13th. It employed a source code propagating method used in the infamous Morris worm, the first computer infection to be labeled as a "blended threat". This program spread so quickly that it infected thousands of servers throughout the world within a matter of days. The Slapper worm took advantage of vulnerabilities in older versions of Apache web servers using peer-to-peer protocol.

Aside from propagating to other machines, the worm has the ability to act as a backdoor on the host computer. This enables a potential intruder to run system commands and launch multiple attacks against other computers, practically giving them complete control of the system. Once created, the backdoor accepts a large number of commands, which may include flooding remote systems with various network packets, downloading binary from a remote system and executing it, sending e-mails, and reporting data on the compromised machine.

3. ***Benevolent worms:*** The widespread use of benevolent worms is a tempting idea for many reasons. One can view it as

a way of fighting off the malicious coders with their own weapons. It could also possibly solve all of those vulnerabilities made visible by the Internet, automatically securing the end-user's system. This could prove to be very useful as today's patching system is not effective as it should be. The fact is that several people, especially home users, simply do not make use of them. In all honesty, efficient all around patching involves a lot of time and labor, something many of us would not find much enjoyment in.

4. ***Lupper worm:*** The Lupper worm spreads by exploiting Apache web servers using PHP/CGI scripts, a programming language known to be more vulnerable than others. This infection is said to be a variant of the Linux Slapper and BSD Scalper worms due to similar propagation techniques. It attacks a web server by transmitting malicious HTTP (Hypertext Transfer Protocol) requests to open ports. The worm downloads and executes itself when the targeted server is running vulnerable scripts at a particular URL. This is enabled by configurations that permit remote file downloads in PHP/CGI and external shell commands. Its most alarming function involves creating a backdoor on the compromised server. The worm then generates URLs, which initiate a scan to seek out other machines for infection. Additionally, the Lupper worm has the ability to harvest e-mail addresses as well.

5. ***Morris worm:*** In 1988, Robert Morris was a 23 years old graduate student at Cornell University. He wrote the first Internet worm in 99 lines of the C language. According to Morris, the program was simply an experiment to enable a single machine to access as many computers as possible. The worm was designed to detect existing copies of itself on infected computers, not to reinfect them. Although the program was not specifically written to destroy files or damage a system, Morris stated that it was designed to break into a system and thieve passwords.

Robert Morris released the worm on November 2, 1988. It was distributed from MIT to disguise the fact that he was a student at Cornell University. Unfortunately, the worm contained a bug, and the part of it that was intended not to reinfect a machine harboring the worm did not function properly. As a result, many systems became infected with numerous copies of the worm, each attempting to break into sensitive accounts and propagate more programs. The infected systems soon crashed or became totally inoperable. Restarting the machines did nothing, and terminating the worm process was useless, as they simply continued to propagate. The only solution was to disconnect the computer from the Internet. It is reported that Morris and his unnamed friend sent an anonymous message describing how the worm could be killed and how to patch vulnerable machines.

6. ***MyDoom worm:*** The MyDoom worm was first discovered on January 26th, 2004. It goes by many different names depending on the antivirus company, including Novag, Shimg or Mimail. Similar to most worms, MyDoom manipulates the e-mail system, which has caused many innocent users to be blamed for distributing it. What contributed to the widespread of the worm was the numerous security alerts sent out by antivirus vendors. The alerting issue arouse from infected e-mails being detected by the Internet Service Provider or the antivirus vendor's domain. Depending on an administrator's configurations, the antivirus solution could send alerts to recipients and the alleged sender.

The problem is that the sender's name was falsified, causing a lot of innocent users to be accused of sending the worm, even if they were never infected. The situation with MyDoom only became more confusing and chaotic as the infection continued spread. Several antivirus products distributed messages infected with the worm to the alleged sender, thus infecting them with MyDoom if they opened the e-mail attachment. The amount of antivirus alerts became so great that it quickly superceded the actual number of MyDoom e-mails. Some have even speculated that these alerts themselves were actually a form of DoS (denial-of-service) attack.

MyDoom distributes itself via e-mail and the popular peer-to-peer network known as KaZaZ. The e-mail is typically spoofed with both a sender name and one of the subject lines: Hi, Hello, Error, Test, Mail Delivery System, Mail Transaction

Failed, Server Report Status. The file attachment comes with a CMD., EXE., PIF. or SCR file extension or it may come as an archived ZIP file.

To hide its activity, MyDoom launches the Notepad application when executed, filling the victim's screen with random text characters. It then secretly drops an infected copy into the Windows System folder as an executable. MyDoom also searches the registry in search of KaZaA. If the program is installed, it drops an infected copy into the KaZaA shared folder using various executable extensions. This enables it to infect KaZaA users who download and unknowingly execute one of the files.

7. ***Nimda worm:*** Nimda is another one of many worms to infect the vulnerable Windows operating system. Its method of propagation is rather unique, as it can be distributed via e-mail or a malware infected website. Nimda also seeks out vulnerable web servers to upload malicious code, giving it the ability to infect an entire network. What makes it more complex is the fact that it is the first worm to behave like a virus by infecting other files. The normal behavior of a worm is to only replicate itself and propagate throughout a hard drive or to other machines via e-mail. Nimda is able to spread quickly inserting its code into EXE. (executable) files on local drives.

TROJAN HORSES

It is a program that masquerades as another common program in an attempt to receive information. A Trojan horse is a harmless-looking program designed to trick you into thinking it is something you want, but which performs harmful acts when it runs. It is typically received through downloads from the Internet. Trojan horses do not spread by themselves like viruses and worms. Most virus protection programs only detect a limited number of Trojan horses.

An example of a Trojan horse is a program that behaves like a system logon to retrieve user names and password information that the writers of the Trojan horse can later use to break into the system. A good way to help protect your computer from Trojan horses is to visit only websites you trust, and avoid downloading things unless you trust the source as well.

A Trojan horse is a hidden program which secretly runs commands, and usually opens up access to the computer running it by opening a backdoor. Like a virus, a Trojan horse is a piece of harmful code placed within a healthy program (like a false file-listing command, which destroys files instead of displaying the list). A Trojan horse may, for example, steal passwords, copy sensitive date, carry out any other harmful operations, etc. The most common Trojan horses open machine ports, allowing their designer to gain entry to your computer over the network by opening a backdoor or backorifice.

Trojan horse attacks pose one of the most serious threats to computer security. Trojans are executable programs, which means that when you open the file, it will perform some action(s). In Windows, executable programs have file extensions like "exe", "vbs", "com", "bat", etc. Some actual Trojan filenames include: "dmsetup.exe" and "LOVE-LETTER-FOR-YOU.TXT.vbs" (when there are multiple extensions, only the last one counts, be sure to unhide your extensions so that you see it). Trojans can be spread in the guise of literally anything people find desirable, such as a free game, movie, song, etc. Victims typically downloaded the Trojan from a WWW or FTP archive, got it via peer-to-peer file exchange using IRC/instant messaging/Kazaa, etc. or just carelessly opened some e-mail attachment. Trojans usually do their damage silently.

Trojan horses are designed to allow a hacker remote access to a target computer system. Once a Trojan horse has been installed on a target computer system it is possible for a hacker to access it remotely and perform operations. Infection by a Trojan horse usually comes after opening a contaminated file containing the Trojan horse and is indicated by the following symptoms:

- ***Abnormal activity by the modem, network adapter or hard drive:*** Data is being loaded without any activity from the user;

- Strange reactions from the mouse;
- Programs opening unexpectedly;
- Repeated crashes.

As a Trojan horse is usually and increasingly intended to open a port on computer machine so that a hacker can gain control of it (such as by stealing personal data stored on the hard drive), the hacker's goal is to first infect your machine by making you open an infected file containing the Trojan and then to access your machine through the opened port. Trojan horses commonly open a port on the infected machine and wait for a connection to open on that port, so that hackers will be able to gain total control over the computer (Table 9.2).

LOGIC BOMBS

A logic bomb is a program which has deliberately been written or modified to produce results when certain conditions are met that are unexpected and unauthorized by legitimate users or owners of the software. Thus, it is a program that masquerades as another common program in an attempt to receive information. The most common activator for a logic bomb is a date. The logic bomb checks the system date and does nothing until a preprogrammed date and time is reached. At that point, the logic bomb activates and executes its code.

A logic bomb could also be programmed to wait for a certain message from the programmer. The logic bomb could, for example, check a website once a week for a certain message. When the logic bomb sees that message, or when the logic bomb stops seeing that message, it activates and executes its code. A logic bomb can also be programmed to activate on a wide variety of other variables, such as when a database grows past a certain size or a user's home directory is deleted.

Logic bombs may reside within stand-alone programs or they may be part of worms (programs that hide their existence and spread copies of themselves within a computer system and through networks) or viruses (programs or code segments which hide within other programs and spread copies of themselves). An example of a logic bomb is any program that

Table 9.2: List of ports commonly used by Trojans

Port	*Trojan*
21	Back construction, Blade runner, Doly, Fore, FTP Trojan, Invisible FTP, Larva, WebEx, WinCrash
23	TTS (Tiny Telnet Server)
25	Ajan, Antigen, E-mail Password Sender, Happy 99, Kuang 2, ProMail Trojan, Shtrilitz, Stealth, Tapiras, Terminator, WinPC, WinSpy
31	Agent 31, Hackers Paradise, Masters Paradise
41	Deep Throat
59	DMSetup
79	FireHotcker
80	Executor, RingZero
99	Hidden port
110	ProMail Trojan
113	Kazimas
119	Happy 99
121	JammerKillah
421	TCP Wrappers
456	Hackers Paradise
531	Rasmin
555	Ini-Killer, NetAdmin, Phase Zero, Stealth Spy
666	Attack FTP, Back Construction, Cain and Abel, Satanz Backdoor, ServeU, Shadow Phyre
911	Dark Shadow
999	Deep Throat, WinSatan
1002	Silencer, WebEx
1010 to 1015	Doly Trojan
1024	NetSpy
1042	Bla
1045	Rasmin
1090	Xtreme
1170	Psyber Stream Server, Streaming Audio Trojan, voice

Contd...

Contd...

1234	Ultor Trojan
port 1234	Ultors Trojan
port 1243	BackDoor-G, SubSeven, SubSeven Apocalypse
port 1245	VooDoo Doll
port 1269	Mavericks Matrix
port 1349 (UDP)	BO DLL
port 1492	FTP99CMP
port 1509	Psyber Streaming Server
port 1600	Shivka-Burka
port 1807	SpySender
port 1981	Shockrave
port 1999	BackDoor
port 1999	TransScout
port 2000	TransScout
port 2001	TransScout
port 2001	Trojan Cow
port 2002	TransScout
port 2003	TransScout
port 2004	TransScout
port 2005	TransScout
port 2023	Ripper
port 2115	Bugs
port 2140	Deep Throat, The Invasor
port 2155	Illusion Mailer
port 2283	HVL Rat5
port 2565	Striker
port 2583	WinCrash
port 2600	Digital RootBeer
port 2801	Phineas Phucker
port 2989 (UDP)	RAT
port 3024	WinCrash
port 3128	RingZero

Contd...

Contd...

port 3129	Masters Paradise
port 3150	Deep Throat, The Invasor
port 3459	Eclipse 2000
port 3700	portal of Doom
port 3791	Eclypse
port 3801 (UDP)	Eclypse
port 4092	WinCrash
port 4321	BoBo
port 4567	File Nail
port 4590	ICQTrojan
port 5000	Bubbel, Back Door Setup, Sockets de Troie
port 5001	Back Door Setup, Sockets de Troie
port 5011	One of the Last Trojans (OOTLT)
port 5031	NetMetro
port 5321	FireHotcker
port 5400	Blade Runner, Back Construction
port 5401	Blade Runner, Back Construction
port 5402	Blade Runner, Back Construction
port 5550	Xtcp
port 5512	Illusion Mailer
port 5555	ServeMe
port 5556	BO Facil
port 5557	BO Facil
port 5569	Robo-Hack
port 5742	WinCrash
port 6400	The Thing
port 6669	Vampyre
port 6670	Deep Throat
port 6771	Deep Throat
port 6776	BackDoor-G, SubSeven
port 6912	Shit Heep (not port 69123!)
port 6939	Indoctrination

Contd...

Contd...

port 6969	GateCrasher, Priority, IRC 3
port 6970	GateCrasher
port 7000	Remote Grab, Kazimas
port 7300	NetMonitor
port 7301	NetMonitor
port 7306	NetMonitor
port 7307	NetMonitor
port 7308	NetMonitor
port 7789	Back Door Setup, ICKiller
port 8080	RingZero
port 9400	InCommand
port 9872	portal of Doom
port 9873	portal of Doom
port 9874	portal of Doom
port 9875	portal of Doom
port 9876	Cyber Attacker
port 9878	TransScout
port 9989	iNi-Killer
port 10067 (UDP)	portal of Doom
port 10101	BrainSpy
port 10167 (UDP)	portal of Doom
port 10520	Acid Shivers
port 10607	Coma
port 11000	Senna Spy
port 11223	Progenic Trojan
port 12076	Gjamer
port 12223	Hack´99 KeyLogger
port 12345	GabanBus, NetBus, Pie Bill Gates, X-bill
port 12346	GabanBus, NetBus, X-bill
port 12361	Whack-a-mole
port 12362	Whack-a-mole
port 12631	WhackJob

Contd...

Contd...

port 13000	Senna Spy
port 16969	Priority
port 17300	Kuang2 The Virus
port 20000	Millennium
port 20001	Millennium
port 20034	NetBus 2 Pro
port 20203	Logged
port 21544	GirlFriend
port 22222	Prosiak
port 23456	Evil FTP, Ugly FTP, Whack Job
port 23476	Donald Dick
port 23477	Donald Dick
port 26274 (UDP)	Delta Source
port 27374	SubSeven 2.0
port 29891 (UDP)	The Unexplained
port 30029	AOL Trojan
port 30100	NetSphere
port 30101	NetSphere
port 30102	NetSphere
port 30303	Sockets de Troie
port 30999	Kuang2
port 31336	Bo Whack
port 31337	Baron Night, BO client, BO2, Bo Facil
port 31337 (UDP)	BackFire, Back Orifice, DeepBO
port 31338	NetSpy DK
port 31338 (UDP)	Back Orifice, DeepBO
port 31339	NetSpy DK
port 31666	Bo Whack
port 31785	Hack´a´Tack
port 31787	Hack´a´Tack
port 31788	Hack´a´Tack
port 31789 (UDP)	Hack´a´Tack

Contd...

Contd...

port 31791 (UDP)	Hack´a´Tack
port 31792	Hack´a´Tack
port 33333	Prosiak
port 33911	Spirit 2001a
port 34324	BigGluck, TN
port 40412	The Spy
port 40421	Agent 40421, Masters Paradise
port 40422	Masters Paradise
port 40423	Masters Paradise
port 40426	Masters Paradise
port 47262 (UDP)	Delta Source
port 50505	Sockets de Troie
port 50766	Fore, Schwindler
port 53001	Remote Windows Shutdown
port 54320	Back Orifice 2000
port 54321	School Bus
port 54321 (UDP)	Back Orifice 2000
port 60000	Deep Throat
port 61466	Telecommando
port 65000	Devil

mysteriously stops working three months after, say, its programmer's name has disappeared from the corporate salary database.

The most dangerous form of the logic bomb is a logic bomb that activates when something does not happen. Imagine a suspicious and unethical system administrator who creates a logic bomb which deletes all of the data on a server if he does not log in for a month. The system administrator programs the logic bomb with this logic because he knows that if he is fired, he won't be able to get back into the system to set his logic bomb. One day on his way to work, our suspicious and unethical system administrator is hit by a bus. Three weeks later, his logic bomb goes off and the server is wiped clean. The system administrator meant for the logic bomb to explode if he was fired; he did not foresee that he would be hit by a bus.

Because a logic bomb does not replicate itself, it is very easy to write a logic bomb program. This also means that a logic bomb will not spread to unintended victims. In some ways, a logic bomb is the most civilized programmed threat, because a logic bomb must be targeted against a specific victim.

SPYWARE

Spyware is a general term used to describe software that performs certain behaviors such as advertising, collecting personal information, or changing the configuration of your computer, generally without appropriately obtaining your consent first. Spyware is often associated with software that displays advertisements (called adware) or software that tracks personal or sensitive information. These programs can change your web browsers home page or search page, or add additional components to your browser you do not need or want. These programs also make it very difficult for you to change your settings back to the way you originally had them.

Spyware is any software designed to collect user personal information and send it out through a background Internet connection without the user's knowledge and consent. Spyware silently tracks user's web browsing habits, records visited websites and logs taken actions. This activity allows spyware vendors to gather data for marketing and advertising purposes. Spyware form and functionality may vary depending on vendor intentions. However, a particular program that uses an Internet connection to transfer data, which can be used to identify the user, is always classified as spyware.

Spyware are programs, cookies, or registry entries that track your activity and send that data off to someone who collects this data for their own purposes. Spyware is usually installed quietly, or even secretly, when you install shareware applications. Many people feel that spyware is a violation of their privacy. Excessive spyware programs can slow down your Internet connection by filling the line with their traffic. They can also slow down your computer by using up available RAM and CPU cycles.

Spyware parasites differ from regular viruses. They do not spread by themselves and usually must be installed as any other software with or without the user's consent. Some rare pests are able to exploit system security vulnerabilities and act similarly to worms. There are three major ways undesirable spyware program can get into the system:

1. Many spyware vendors deceive the user by presenting a particular spyware program as a useful tool, for example, a powerful web search service, fast download manager or reliable Internet accelerator. Users download and install such programs. However, practically all of them appear to be either completely useless or ineffective. Although in most cases users can uninstall such programs, spyware components stay in the system and remain fully functional.

2. Lots of free, ad-supported or shareware products are bundled with small add-ons needed by the host program to work properly. These add-ons actually are third-party spyware parasites. Uninstalling the host application not always removes bundled spyware.

3. Most widely spread spyware programs get into the system using Internet Explorer ActiveX controls or exploiting certain web browser vulnerabilities. Their vendors run insecure web-sites filled with malicious code or distribute unsafe advertising pop-ups. Whenever the user visits such a site or clicks on such a pop-up, harmful scripts instantly install spyware. The user cannot notice anything suspicious, as parasites do not display any setup wizards, dialogs or warnings.

There are thousands of different spyware parasites. The following examples illustrate how treacherous and harmful spyware can be.

- CoolWebSearch is the entire family of browser hijackers that all attempt to redirect a web browser to the coolwebsearch.com domain. Most of these threats display advertisements, change web browser's default start and search pages and modify security settings. From the first sight,

CoolWebSearch parasites are relatively harmless. However, some variants are able to steal user passwords, bank account details and other identity data. These pests are virtually impossible to remove.

- Gator spyware made the headlines because of its enormous prevalence. Various Gator variants are still bundled with ad-supported software and can get into the system from insecure websites. Parasites display numerous advertisements and install additional spyware components without user consent. Most of their victims noticed increased frequency of web browser crashes and overall system instability. Practically all Gator variants include parts that stay active even after a user uninstalls the pest.
- BonziBuddy spyware is targeted at children. Its description says that the program displays an animated on-screen ape that helps kids to surf the web and use e-mail. However, BonziBuddy also silently installs several additional spyware parasites that not only violate user privacy, but also affect computer's performance and security.

ADWARE

Adware is any software package which automatically plays, displays, or downloads advertisements to a computer after the software is installed on it or while the application is being used. Some types of adware are also spyware and can be classified as privacy-invasive software.

Adware is a close relative of spyware. Adware is software that is installed on your computer to show you advertisements. Adware can slow your PC by using RAM and CPU cycles. Adware can also slow your Internet connection by using bandwidth to retrieve advertisements. In addition, adware can increase the instability of your system because many adware applications are not programmed well.

Not all adware is bad. Many useful programs are able to be distributed for free because the ads they display pay for their development. The Opera web browser and the KaZaA peer-to-peer file sharing clients are good examples of such applications. Good adware only installs itself on your system if you give it permission to do so. Bad adware installs itself without your permission. Good adware allows itself to be uninstalled, often through the Add and Remove button in the Microsoft Windows control panel. Bad adware makes it difficult or even impossible for you to uninstall it. Good adware displays unobtrusive ads inside the applications which it comes packaged with. Bad adware installs itself within other applications and often hijacks your web browser settings to display more ads.

SPAM

Spam is unsolicited e-mail which is sent in massive quantities to unsuspecting Internet e-mail users. Most spam tries to sell products and services such as mortage refinancing, memberships to pornograpic websites, and drugs such as Viagra. A more dangerous category of spam tries to convince the recipient to share their bank account numbers, credit card numbers, or logins and passwords to their online banking systems or services such as eBay and PayPal. Not all spam is commercial. Some spam is simply criminal, while other spammers send unrequested e-mails attempting to share their political or religious views.

There are a number of ways spammers harvest your e-mail address. Here are some of the more common ways:

- Message boards
- Guest books
- Forwarding e-mail
- Webmaster address on site
- Form mailers
- Registrar records
- Common e-mail addresses
- Auto responders/vacation messages.

A spam filter is a software application which is installed either on a mail server or a mail client. E-mail administrators typically install spam filtering software on mail servers. By far the best spam filtering software for mail servers is Spam

Assassin. Spam Assassin is a free product of the Apache Project. Microsoft Outlook is currently the most popular e-mail client software in use. As of Outlook 2003, Outlook now ships with a reasonably good spam filter. Many companies sell software designed to improve the Microsoft Outlook spam filter.

ROOTKITS

Rootkits can be named the most technically sophisticated form of malicious code (malware) and one of the most difficult to discover and eliminate. Of all types of malware, probably viruses and worms get the most publicity because they are generally widespread. Many people are known to have been affected by a virus or a worm, but this definitely does not mean that viruses and worms are the most destructive variety of malware. There are more dangerous types of malware, because as a rule they operate in stealth mode, are difficult to detect and remove and can go unnoticed for very long periods of time, silently gaining access, stealing data, and modifying the files on the victim's machine.

An example of such a stealthly enemy is rootkits, i.e. a collection of tools that can replace or change executable programs, or even the kernel of the operating system itself, in order to gain administrator-level access to the system, which can be used for installing spyware, keyloggers and other malicious tools. Essentially, a rootkit allows an attacker to gain complete access over the victim's machine (and possibly to the whole network the machine belongs to).

Similar to Trojan horses, viruses and worms, rootkits install themselves by exploiting flaws in the network security and operating system, often with no user interaction. Although there are rootkits that can come as an e-mail attachment or in a bundle with a legitimate software programs, they are harmless until the user opens the attachment or installs the program. But unlike less sophisticated forms of malware, rootkits infiltrate very deep into the operating system and make special efforts to disguise their presence, for instance, by modifying system files.

Basically, there are two types of rootkits:

1. ***Kernel level rootkits:*** They add code to or modify the kernel of the operating system. This is achieved by installing a device driver or a loadable module, which alters system calls to hide the presence of an attacker. Thus, if you look in your log files, you will see no suspicious activity on the system.

2. ***Application level rootkits:*** They are less sophisticated and generally are easier to detect because they modify the executables of applications, rather than the operating system itself. Since Windows 2000 reports every change of an executable file to the user, it makes it more difficult for the attacker to go unnoticed.

Rootkits can act as a backdoor and are usually not alone in their mission; they are often accompanied by spyware, Trojan horses or viruses. The aims of a rootkit can vary from simple malicious joy of penetrating somebody else's computer (and hiding the traces of foreign presence) to building a whole system for illegally obtaining confidential data.

PROTECTION OF COMPUTER AND NETWORK FROM MALWARES

An unprotected computer is a vulnerable computer, plain and simple. Every year there are hundreds of viruses, Trojans, worms and other malware, released into cyberspace designed to harm your computer. Antivirus companies are beginning to pay attention to malware.

Network security is a level of guarantee that all the machines in a network are working optimally and the users of these machines only possess the rights that were granted to them. This can include:

- Preventing unauthorized people from acting on the system maliciously.
- Preventing users from performing involuntary operations that are capable of harming the system.
- Securing data by anticipating failures.
- Guaranteeing that services are not interrupted.

1. ***Protection and removal of computer viruses:*** The best way to protect your system from these viruses and virus writers is to be aware. Upload and use antivirus software programs to keep your computer safe and secure. When you receive e-mails, be aware of what you open even if it is from people you know. A majority of viruses are transmitted via e-mails and you should take great precaution when you receive attachments and forwarded e-mails. If you were not expecting an e-mail or receive an e-mail from someone whom you do not recognize, delete it right away.

Another way to protect your computer from viruses is to check for updates for all your antivirus software programs regularly. It is very important that you update your antivirus software so that it can recognize new viruses. If you do not update, your program will not recognize new viruses. So, updating your software regularly is very important if you want your computer to be free from viruses.

Finally, be sure to check if you have installed your antivirus software correctly on your computer. Many people fail to check and sometimes find that their programs do not work at all on their computer.

2. ***Protection from computer worms:*** From updating your security software to being aware of the e-mails in your inbox, there are many steps you can take to protect yourself and your computer from worms and viruses. One of the most important and simplest ways to protect yourself from computer worms is by being careful and aware of what kind of e-mails and attachments you receive what you open and whom it is from.

If you are not expecting an e-mail or do not recognize the person, then the best idea would be to delete it right away and forget about it. Another step you can take to protect your computer is to regularly update your antivirus software. Make sure that you are using the most up-to-date and enhanced version of your software, so it can catch all those new viruses and worms out there. Also, make sure to check if your software is installed correctly. Finally, when you use e-mail programs, use the ones that have built in spam filters, for instance, Outlook

Express, Windows Hotmail and so on. This way, not only will the e-mail be tracked and filtered for viruses, but you will also feel secure that your computer is free from worms and viruses.

3. ***Protection and removal of Trojan horse:*** Installing a firewall (a program which filters data entering and leaving your machine) is enough to protect you from this kind of intrusion. A firewall monitors both data leaving your machine (normally initiated by the programs you are using) and data entering it. However, the firewall may detect unknown outside connections even if a hacker is not specifically targeting you. They may be tests carried out by your Internet service provider, or a hacker randomly scanning a range of IP addresses. For Windows systems, there are two free high-performance firewalls:

- Zone Alarm.
- Tiny personal firewall.

Antivirus software is designed to detect and delete Trojan horses ideally preventing them from ever being installed. It may be possible to remove a Trojan horse manually given a full understanding of how that particular Trojan horse operates, however, if it is possible that a Trojan horse has been used by a hacker to access a computer system it will be difficult to know what damage has been done and what other problems have been introduced. In situations where the security of the computer system is critical it is advisable to rebuild it from known good software.

If a program whose origins you are unsure of, attempts to open a connection, the firewall will ask you to confirm it before initiating the connection. It is important not to authorize connections for a program you do not recognize, because it might very well be a Trojan horse. If this reoccurs, it may be helpful to check that your computer is not affected by a Trojan, by using a program that detects and deletes them (called an anti-Trojan). One example is The Cleaner.

4. ***Protection and removal of spyware:*** One of the ways to defend against spyware is to use a third party firewall. Although the current version of Windows XP comes with a

firewall it is not effective at stopping spyware as of this writing. Third party firewalls can block unwanted traffic from passing to and from the internet to your computer. Some of the better third party firewalls are listed below:

- Kerio Personal Firewall.
- Zone Alarm Firewall.
- Sygate Firewall.

Firewalls are effective at stopping many spyware programs as well as other potential problems but they are not a cure all. To be more effective you will want to use antispyware software along with your firewall.

Some of the top antispyware programs are Webroot Spy Sweeper, Spyware Doctor, Ad-Aware SE Personal Edition, GIANT Antispyware and Spybot-Search and Destroy. Major antivirus firms such as Symantec, McAfee and Sophos have come later to the table, adding antispyware features to their existing antivirus products. Microsoft Antispyware, in real-time protection blocks an instance of the AlwaysUpdateNews from being installed.

Antispyware programs can combat spyware in two ways:

- They can provide real time protection against the installation of spyware software on your computer. This type of spyware protection works the same way as that of antivirus protection in that the antispyware software scans all incoming network data for spyware software and blocks any threats it comes across.

- Antispyware software programs can be used solely for detection and removal of spyware software that has already been installed onto your computer. This type of spyware protection is normally much easier to use and more popular. With this spyware protection software you can schedule weekly, daily, or monthly scans of your computer to detect and remove any spyware software that has been installed on your computer. This type of antispyware software scans the contents of the windows registry, operating system files, and installed programs on your computer and will provide a list of any threats found, allowing you to choose what you want to delete and what you want to keep.

5. ***Detection and removal of rootkits:*** Not those other types of malware are easy to detect and remove, but kernel level rootkits are a particular disaster. In a sense, it is a Catch 22, if you have a rootkit, then the system files needed by the anti-rootkit software are likely to be modified and therefore, the results of the check cannot be trusted. What's more, if a rootkit is running, it can successfully modify the list of files or list of running processes that antivirus programs rely on, thus providing fake data. Also, a running rootkit can simply unload antivirus program processes from memory, causing the application to shutdown or terminate unexpectedly. However, by doing this it indirectly shows its presence, so one can get suspicious when something goes wrong, especially with software that maintains system security.

A recommended way for detection of the presence of a rootkit is to boot from an alternative medium, which is known to be clean (i.e. a backup, or rescue CD-ROM) and check the suspicious system. The advantage of this method is that the rootkit will not be running (therefore, it will not be able to hide itself) and the system files will not be actively tampered.

ANTIVIRUS SOFTWARE

Characteristics of Antivirus Software

Malware is an umbrella term for all malicious software. The most common are viruses and spyware. An antivirus program is software which can detect the presence of a virus on a computer and, to the best of its abilities, remove the virus. Eradicating a virus is the term used for cleaning out a computer. There are several methods of eradication:

- Removing the code in the infected file which corresponds to the virus.
- Removing the infected file.
- Quarantining the infected file, which involves moving it to a location where it cannot be run.

Antivirus software should be easy enough for a computer user to both install and uninstall. The software should effectively seek out and identify virus threats, as well as clean or isolate infected files. There should be understandable reporting available for each scan and plenty of help support available, so you can be well-informed of the software's activities and capabilities. The following are the important characteristics that antivirus software should possess:

1. ***Ease of use:*** Antivirus software is simple to use, regardless of a user's computer experience or knowledge of viruses. The software should be easy to install and configure. The best antivirus software is the kind you simply install on your system and then let it do its work.

2. ***Effective at identifying viruses and worms:*** The best antivirus software identifies infected files quickly through real-time scanning, searching for viruses in a multitude of sources, including e mail, instant message applications, web browsing, etc. Scanning speed is also important. Slow antivirus software will tend to interfere with your work or gaming, and if it is very slow or you are particularly impatient, you might have the tendency to stop or pause the scan, rendering the software useless. Generally, antivirus software scans hard drive and files looking for known viruses.

3. ***Effective at cleaning or isolating infected files:*** Truly capable antivirus software thoroughly cleans, deletes or quarantines infected files, keeping them from spreading throughout the hard drive or network. Proactive/heuristic testing enables the antivirus software to detect and quarantine code that looks and acts like a virus even before it has been reported. This could be critical in protecting you on a "Day Zero" attack and spare you from being one of the first casualties.

4. ***Activity reporting:*** Antivirus programs should give immediate notification of viruses found by real-time scanners and should provide an easy to read report of scan results, including what was found and what was done with infected files.

5. ***Feature set:*** A well-rounded feature set allows antivirus software to provide absolute protection. The best programs

are those that offer a wide variety of tools, from basic real-time scanning to more advanced heuristic scanning and script blocking. When it comes to virus protection, the more options the better. Many of the best antivirus packages now include multiple protection schemes at no extra cost. These include antispyware, antimalware, rootkit detection, parental controls and e-mail screening, as many of the new threats are not literally viruses, but rather a variety of malware.

6. ***Ease of installation and setup:*** Antivirus programs should be a breeze to install, making it easy to go from installation to initial scan in just a couple clicks of the mouse.

7. ***Help documentation:*** High-end antivirus software comes with plenty of help, including support via e-mail, online chat or via telephone. There should also be online resources, such as knowledge bases and FAQs available for quick and convenient help.

Detecting a Virus by Software

Viruses reproduce by infecting "host application" meaning that they copy a portion of executable code into an existing program. So to ensure that they work as planned; viruses are programmed to not infect the same file multiple times. To do so, they include a series of bytes in the infected application to check if has already been infected: This is called a virus signature.

Antivirus programs rely on this signature, which is unique to each virus, in order to detect them. This method is called signature scanning, the oldest method used by antivirus software.

This method is only reliable if the antivirus program's virus database is up-to-date and includes signatures for all-known viruses. However, this method cannot detect viruses which have not been archived by the publishers of the antivirus software. What is more, virus programmers have often given them camouflage features, making their signature hard to detect, if not undetectable such as polymorphic viruses.

Some antivirus programs use an integrity checker to tell if the folders have been changed. The integrity checker builds a database containing information on the executable files on the system (date modified, file size, and possibly a checksum). That way, when an executable file's characteristics change, the antivirus program warns the machine's user.

The heuristic method involves analyzing the behaviour of applications in order to detect activity similar to that of a known virus. This kind of antivirus program can, therefore, detect viruses even when the antivirus database has not been updated. On the other hand, they are prone to triggering false alarms.

Installing trusted antivirus / spyware tools and keeping them and their signatures current is an important part of defensive computer security. Using real-time antivirus and antispyware tools and scanning applications manually prior to their execution can help locate and identify many threats before they are able to infect systems and become problems. Table 9.3 lists examples of antivirus software.

Features of Some Antivirus Software

1. ***AVG antivirus pro:*** AVG is focused on providing home and business computer users with the most comprehensive and proactive protection against computer security threats. This gives you maximum protection with real-time scanning, automatic updates, low-impact background scanning for online threats, and instant quarantining or removal of infected files ensures maximum protection. With AVG software on your system, you can safely surf the net, create online profiles, shop, bank online, download files, store data, chat, and e-mail, safe in the knowledge that your personal and professional information will not be stolen or misused.

- ***Antivirus and antispyware:*** Protection against viruses, spyware, adware and Trojans.
- ***LinkScanner active surf-shield:*** Protects in real-time against poisoned web pages while you are surfing.
- ***LinkScanner search-shield:*** Real-time safety ratings for all search results in Google, Yahoo and MSN / Live search.

Table 9.3: Examples of antivirus software

Antivirus software	*Windows*	*Mac OS X*	*Linux*	*Free BSD*	*Unix*	*On-demand scan*	*On-access scan*	*Boot-time scan*
AOL Active Virus Shield	Yes	No	No	No	No	Yes	Yes	No
Avast! Home Edition	Yes	No	Yes	No	No	Yes	Yes	Yes
Avast! Professional Edition	Yes	Yes	Yes	No	No	Yes	Yes	Yes
AVG Antivirus	Yes	No	Yes	Yes	No	Yes	Yes	No
Avira Antivir Premium	Yes	No	Yes	Yes	Yes	Yes	Yes	No
BitDefender	Yes	Yes (beta)	Yes	Yes	No	Yes	Yes	No
BullGuard	Yes	No	No	No	No	Yes	Yes	No
CA Antivirus	Yes	Yes	Yes	No	Yes	Yes		No
Clam Antivirus	Yes	Yes	Yes	Yes	Yes	Yes	Only on Free BSD and Linux	No
Comodo Antivirus	Yes	No	No	No	No	Yes	Yes	Yes
Dr. Web	Yes	Yes	Yes	Yes	Yes	Yes	Yes	No
F-Prot	Yes	No	Yes	Yes	Yes	Yes	Yes	No
F-Secure	Yes	No	Yes	No	No	Yes	Yes	No
Fortinet FortiClient End Point Security	Yes	No	No	No	No	Yes	Yes	No

Contd...

Contd...

G DATA Software	Yes	No	No	No	No	Yes	Yes	No
Kaspersky Antivirus	Yes	Yes (beta)	Yes	Yes	Yes	Yes	Yes	No
McAfee VirusScan	Yes	Yes	Yes	Yes	Yes	Yes	Yes	No
ESET NOD32	Yes	No	Yes	Yes	Yes	Yes	Yes	No
Norman	Yes	No	Yes	No	No	Yes	Yes	No
Panda Antivirus	Yes	No	Yes	No	No	Yes	Yes	No
Panda Cloud Antivirus	Yes	No	Yes	No	No	Yes	Yes	No
PC Tools Antivirus	Yes	Yes	No	No	No	Yes	Yes	No
Sophos Antivirus	Yes	Yes	Yes	Yes	Yes	Yes	Yes	No
Symantec Norton AntiVirus/Norton 360	Yes	Yes	Yes	Yes	Yes	Yes	Yes	No
Trend Micro Internet Security	Yes	Yes	No	No	No	Yes	Yes	Yes
The Hacker	Yes	No	Yes	No	Yes	Yes	Yes	Yes
Vba32Antivirus	Yes	No	Yes	Yes	No	Yes	Only on Windows	No
Sunbelt Software VIPRE Antivirus + Antispyware	Yes	No	No	No	No	Yes	Yes	No
VirusBuster	Yes	No	Yes	Yes	Yes	Yes	Yes	No
ZoneAlarm Antivirus	Yes	No	No	No	No	Yes	Yes	No

- ***AVG security toolbar:*** Easy access to LinkScanner tools, built-in search capability.
- ***Web shield:*** Screens your downloads and prevents accidental infections through IM chats.
- ***Anti-rootkit:*** Protection against hidden threats that deliver malicious content.
- ***Free support:*** Free support and service around the clock and across the globe.

2. ***Avast! Antivirus Home Edition:*** It is a full-featured antivirus package designed exclusively for non-commercial and home use only. Antivirus Home Edition includes antispyware protection, certified by the West Coast Labs Checkmark process, and anti-rootkit detection based on the best-in class GMER technology.

- Antispyware built-in
- Anti-rootkit built-in
- Strong self-protection
- Antivirus kernel
- Simple user interface
- Standard resident protection
- Network shield
- Web shield
- Automatic updates
- Virus chest
- System integration
- Virus cleaner
- Support for 64-bit windows
- It is offered in over 30 language versions.

3. ***BitDefender:*** BitDefender provides security solutions to satisfy the protection requirements of today's computing environment, delivering effective threat management in more than 100 countries.

- Features antivirus, firewall, antispyware, antispam and parental control for corporate and home users.

- Minimal impact on system performance.
- Easy to use, with an installation wizard that guides users through the installation process.
- Lightning fast response time to new computer attacks.
- Best detection rate.
- Hourly Internet updates of virus signatures—automatic or scheduled actions offering protection against the newest viruses.
- Round the clock customer care.
- Worldwide distribution, products available in 18 languages.

4. ***Symantec Norton Antivirus/Norton 360:*** It is a comprehensive, automated antivirus and antispyware protection software.

- Antivirus
- Spyware protection
- Antiphishing
- Network security
- Botnet protection
- Rootkit detection
- Browser protection
- Internet worm protection
- Antispam
- Recovery tool
- Norton protection system
- OS and application protection.

5. ***Kaspersky Antivirus:*** It offers real-time automated protection from a range of IT threats:

- Real-time scanning of files, web pages and e-messages.
- Basic identity theft protection.
- Color-coding of links to unsafe websites.
- Disabling of links to malicious websites.
- Blocking of suspicious programs based on their behaviour.

- Protection from hijacking of your PC.
- Self-protection from malware.
- Regular and emergency updates for always-on protection.

6. ***McAfee Virus Scan:*** It offers you and your family the ultimate PC security with accelerated performance, for online activities, personal files and home networking.

- Antivirus, antispyware, antispam, and SiteAdvisor protect you from malicious software.
- QuickClean safely removes junk files that slow your PC and take up space on your hard drive.
- Advanced website safety ratings.
- Identity theft protection, antiphishing, and SiteAdvisor all help keep your identity safe.
- Local backup protects your electronic files if they are deleted or lost.

FIREWALL

Firewall is a system that protects a computer or a computer network against intrusions coming from a third-party network, generally the Internet. A firewall is a system that filters data packets that are exchanged over the network (Fig. 9.1). Therefore, it is a filtering gateway that comprises at least the following network interfaces:

- An interface for the network being protected (internal network).
- An interface for the external network.

The firewall system is a software system, often supported by dedicated network hardware, forming an intermediary between the local network (or the local computer) and one or more external networks. A firewall system can be set up on any computer that uses any system as long as:

- The machine is powerful enough to process the traffic.
- The system is secure.
- No other service than the packet filtering service is running on the server.

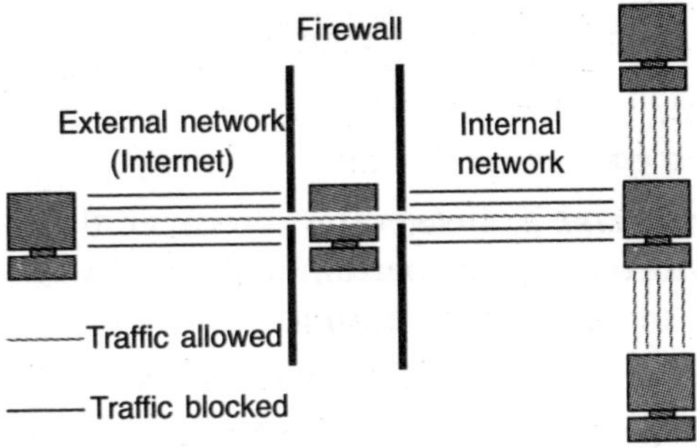

Fig. 9.1: Concept of firewall

Firewall system contains a set of predefined rules that allow the system to:

- Authorize the connection (allow).
- Block the connection (deny).
- Reject the connection request without informing the issuer (drop).

All of these rules implement a filtering method that depends on the security policy that was adopted by the organization.

1. ***Stateless packet filtering:*** A firewall system operates on the principle of simple packet filtering, or stateless packet filtering. It analyses the header of each data packet (datagram) exchanged between an internal network computer and an external computer.

Thus, the data packets exchanged between an external network computer and an internal network computer pass through the firewall and contain the following headers, which are systematically analyzed by the firewall:

- The IP address of the computer sending the packets.
- The IP address of the computer receiving the packets.
- The type of packet (TCP, UDP, etc.).
- The port number (reminder: a port is a number associated with a service or a network application).

The IP addresses contained in the packets allow you to identify the computer that is sending the packets and the target computer, while the type of packet and the port number indicate the type of service being used. Most firewall devices are at least configured to filter communications according to the port being used. It is generally recommended to block all ports that are not essential.

2. ***Dynamic packet filtering:*** The system of dynamic packet filtering is based on the inspection of layers 3 and 4 of the OSI model, allowing for full monitoring of the transactions between the client and the server. Firewall device is able to ensure the monitoring of exchanges, meaning that it takes into account the status of previous packets when defining filtering rules. Even if dynamic filtering is more effective than basic packet filtering, that does not mean that it protects against hackers taking advantage of application vulnerabilities.

3. ***Application filtering:*** Application filtering allows you to filter communications application by application. Application filtering operates at level 7 (the application layer) of the OSI model, contrary to simple packet filtering (level 4). Application filtering implies knowledge of the protocols used by each application. As the name indicates, application filtering allows you to filter communications application by application. Application filtering implies knowledge of the applications on the network and notably of the way in which it structures the exchanged data (ports, etc.).

The term personal firewall is used to describe the case where the protected area is limited to the computer on which the firewall is installed. A personal firewall allows you to control access to the network of applications installed on the computer and notably to prevent attacks like Trojan horses, i.e. harmful programs that breach the system in order to allow a hacker to remotely take control of the computer. Personal firewalls allow you to repair and prevent breaches by applications that are not authorized to connect to your computer.

Overview of Bioinformatics and eHealth

FUNDAMENTALS OF BIOINFORMATICS

Biology is in the middle of a major paradigm shift driven by computing technology. Although it is already an informational science in many respects, the field has been rapidly becoming much more computational and analytical. Rapid progress in genetics and biochemistry research combined with the tools provided by modern biotechnology has generated massive volumes of genetic and protein sequence data.

Bioinformatics has been defined as a means for analyzing, comparing, graphically displaying, modeling, storing, systemizing, searching, and ultimately distributing biological information, which includes sequences, structures, function, and phylogeny. Thus bioinformatics may be defined as a discipline that generates computational tools, databases, and methods to support genomic and postgenomic research. It comprises the study of DNA structure and function, gene and protein expression, protein production, structure and function, genetic regulatory systems, and clinical applications.

The National Center for Biotechnology Information (NCBI, 2001) defines bioinformatics as: "Bioinformatics is the field of science in which biology, computer science, and information technology merge into a single discipline". There are three important sub-disciplines within bioinformatics: the development of new algorithms and statistics with which to assess relationships among members of large data sets; the analysis and interpretation of various types of data including nucleotide and amino acid sequences, protein domains, and protein structures; and the development and implementation of tools that enable efficient access and management of different types of information.

The three terms bioinformatics, computational biology and bioinformation infrastructure are oftentimes used interchangeably. These three may be defined as follows:

1. Bioinformatics refers to database-like activities, involving persistent sets of data that are maintained in a consistent state over essentially indefinite periods of time.
2. Computational biology encompasses the use of algorithmic tools to facilitate biological analyses.
3. Bioinformation infrastructure comprises the entire collective of information management systems, analysis tools and communication networks supporting biology. Thus the latter may be viewed as a computational scaffold of the former two.

Bioinformatics is the application of information technology to the field of molecular biology. The term bioinformatics was coined by Paulien Hogeweg in 1979 for the study of informatic processes in biotic systems. Bioinformatics now entails the creation and advancement of databases, algorithms, computational and statistical techniques, and theory to solve formal and practical problems arising from the management and analysis of biological data. Over the past few decades rapid developments in genomic and other molecular research technologies and developments in information technologies have combined to produce a tremendous amount of information related to molecular biology. It is the name given to these mathematical and computing approaches used to glean understanding of biological processes. Common activities in bioinformatics include mapping and analyzing DNA and protein sequences, aligning different DNA and protein sequences to compare them and creating and viewing 3-D models of protein structures.

Bioinformatics is the analysis of biological information using computers and statistical techniques; the science of developing and utilizing computer databases and algorithms to accelerate and enhance biological research. Bioinformatics is more of a tool than a discipline, the tools for analysis of biological data. Specifically, it is the science of developing computer databases and algorithms to facilitate and expedite biological research. Bioinformatics was being used largely in the field of human genome research by the Human Genome Project that has been determining the sequence of the entire human genome (about 3 billion base pairs) and is essential in using genomic information to understand diseases. The science of bioinformatics, which is the melding of molecular biology with computer science, is essential to the use of genomic information in understanding human diseases and in the identification of new molecular targets for drug discovery. In recognition of this, many universities, government institutions and pharmaceutical firms have formed bioinformatics groups, consisting of computational biologists and bioinformatics computer scientists. Such groups will be key to unraveling the mass of information generated by large scale sequencing efforts underway in laboratories around the world. It is also used largely for the identification of new molecular targets for drug discovery.

Major research areas in bioinformatics are:

- Sequence analysis
- Genome annotation
- Computational evolutionary biology
- Biodiversity
- Analysis of gene expression
- Analysis of regulation
- Analysis of protein expression
- Analysis of mutations in cancer
- Prediction of protein structure
- Comparative genomics
- Modeling biological systems
- High-throughput image analysis
- Protein-protein docking.

The primary goal of bioinformatics is to increase our understanding of biological processes. What sets it apart from other approaches, however, is its focus on developing and applying computationally intensive techniques (e.g. data mining, machine learning algorithms and visualization) to achieve this goal. Major research efforts in the field include sequence alignment, gene finding, genome assembly, protein structure alignment, protein structure prediction, prediction of gene expression and protein-protein interactions, genome-wide association studies and the modeling of evolution.

With the confluence of biology and computer science, the computer applications of molecular biology are drawing a greater attention among the life science researchers and scientists these days. As it becomes imperative for biologists to seek the help of information technology professionals to accomplish the ever growing computational requirements of a host of exciting and needy biological problems, the synergy between modern biology and computer science is to blossom in the days to come. Thus, the research scope for all the mathematical techniques and algorithms coupled with software programming languages, software development and deployment tools is to get a real boost. In addition, information technologies such as databases, middleware, graphical user interface (GUI) design, distributed object computing, storage area networks (SAN), data compression, network and communication and remote management are all set to play a very critical role in taking forward the goals for which the bioinformatics field came into existence. Table 10.1 gives a historical sequence of events.

BIOINFORMATICS TOOLS

The tools of computer science, statistics, and mathematics are very critical for studying biology as an informational science subject.

Some of the recent advances happened include improved DNA sequencing methods, new approaches to identify protein structure, and revolutionary methods to monitor the expression of many genes in parallel. The design of techniques able to deal with different sources of incomplete and noisy data has become another crucial goal for the bioinformatics community.

Table 10.1: Bioinformatics events

1665	Robert Hooke published Micrographia, described the cellular structure of cork. He also described microscopic examinations of fossilized plants and animals, comparing their microscopic structure to that of the living organisms they resembled. He argued for an organic origin of fossils, and suggested a plausible mechanism for their formation.
1683	Antoni van Leeuwenhoek discovered bacteria.
1686	John Ray, in his book "Historia Plantarum" catalogued and described 18,600 kinds of plants. His book gave the first definition of species based upon common descent.
1843	Richard Owen elaborated the distinction of homology and analogy.
1864	Ernst Haeckel (Häckel) outlined the essential elements of modern zoological classification.
1865	Gregor Johann Mendel Austria, established the theory of genetic inheritance.
1902	The chromosome theory of heredity was proposed by Sutton and Boveri, working independently.
1962	Pauling's theory of molecular evolution introduced.
1905	The word "genetics" was coined by William Bateson.
1913	First ever linkage map created by Columbia undergraduate Alfred Sturtevant along with T.H. Morgan.
1930	Tiselius, Uppsala Sweden introduced a new technique electrophoresis for separating proteins in solution.
1946	Genetic material can be transferred laterally between bacterial cells, was shown by Lederberg and Tatum.
1952	Alfred Day Hershey and Martha Chase proved that the DNA alone carries genetic information. This was proved on the basis of their bacteriophage research.
1961	Sidney Brenner, François Jacob and Matthew Meselson identified messenger RNA.
1965	Margaret Dayhoff's released atlas of protein sequences.
1970	Needleman-Wunsch algorithm was developed.
1977	Software developed to analyze DNA sequencing.
1982	GenBank release made public.
1982	Phage lambda genome was sequenced.

Contd...

Contd...

1983	Sequence database searching algorithm was developed.
1985	FASTP/FASTN: fast sequence similarity searching technique was developed.
1988	National Center for Biotechnology Information (NCBI) was created at NIH/NLM.
1988	EMBnet network for database distribution.
1990	BLAST: fast sequence similarity searching program.
1991	EST: expressed sequence tag sequencing program.
1995	First bacterial genomes was completely sequenced.
1996	Yeast genome was completely sequenced.
1997	PSI-BLAST software was released.
1998	Worm (multicellular) genome was completely sequenced.
1999	Fly genome was completely sequenced.
2000	The genome for *Pseudomonas aeruginosa* (6.3 Mbp) was published.
2000	The *A. thaliana* genome (100 Mb) was secquenced.
2001	The human genome (3 Giga base pairs) was published.

In addition, there is the need to implement computational solutions based on theoretical frameworks to allow scientists to perform complex inferences about the phenomena under study.

Genomics in the recent past has triggered the development of high-throughput instrumentation for DNA sequencing, DNA arrays, genotyping, proteomics, etc. These instruments have catalyzed a new type of science for biology termed discovery science.

Bioinformatics tools are the software programs for the saving, retrieving and analysis of biological data and extracting the information from them.

Classification of Bioinformatics Tools

Bioinformatics tools may be categorized into following categories:

- Homology and similarity tools
- Protein function analysis
- Structural analysis
- Sequence analysis

1. ***Homology and similarity tools:*** The term homology implies a common evolutionary relationship between two traits—whether they are DNA sequences or bristle patterns on a fly's nose. Homologous sequences are sequences that are related by divergence from a common ancestor. Thus, the degree of similarity between two sequences can be measured while their homology is a case of being either true of false. This set of tools can be used to identify similarities between novel query sequences of unknown structure and function and database sequences whose structure and function have been elucidated.

2. ***Protein function analysis:*** Function analysis is identification and mapping of all functional elements (both coding and non-coding) in a genome. This group of programs allows you to compare your protein sequence to the secondary (or derived) protein databases that contain information on motifs, signatures and protein domains. Highly significant hits against these different pattern databases allow you to approximate the biochemical function of your query protein.

3. ***Structural analysis:*** This set of tools allows you to compare structures with the known structure databases. The function of a protein is more directly a consequence of its structure rather than its sequence with structural homologs tending to share functions. The determination of a protein's 2D/3D structure is crucial in the study of its function.

4. ***Sequence analysis:*** This set of tools allows you to carry out further more detailed analysis on your query sequence including evolutionary analysis, identification of mutations, hydropathy regions, CpG islands and compositional biases. The identification of these and other biological properties are all clues that aid the search to elucidate the specific function of your sequence.

Examples of Bioinformatics Software Programs

1. ***BLAST:*** The Basic Local Alignment Search Tool (BLAST) for comparing gene and protein sequences against others in public databases now comes in several types including PSI-BLAST, PHI-BLAST, and BLAST 2 sequences. Specialized BLASTs are also available for human, microbial, malaria, and other genomes, as well as for vector contamination, immunoglobulin, and tentative human consensus sequences.

2. ***FASTA:*** A database search tool used to compare a nucleotide or peptide sequence to a sequence database. The program is based on the rapid sequence algorithm described by Lipman and Pearson. It was the first widely used algorithm for database similarity searching. The program looks for optimal local alignments by scanning the sequence for small matches called "words". Initially, the scores of segments in which there are multiple word hits are calculated ("init1"). Later the scores of several segments may be summed to generate an "initn" score. An optimized alignment that includes gaps is shown in the output as "opt". The sensitivity and speed of the search are inversely related and controlled by the "k-tup" variable which specifies the size of a "word".

3. ***EMBOSS:*** European Molecular Biology Open Software Suite (EMBOSS) is a new, free open source software analysis package specially developed for the needs of the molecular biology user community. Within EMBOSS you will find around 100 programs (applications) for sequence alignment, database searching with sequence patterns, protein motif identification and domain analysis, nucleotide sequence pattern analysis, codon usage analysis for small genomes, and much more. A list of applications that are included with the EMBOSS package can be found in http://www.hgmp.mrc.ac.uk/Software/EMBOSS/Apps/.

4. ***ClustalW:*** ClustalW is a general purpose multiple sequence alignment program for DNA or proteins. It produces biologically meaningful multiple sequence alignments of divergent sequences, calculates the best match for the selected

sequences, and lines them up so that the identities, similarities and differences can be seen.

5. ***RasMol:*** It is a powerful research tool to display the structure of DNA, proteins and smaller molecules. Protein Explorer, a derivative of RasMol, is an easier-to-use program.

Examples of Application Programs

1. ***JAVA in bioinformatics:*** Due to platform independence nature of Java, it is emerging as a key player in bioinfor-matics. Physiome sciences computer-based biological simulation technologies and bioinformatics Solutions Pattern Hunter are two examples of the growing adoption of Java in bioinformatics.
2. ***Perl in bioinformatics:*** Perl is also being used in the processing of biological data. One example of perl project is BioPerl project.

Examples of Bioinformatics Projects

1. ***BioJava:*** The BioJava project is providing the Java tool for the processing of data in Java.
2. ***BioPerl:*** The BioPerl project many modules for biological data processing.
3. ***BioXML:*** A part of the BioPerl project, this is a resource to gather XML documentation, DTDs and XML aware tools for biology in one location.

BIOLOGICAL DATABASES

There are mainly two types of biological information:

- The information of genes or proteins, which are the molecular machines of life.
- The information of the regularity networks that coordinate and specify the expression patterns of the genes and proteins.

All of these paradigm shift lead to the view that the major challenges for biology and medicine in this new century will be the study of complex systems and the approach necessary for studying these biological complexities. Here comes a viable approach:

- Identify all elements, such as sequence of genomes in the system with currently available discovery tools.
- Use current knowledge of the system to formulate a model predicting its behaviour.
- Perturb the system in a model organism using biological, genetic or environmental perturbations, capture information at all relevant levels, such as DNA, mRNA, protein, protein interactions, etc. and integrate the collected information.
- Compare theoretical predictions and experimental data, carry out additional perturbations to bring theory and experiment into closer apposition, and integrate new data into model.
- Iterate the above third and fourth steps till the mathematical model can predict the structure of the system and its systems or emergent properties given particular perturbations.

Biological database contains the sequence data of DNA, RNA, etc. These databases are organized for optimal retrieval and analysis. The following are examples of biological databases:

1. ***National center for biotechnology information (NCBI):*** It was established in 1988 as a national resource for molecular biology information, NCBI creates public databases, conducts research in computational biology, develops software tools for analyzing genome data, and disseminates biomedical information; all for the better understanding of molecular processes affecting human health and disease.

2. ***Entrez search and retrieval system:*** Entrez programming utilities are tools that provide access to Entrez data outside of the regular web query interface and may be helpful for retrieving search results for future use in another environment.

3. ***Kyoto encyclopedia of genes and genomes (KEGG):*** A grand challenge in the post-genomic era is a complete computer

representation of the cell and the organism, which will enable computational prediction of higher-level complexity of cellular processes and organism behaviors from genomic information. Towards this end a bioinformatics resource named KEGG is being developed, as part of the research projects in the Kanehisa Laboratory of Kyoto University Bioinformatics Center.

4. ***TIGR gene indices:*** The TIGR gene index project is supported in part by funding from the US Department of Energy and the US National Science Foundation. Additional funds are provided by the US National Science Foundation.

5. ***Gramene:*** Gramene is a curated, open-source, web-accessible data resource for comparative genome analysis in the grasses. Our goal is to facilitate the study of cross-species homology relationships using information derived from public projects involved in genomic and EST sequencing, protein structure and function analysis, genetic and physical mapping, interpretation of biochemical pathways, gene and QTL localization and descriptions of phenotypic characters and mutations.

6. ***MaizeDB:*** The goals of this project are to provide a central repository for public maize information and present it in a way that creates intuitive biological connections for the researcher with minimal effort as well as provide a series of computational tools that directly address the questions of the biologist in an easy-to-use form.

7. ***Barley genomics:*** Areas of research include genome mapping, map-based cloning, molecular breeding, mutant isolation and characterization, functional genomics, BAC address calculator, and developmental mutants.

8. ***European bioinformatics institute:*** The European Bioinformatics Institute (EBI) is a non-profit academic organization that forms part of the European Molecular Biology Laboratory (EMBL). The EBI is a centre for research and services in bioinformatics. The institute manages databases of biological data including nucleic acid, protein sequences and macromolecular structures.

9. ***Catalog of genes for plant glycerol lipid biosynthesis:*** The current version of this catalog contains more than 2600 sequence

files, many of them with annotation and results of our analysis. This version is updated as of Aug. 1999 and includes essentially all publicly available genomic, cDNA, EST and GSS sequences for 62 plant polypeptides involved in lipid metabolism in higher plant species. An important feature of the catalog is the multiple alignments of amino acid sequences deduced from genomic and EST sequences. This version of the dataset accounts for approximately 70% of the Arabidopsis genome.

10. ***GrainGenes:*** A small grains and sugarcane database. GBrowse, developed by the GMOD group is a genome browser that provides a wealth of genome annotation for maps in the GrainGenes collection. Users can easily manipulate the view of the chromosome and type of data displayed.

11. ***PathDB pathways:*** PathDB is a beta level research tool for scientists interested in analyzing their experimental or computational data in the context of biological pathways and networks.

12. ***Enzymes and metabolic pathways database (EMP):*** EMP is a unique and most comprehensive electronic source of biochemical data. It covers all aspects of enzymology and metabolism and represents the whole factual content of original journal publications.

13. ***ExPASy molecular biology server:*** The ExPASy (Expert Protein Analysis System) proteomics server of the Swiss Institute of Bioinformatics (SIB) is dedicated to the analysis of protein sequences and structures as well as 2-D page.

14. ***Nucleic acids research database:*** Nucleic Acids Research (NAR) publishes the results of leading edge research into physical, chemical, biochemical and biological aspects of nucleic acids and proteins involved in nucleic acid metabolism and/or interactions. It enables the rapid publication of papers under the following categories: chemistry, computational biology, genomics, molecular biology, RNA and structural biology. A Survey and Summary section provides a format for brief reviews. The first issue of each year is devoted to biological databases, and an issue in July is devoted to papers describing web-based software resources of value to the biological community.

15. ***Yeast protein database:*** Six database volumes of biological information about proteins comprise Incyte's Proteome BioKnowledge Library. Each volume focuses on a different organism important in pharmaceutical research.

16. ***Saccharomyces genome database:*** SGDTM is a scientific database of the molecular biology and genetics of the yeast *Saccharomyces cerevisiae,* which is commonly known as bakers or budding yeast.

17. ***Breast cancer gene database:*** A database of genes involved in breast cancer. It is similar to the tumor gene database (below) but limited in scope to those genes involved in human breast cancer and thus will be able to go into greater depth. The criteria for a gene to be included in this database are that it has been shown to be involved in human breast cancer (rather than an animal model) and that there is some evidence that it plays a functional role in the induction or progression of breast cancer.

18. ***Mammary transgene interactive database:*** This is an interactive database of literature on research designed to target transgene proteins to the mammary gland. Current emphasis is on biotechnology applications. Addition of tumor model and developmental model literature is planned.

19. ***Small RNA database:*** Small RNAs are broadly defined as the RNAs not directly involved in protein synthesis. These are grouped under three categories:

   i. Capped small RNAs;

   ii. Noncapped small RNAs; and

   iii. Viral small RNAs. Sequences and references are included, and you can do WAIS searching with a keyword.

20. ***Tumor gene database:*** A database of genes associated with tumorigenesis and cellular transformation. This database includes oncogenes, proto-oncogenes, tumor suppressor genes / anti-oncogenes, regulators and substrates of the above, regions believed to contain such genes such as tumor-associated chromosomal break points and viral integration sites, and other genes and chromosomal regions that seem relevant.

Table 10.2: URL of important biological databases

Name of database	*URL*
NCBI	http://www.ncbi.nlm.nih.gov/
Entrez Search and Retrieval System	www.ncbi.nlm.nih.gov/Entrez
Kyoto Encyclopedia of Genes and Genomes	http://www.genome.ad.jp/kegg/
TIGR Gene Indices	http://www.tigr.org/tdb/tgi.shtml
Gramene	http://www.gramene.org/
MaizeDB	http://www.maizegdb.org/
Barley Genomics	http://barleygenomics.wsu.edu/
European Bioinformatics Institute	http://www2.ebi.ac.uk/
Catalog of Genes for Plant Glycerol Lipid Biosynthesis	http://www.canr.msu.edu/lgc
GrainGenes	http://wheat.pw.usda.gov/
PathDB Pathways Enzymes and Metabolic	http://www.ncgr.org/pathdb/index.html
Pathways Database	http://www.empproject.com/about
Expasy Molecular Biology Server	http://www.expasy.ch/
Nucleic Acids Research Database	http://nar.oupjournals.org/cgi/content/full/28/1/1/DC1
Yeast Protein Database	http://www.proteome.com/YPDhome.html
Saccharomyces	http://genome-www.stanford.edu/
Genome Database	Saccharomyces/
Breast Cancer Gene Database	http://condor.bcm.tmc.edu/ermb/bcgd/bcgd.html
Mammary Transgene Interactive Database	http://mbcr.bcm.tmc.edu/ermb/mtdb/mtdb.html
Small RNA Database	http://mbcr.bcm.tmc.edu/smallRNA/smallrna.html
Tumor Gene Database	http://condor.bcm.tmc.edu/ermb/tgdb/tgdb.html

BIOINFORMATICS RESOURCES ON WEB

The following is some of bioinformatics resources on the Internet:

- ***Search databases:*** Different searches against different databases.
- ***General nucleotide sequence databases:*** Some general nucleotide sequence databases.
- ***Specific human genome databases:*** Collection of human genome databases.
- ***Specific genome databases of all other species:*** Collection of genome databases of all other species.
- ***Online tools and protocols:*** Online tools and protocols links.
- ***Bio-Journals:*** This is a combination of Pedro's Collection, Springer, Oxford, and APNet.
- ***NCBI:*** Established in 1988 as a national resource for molecular biology information, NCBI creates public databases, conducts research in computational biology, develops software tools for analyzing genome data, and disseminates biomedical information—all for the better understanding of molecular processes affecting human health and disease (Table 10.2).
- ***EBI:*** The European Bioinformatics Institute (EBI) is a non-profit academic organization that forms part of the European Molecular Biology Laboratory (EMBL).
- ***DDBJ:*** DNA Data Bank of Japan (DDBJ) began DNA data bank activities in earnest in 1986 at the National Institute of Genetics (NIG). DDBJ has been functioning as the international nucleotide sequence database in collaboration with EBI/EMBL and NCBI/GenBank. DNA sequence records organismic evolution more directly than other biological materials and thus is invaluable not only for research in life sciences but also human welfare in general. The databases are, so to speak, a common treasure of human beings.
- ***Feature table definition:*** The format of entries in these databases is DNA Data Bank of Japan, EMBL Nucleotide

Sequence Database, Cambridge, UK.GenBank, NCBI, Bethesda, MD, USA.

APPLICATIONS OF BIOINFORMATICS

Bioinformatics is the use of IT in biotechnology for the data storage, data warehousing and analyzing the DNA sequences. In bioinformatics knowledge of many branches is required like biology, mathematics, computer science, laws of physics and chemistry, and of course sound knowledge of IT to analyze biotech data. Bioinformatics is not limited to the computing data, but in reality it can be used to solve many biological problems and find out how living things work.

It is the comprehensive application of mathematics (e.g. probability and statistics), science (e.g. biochemistry), and a core set of problem-solving methods (e.g. computer algorithms) to the understanding of living systems.

The aims of bioinformatics are threefold. First, at its simplest bioinformatics organizes data in a way that allows researchers to access existing information and to submit new entries as they are produced, e.g. the Protein Data Bank for 3D macromolecular structures. While data-creation is an essential task, the information stored in these databases is essentially useless until analyzed. Thus the purpose of bioinformatics extends much further. The second aim is to develop tools and resources that aid in the analysis of data. For example, having sequenced a particular protein, it is of interest to compare it with previously characterized sequences. This needs more than just a simple text-based search and programs such as FASTA and PSI-BLAST must consider what comprises a biologically significant match. Development of such resources dictates expertise in computational theory as well as a thorough understanding of biology. The third aim is to use these tools to analyze the data and interpret the results in a biologically meaningful manner. Traditionally, biological studies examined individual systems in detail, and frequently compared those with a few that are related. In bioinformatics, we can now conduct global analyses of all the available data with the aim of uncovering common principles that apply across many systems and highlight novel features.

Bioinformatics is being used in following fields:

- Molecular medicine
- Personalized medicine
- Preventative medicine
- Gene therapy
- Drug development
- Microbial genome applications
- Waste cleanup
- Climate change studies
- Alternative energy sources
- Biotechnology
- Forensic analysis of microbes
- Evolutionary studies
- Crop improvement
- Insect resistance
- Improve nutritional quality
- Development of drought-resistant varieties
- Veterinary science
- Bio-weapon creation.

One of the earliest medical applications of bioinformatics has been in aiding rational drug design. Sequence search techniques can then be used to find homologues in model organisms, and based on sequence similarity; it is possible to model the structure of the human protein on experimentally characterized structures. Finally, docking algorithms could design molecules that could bind the model structure, leading the way for biochemical assays to test their biological activity on the actual protein.

With the current deluge of data, computational methods have become indispensable to biological investigations. Originally developed for the analysis of biological sequences, bioinformatics now encompasses a wide range of subject areas including structural biology, genomics and gene expression studies.

Two principal approaches underpin all studies in bioinformatics. First is that of comparing and grouping the data according to biologically meaningful similarities and second, that of analyzing one type of data to infer and understand the observations for another type of data. These approaches are reflected in the main aims of the field, which are to understand and organize the information associated with biological molecules on a large scale. As a result, bioinformatics has not only provided greater depth to biological investigations, but added the dimension of breadth as well. In this way, we are able to examine individual systems in detail and also compare them with those that are related in order to uncover common principles that apply across many systems and highlight unusual features that are unique to some.

Most recent applications in the medical sciences have centered on gene expression analysis. This usually involves compiling expression data for cells affected by different diseases, e.g. cancer and arteriosclerosis, and comparing the measurements against normal expression levels. Identification of genes that are expressed differently in affected cells provides a basis for explaining the causes of illnesses and highlights potential drug targets.

Further advances in bioinformatics combined with experimental genomics for individuals are predicted to revolutionalize the future of healthcare. A typical scenario for a patient may start with post-natal genotyping to assess susceptibility or immunity from specific diseases and pathogens. With this information, a unique combination of vaccines could be prescribed, minimizing the healthcare costs of unnecessary treatments and anticipating the onslaught of diseases later in life. Regular lifetime screenings could lead to guidance for nutrition intake and early detections of any illnesses. In addition, drug-based treatments could be tailored specifically to the patient and disease, thus providing the most effective course of medication with minimal side-effects. Given the present rate of development, such a scenario in healthcare appears to be possible in the not too distant future.

WHAT IS eHEALTH?

eHealth is a relatively recent term for healthcare practice which is supported by electronic processes and communication. The term can encompass a range of services that are at the edge of medicine/healthcare and information technology:

1. ***Electronic health records:*** It enable easy communication of patient data between different healthcare professionals (GPs, specialists, care team, pharmacy).
2. ***Telemedicine:*** It includes all types of physical and psychological measurements that do not require a patient to travel to a specialist. When this service works, patients need to travel less to a specialist or conversely the specialist has a larger catchment area.
3. ***Consumer health informatics:*** It includes both healthy individuals and patients want to be informed on medical topics.
4. ***Health knowledge management:*** For example, an overview of latest medical journals, best practice guidelines or epidemiological tracking. Examples include physician resources such as Medscape and MDLinx.
5. ***Virtual healthcare:*** It consists of healthcare professionals who collaborate and share information on patients through digital equipment (for transmural care).
6. ***mHealth:*** It includes the use of mobile devices in collecting aggregate and patient level health data, providing healthcare information to practitioners, researchers, and patients, real-time monitoring of patient vitals, and direct provision of care (via mobile telemedicine).
7. ***eHealth grids:*** Medical research uses eHealth Grids that provide powerful computing and data management capabilities to handle large amounts of heterogeneous data.
8. ***Healthcare information systems:*** It is also often refers to software solutions for appointment scheduling, patient data

management, work schedule management and other administrative tasks surrounding health. Whether these tasks are part of eHealth depends on the chosen definition, they do, however, interface with most eHealth implementations due to the complex relationship between administration and healthcare at Health Care Providers.

ELECTRONIC HEALTH RECORD

An electronic health record (EHR) refers to an individual patient's medical record in digital format. Electronic health record systems coordinate the storage and retrieval of individual records with the aid of computers. EHRs are usually accessed on a computer, often over a network. It may be made up of electronic medical records (EMRs) from many locations and/or sources. Among the many forms of data often included in EMRs are patient demographics, medical history, medicine and allergy lists (including immunization status), laboratory test results, radiology images, billing records and advanced directives. EHR systems increase physician efficiency and reduce costs, as well as promote standardization of care.

The EHR has the ability to generate a complete record of a clinical patient encounter as well as supporting other care-related activities directly or indirectly via interface including evidence-based decision support, quality management, and outcomes reporting.

Advantages of electronic health records include:

1. ***Improve quality of care:*** An EHR system can help reduce medical errors by providing healthcare workers with decision support. Fast access to medical literature and current best practices in medicine enable proliferation of ongoing improvements in healthcare efficacy.

2. ***Reduce healthcare costs:*** One of the major sources of rapid growth in healthcare costs comes from medical imaging. Access to a patient's images in an EHR is an effective way to avoid duplicating expensive imaging procedures. Another high cost to healthcare is the printing and mailing of checks. Other cost

savings include the reduction of medical errors that can otherwise lead to further expensive care.

3. ***Promote evidence-based medicine:*** EHRs provide access to unprecedented amounts of clinical data for research that can accelerate the level of knowledge of effective medical practices. These benefits may be realized in a realistic sense only if the EHR systems are interoperable and widespread (e.g. national) so that various systems can easily share information. Also, to avoid failures that can cause injury to the patient and violations to privacy, the best practices in software engineering and medial informatics must be deployed. EHRs also have the advantages of electronic medical records (EMR). EMRs can be continuously updated. In general, medical records may be on "physical" media such as film (X-rays), paper (notes), or photographs, often of different sizes and shapes. Physical storage of documents is problematic, as not all document types fit in the same size folders or storage spaces. Handwritten paper medical records can be associated with poor legibility, which can contribute to medical errors.

TELEMEDICINE

Telemedicine is a rapidly developing application of clinical medicine where medical information is transferred through the phone or the Internet and sometimes other networks for the purpose of consulting, and sometimes remote medical procedures or examinations.

Telemedicine may be as simple as two health professionals discussing a case over the telephone, or as complex as using satellite technology and video-conferencing equipment to conduct a real-time consultation between medical specialists in two different countries. Telemedicine generally refers to the use of communications and information technologies for the delivery of clinical care.

Telemedicine is practised on the basis of concepts of:

- Real-time (synchronous)
- Store-and-forward
- Home health (asynchronous).

1. ***Real-time telemedicine:*** It could be as simple as a telephone call or as complex as robotic surgery. It requires the presence of both parties at the same time and a communication link between them that allows a real-time interaction to take place. Video-conferencing equipment is one of the most common forms of technologies used in synchronous telemedicine. There are also peripheral devices which can be attached to computers or the video-conferencing equipment which can aid in an interactive examination. For instance, a tele-otoscope allows a remote physician to 'see' inside a patient's ear; a tele-stethoscope allows the consulting remote physician to hear the patient's heartbeat. Medical specialties conducive to this kind of consultation include psychiatry, family practice, internal medicine, rehabilitation, cardiology, pediatrics, obstetrics, gynecology, neurology, speech-language pathology and pharmacy.

2. ***Store-and-forward telemedicine:*** It involves acquiring medical data (like medical images, bio-signals, etc.) and then transmitting this data to a doctor or medical specialist at a convenient time for assessment offline. It does not require the presence of both parties at the same time. Dermatology, radiology, and pathology are common specialties that are conducive to asynchronous telemedicine. A properly structured medical record in electronic form should be a component of this transfer.

3. ***Home health telemedicine:*** When a patient is in the hospital and he is placed under general observation after a surgery or other medical procedure, the hospital is usually losing a valuable bed and the patient would rather not be there as well. Home health allows the remote observation and care of a patient. Home health equipment consists of vital signs capture, video-conferencing capabilities, and patient states can be reviewed and alarms can be set from the hospital nurse's station, depending on the specific home health device usually low bandwidth analog Plain Old Telephone System (POTS). Some newer systems do support higher bandwidth capabilities.

Telemedicine is most beneficial for populations living in isolated communities and remote regions and is currently being applied in virtually all medical domains. Specialties that use telemedicine often use a "tele" prefix; for example, telemedicine as applied by radiologists is called teleradiology. Similarly telemedicine as applied by cardiologists is termed as tele-cardiology, etc. Telemedicine is also useful as a communication tool between a general practitioner and a specialist available at a remote location.

HEALTH INFORMATICS

Health informatics is the intersection of information science, computer science, and health care. It deals with the resources, devices, and methods required to optimize the acquisition, storage, retrieval, and use of information in health and biomedicine. Health informatics tools include not only computers but also clinical guidelines, formal medical terminologies, and information and communication systems. It is applied to the areas of nursing, clinical care, dentistry, pharmacy, public health and biomedical research. It includes the following:

- Architectures for electronic medical records and other health information systems used for billing, scheduling, and research.
- Decision support systems in healthcare, including clinical decision support systems.
- Standards and integration profiles to facilitate the exchange of information between healthcare information systems, these specifically define the means to exchange data, not the content.
- Controlled medical vocabularies such as the systematized nomenclature of medicine, clinical terms, logical observation identifiers, names and codes are used to allow a standard, accurate exchange of data content between systems and providers.
- Use of hand-held or portable devices to assist providers with data entry / retrieval or medical decision-making, sometimes called mHealth.

mHEALTH

mHealth is a term for medical and public health practice supported by mobile devices, such as mobile phones, patient monitoring devices, PDAs, and other wireless devices. mHealth applications include the use of mobile devices in collecting community and clinical health data, delivery of healthcare information to practitioners, researchers, and patients, real-time monitoring of patient vital signs, and direct provision of care (via mobile telemedicine). It is emerging mobile communica-tions and network technologies for health care. mHealth broadly encompasses the use of mobile telecommunication and multimedia technologies as they are integrated within increasingly mobile and wireless health care delivery systems and is part of a movement towards citizen-centered health service delivery. Mobile technologies by nature lend themselves to more decentralized health service delivery. Key mobile communication technologies relevant to mHealth include:

- Mobile phones.
- PDAs and smart phones.
- Patient monitoring devices.
- Mobile telemedicine/telecare devices.
- MP3 players for mLearning.
- Microcomputers.

The recent advances in information and communication technologies (ICT) enable technically the continual monitoring of health-related parameters with wireless sensors, wherever the user happens to be. Mobile phones or personal digital assistants (PDAs) with wireless networking capabilities may serve as gateways that process, store, and transfer measured parameters to clinicians for further analysis or diagnosis. The applications can be summarized as follows:

- Education and awareness.
- Data collection (for public health or clinical domains).
- Remote monitoring.
- Communication and training for health care workers.

- Disease surveillance and epidemic outbreak tracking (Malaria, HIV/AIDS, TB, etc.).
- Diagnostics and treatment support.

Ministries of Health in low and middle income countries and policy makers are eager to explore the use of mobile phones and other ICT to promote health, the lack of a comprehensive model, knowledge base, and published data on the health benefits poses significant barriers. Three key areas in which early and rapid gains can be achieved through technology design and integration are the areas of safe motherhood, routine immunization and integrated management of childhood illness, and in addressing the diseases of poverty, namely HIV and AIDS, malaria, and TB where significant resources have been mobilized to reduce the disease burden in low and middle income countries.

Emerging trends of interest in mHealth include the use of technologies in the following areas:

- Emergency response systems (e.g. road traffic accidents, emergency obstetric care).
- Human resources coordination, management, and supervision.
- Mobile synchronous (voice) and asynchronous (SMS) telemedicine diagnostic and decision support to remote clinicians.
- Clinician-focused, evidence-based formulary, database and decision support information available at the point-of-care.
- Clinical care and remote patient monitoring.
- Health extension services.
- Health services monitoring and reporting.
- Health-related mLearning for the general public.
- Training and continuing professional development for health care workers.
- Health promotion and community mobilization.

Technology integration within the health sector has great potential to promote healthy lifestyles, improve decisions by health professionals as well as patients, and enhance health care quality by improving access to medical and health information and facilitating instantaneous communication in places where this was not previously possible. The increased use of technology can help reduce health care costs by improving efficiencies in the health care system and promoting prevention through behavior change communication. It also has the potential to advance clinical care and public health services by facilitating health professional practice and communication and reducing health disparities by applying new approaches to improve the health of isolated populations.

Appendices

Computer Terminology

Access time: The performance of a hard drive or other storage device—how long it takes to locate a file.

Active program or window: The application or window at the front (foreground) on the monitor.

Alert: A message that appears on screen, usually to tell you something went wrong.

Antivirus application: An application that scans a computer's disks and memory for viruses and removes any that are found.

Application files: Program files environment where you can create and edit the kind of document that application makes.

Application menu: On the right side of the screen header. Lists running applications.

ASCII: American Standard Code for Information Interchange. A commonly used data format for exchanging information between computers or programs.

Backup: A copy of a file or disk you make for archiving purposes.

Binary: This is a basic system of numbering using ones and zeros.

Bit: The smallest piece of information used by the computer. Derived from "binary digit".

Boot: To start up a computer.

Bug: A programming error that causes a program to behave in an unexpected way.

Bus: An electronic pathway through which data is transmitted between components in a computer.

Byte: A piece of computer information made up of eight bits.

C: A programming language developed at AT and T.

Card: A printed circuit board that adds some feature to a computer.

Cartridge drive: A storage device, like a hard drive, in which the medium is a cartridge that can be removed.

CD-ROM: An acronym for Compact Disc-Read Only Memory.

Chooser: A desk accessory used to select a printer, or other external device, or to log onto a network.

Click: To select an object by pressing the mouse button when the cursor is pointing to the required menu option, icon or hypertext link.

Clipboard: It is used to hold information which is to be moved, as in word processing where text is "cut" and then "pasted".

Clock rate: The instruction processing speed of a computer measured in millions of cycles per second (i.e. 200 MHz).

Close: To close a window that has been opened for viewing and/or editing.

COBOL: Stands for Common Business Oriented Language.

Command: The act of giving an instruction to your Mac either by menu choice or keystroke.

Compiler: A program that converts programming code into a form that can be used by a computer.

Compression: A technique that reduces the size of a saved file by elimination or encoding redundancies (i.e. JPEG, MPEG, LZW, etc.)

Computer: A general-purpose machine that processes data according to a set of instructions that are stored internally either temporarily or permanently.

Control key: Seldom used modifier key on the Mac.

Control panel: A program that allows you to change settings in a program or change the way a Mac looks and/or behaves.

CPU: The Central Processing Unit. The processing chip that is the "brains" of a computer.

Crash: A system malfunction in which the computer stops working and has to be restarted.

Creating a file: Storing data as a file with an assigned file name that is unique within the directory it resides in.

Cursor: The pointer, usually arrow or cross-shaped, which is controlled by the mouse.

Daisy chaining: The act of stringing devices together in a series (such as SCSI).

Data: Information processed by a computer.

Database: An electronic list of information that can be sorted and/or searched.

Defragment: To concatenate fragments of data into contiguous blocks in memory or on a hard drive.

Delete: To remove an item of data from a file or to remove a file from the disk.

Desktop file: An invisible file in which the finder stores a database of information about files and icons.

Desktop: An on-screen representation of a desktop such as used in the Macintosh and Windows operating systems.

Dialog boxes: Takes over your screen and allows you to "dialog" with the computer.

Digitize: To convert linear, or analog, data into digital data which can be used by the computer.

Directory: Allows you to organize files and other folders.

Disk drive: The machinery that writes the data from a disk and/or writes data to a disk.

Disk space: This is the place where your files live. The greater the disk space the more files you can keep.

Disk window: The window that displays the contents or directory of a disk.

Disk: A spinning platter made of magnetic or optically etched material on which data can be stored.

Document files: Files we care about (memos, letters, pictures, etc.)

Document: A file you create, as opposed to the application which created it.

Domain name: A domain name is a dot com (.com) name. Domain Names are normally used by website owners.

DOS: Acronym for Disk Operating System; used in PCs.

Double click: To press the mouse button twice in rapid succession without moving the mouse between clicks.

Download: To transfer data from one computer to another. If you are on the receiving end, you are downloading.

DPI: Acronym for Dots Per Inch; a gauge of visual clarity on the printed page or on the computer screen.

Drag and drop: It allows one to drag the icon for a document on top of the icon for an application, thereby launching the application and opening the document.

Drag: To move the mouse while its button is being depressed.

Drive: A drive is a piece of hardware that is normally used to read/write data from/onto its storage media.

Driver: A file on a computer which tells it how to communicate with an add-on piece of equipment (like a printer).

e-Commerce: Conducting business transactions through electronic transmissions between computers.

Edit: To make a change to existing data.

Ethernet: A protocol for fast communication and file transfer across a network.

Expansion slot: A connector inside the computer which allows one to plug in a printed circuit board that provides new or enhanced features.

Extension: A startup program that runs when you start the Mac and then enhances its function.

File: The generic word for an application, document, control panel or other computer data.

Firewall: Hardware and/or software used to divide a LAN into two or more parts for security reasons.

Floppy: A 3.5 inch square rigid disk which holds data.

Folder: An electronic subdirectory which contains files.

Font: A typeface that contains the characters of an alphabet or some other letter forms.

Footprint: The surface area of a desk or table which is occupied by a piece of equipment.

Fragmentation: The breaking up of a file into many separate locations in memory or on a disk.

Freeze: A system error which causes the cursor to lock in place.

Get info: A finder file menu command that presents an information window for a selected file icon.

Gig: A gigabyte = 1024 megabytes.

Hard drive: A large capacity storage device made of multiple disks housed in a rigid case.

Hardware: These are the physical items including your computer and floppy discs.

High density disk: A 1.4 MB floppy disk.

Highlight: To select by clicking once on an icon or by highlighting text in a document.

HTML (HyperText Markup Language): Common language used to write documents on World Wide Web.

HTTP (HyperText Transport Protocol): Common protocol used to communicate between World Wide Web Servers.

Icon view: Allows you to see icons of folders and files primarily as icons with little information.

Icons: In a graphical user interface (GUI), a small, pictorial, on screen representation of an object, such as a document, program, folder or disk drive.

Initialize: To format a disk for use in the computer; creates a new directory and arranges the tracks for the recording of data.

Internet: A conglomeration of networks connected together forming a worldwide network.

Insertion point: In word processing, the short flashing marker which indicates where your next typing will begin.

Installer: Software used to install a program on your hard drive.

Interrupt button: A tool used by programmers to enter the debugging mode. The button is usually next to the reset button.

Java: Java is an object oriented program developed by James Gosling at Sun Microsystems.

K: Short for kilobyte. 1 kilobyte = 1024 bytes.

Keyboard shortcut: A combination of keystrokes that performs some function otherwise found in a pulldown menu.

Keyboard: This is primary text input device. It contains certain standard function keys, such as the escape key, tab, and arrow keys, shift and control keys.

LAN (Local Area Network): A communication network that links PCs and other devices in a single office or small campus.

Landscape: In printing from a computer to print sideways on the page.

Launch: Start an application.

List view: Shows the icons but also orders the icons (often by name, but can sort the list in other ways) and shows more information about them.

Macintosh: The brand name of a family of personal computers (hardware) and an operating system (software) from Apple, introduced in 1984.

Mb: Short for megabyte. 1 megabyte = 1024 kilobytes.

Megabytes (Mb): Mega = million so 1 Mb = 1,000,000 bytes.

Megahertz (MHz): This stands for megahertz. 1 megahertz = 1,000,000 cycles per second.

Memory: The temporary holding area where data is stored while it is being used or changed; the amount of RAM a computer has installed.

Menu bar: The horizontal bar across the top of the monitor screen that lists the menus.

Menu: A list of program commands listed by topic, some with images next to them.

Modem: A telecommunication peripheral device that allows computer to communicate with one another via conventional telephone lines.

Modifier keys: Keys that change the meaning of what you type.

Motherboard: The circuit board on which most of the major electronic components are situated.

Mouse: Pointing device that allows you to tell the computer what to do.

Multi-tasking: Running more than one application in memory at the same time.

Operating system: The instructions that allow the computer to start working and permit it to run other programs.

Optical disk: A high-capacity storage medium that is read by a laser light.

Packet: An individual bundle of data that is transmitted across the network.

Palette: A small floating window that contains tools used in a given application.

Partition: A subdivision of a hard drive's surface that is defined and used as a separate drive.

Paste: To insert text, or other material, from the clipboard or copy buffer.

PC: Acronym for Personal Computer.

PCI: Acronym for Peripheral Component Interchange—the newer, faster bus architecture.

Peripheral device: Any device that is connected to the computer in addition to the basic CPU–Monitor–Keyboard–Mouse configuration.

Printer: A peripheral device that allows the computer user to produce paper copies of the information processed by the computer.

Pointer: The name of the arrow (or other shape) that tracks across the screen as you move the mouse (or other pointing device) around.

Pop-up menu: Any menu that does not appear at the top of the screen in the menu bar (may pop up or down).

Port: A connection socket.

Program: A complex set of instructions that allow the computer user to process data.

Random Access Memory (RAM): Volatile memory which can be written and read.

Recycle bin: Place where you put files and folders that you may later want to delete or get rid of. Compare trash.

Resize box: The small square at the lower right corner of a window which, when dragged, resizes the window.

Right click: To press the right button on the mouse.

Read Only Memory (ROM): Non-volatile memory that can only be read and not written, i.e. cannot be altered.

Root directory: The main hard drive window.

Router: A computer or network device which transfers packets of data from one network to another

Save as: To save a previously saved file in a new location and/ or with a new name.

Save: Tell the computer to create a file on disk that has the information you have put into the document (usually typing).

Scroll bar: A bar at the bottom or right side of a window that contains the scroll box and allows scrolling.

Scroll box: The box in a scroll bar that is used to navigate through a window.

Scroll: To shift the contents of a window to bring hidden items into view.

SCSI address: A number between zero and seven that must be unique to each device in a SCSI chain.

SCSI port: A 25 pin connector on the back used to connect SCSI devices to the CPU.

SCSI terminator: A device placed at the end of a SCSI chain to complete the circuit.

SCSI: Acronym for Small Computer System Interface.

Serial port: A port that allows data to be transmitted in a series (one after the other), such as the printer and modem ports on a Mac.

Server: A central computer dedicated to sending and receiving data from other computers (on a network).

Shut down: To quit all applications and turn off the computer.

Software: Files on disk that contain instructions for a computer.

Software: Instructions that tell the computer what to do.

Spreadsheet: A program designed to look like an electronic ledger.

Start up disk: The disk containing system software and is designated to be used to start the computer.

System folder: An all-important folder that contains at least the System file and the Finder.

Title bar: The horizontal bar at the top of a window which has the name of the file or folder it represents.

Trash: Place where you put files and folders that you want to delete or get rid of.

Uninterruptible Power Source (UPS): A constantly charging battery pack which powers the computer.

Upload: To send a file from one computer to another through a network.

Virus: It is a destructive program that infects the operation of a computer system.

Virtual memory: Using part of your hard drive as though it were "RAM".

Website: A website is the term used to describe the whole contents of a folder that is stored on a Hosting Server.

Worm: It is a destructive routine in a program designed to adulterate a program or database either all at once or over a period of time.

Windows: The most widely used operating system for personal computers from Microsoft.

Zoom box: A small square in the upper right corner of a window which, when clicked, will expand the window to fill the whole screen.

Shortcut Keys

Document Actions	
Open	CTRL+O
New	CTRL+N
Save As	F12
Save	CTRL+S
Print	CTRL+P
Help	F1
Editing and Formatting Text	
Select All	CTRL+A
Copy	CTRL+C
Cut	CTRL+X
Paste	CTRL+V
Undo	CTRL+Z
Redo	CTRL+Y
Find	CTRL+F
Replace	CTRL+H
Go to	CTRL+G
Bold	CTRL+B
Italics	CTRL+I
Underline	CTRL+U
Left Justified	CTRL+L

Center Justified	CTRL+E
Right Justified	CTRL+R
Apply larger font size	CTRL+]
Apply smaller font size	CTRL+[
Line Spacing	ALT+O S
Bullets and Numbering	ALT+O N
Header and Footer	ALT+V H
Background	ALT+O K
Insert Comment	ALT+I M
Insert Symbol	ALT+I S
Spelling and Grammar	F7
Insert Object	ALT+I O
Remove paragraph or character formatting	CTRL+SPACEBAR
Insert Hyperlink	CTRL+K
Macros	ALT+F8
Autocorrect	ALT+T A
Presentation Actions	
Begin Slide Show	F5
Next Slide	ENTER or Down arrow key
Previous Slide	BACKSPACE or Up arrow key
Activate Pen Tool	CTRL+P
Erase Pen Strokes	E
Deactivate Pen Tool	CTRL+A
Show/Hide Black Screen	B
Show/Hide White Screen	W
Show/Hide Pointer and button	A

End slide show	ESC
Insert a Hyperlink	CTRL+K
Custom Animation	ALT+D M
Custom Shows	ALT+D C
Close the Presentation	CTRL+W
Animation Preview	ALT+D E
Preset Animation	ALT+D P
Slide Master View	ALT+V M S
Slide Show View	ALT+V W
Slide Color Scheme	ALT+O C
Start a New Presentation	CTRL+N
Record Narration	ALT+D N
Rehearse Timings	ALT+D R
Repeat the last action	CTRL+Y
Excel Keys	
Insert a new worksheet	SHIFT+F11 or ALT+SHIFT+F1
Rename the current worksheet	ALT+O H R
Move or Copy the current sheet	ALT+E M
Delete the current sheet	ALT+E L
Select the current and next sheet	SHIFT+CTRL+PAGE DOWN
Select the entire column	CTRL+SPACEBAR
Select the entire row	SHIFT+SPACEBAR
Select the entire worksheet	CTRL+A
Select the current region around the active cell	CTRL+SHIFT+*

Select the array containing the active cell	CTRL+/
Select cells that contain formulas that directly refer to the active cell	CTRL+]
Delete the selected cells	CTRL+HYPHEN
Insert blank cells	CTRL+SHIFT+PLUS SIGN
Apply the General number format	CTRL+SHIFT+~
Apply the Percentage format with no decimal places	CTRL+SHIFT+%
Apply the Exponential number format with two decimal places	CTRL+SHIFT+^
Hide the selected rows	CTRL+9
Move the selected field into the row area	ALT+R
In a formula, display the Insert Function dialog box	SHIFT+F3
Insert an AutoSum formula with the SUM function	ALT+=
Copy a formula from the cell above the active cell into the cell or the Formula Bar	CTRL+'
Display the Pivot Table Field dialog box for the selected field.	ALT+L
Create a chart of the data in the current range	F11 or ALT+F1
Inserts a Microsoft Excel macro sheet	CTRL+F11

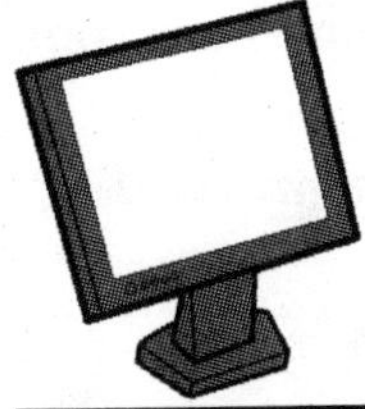

Revision Questions

Introduction to Computers

1. What is a computer? List various applications of computers.
2. How can computers be classified?
3. List and explain important characteristics of a computer.
4. Who is known as the father of computers and why?
5. Distinguish between analog and digital computers.
6. Describe the generations of computer with reference to their electronic components.
7. What are the basic components of a computer system?
8. Draw a block diagram to illustrate the basic organization of a computer system and explain the functions of the various units.
9. Describe the functioning of CPU, Input unit and Output unit.
10. Which component of a computer system executes the program and how?
11. What does MICR stand for? Name the field in which MICR is extensively used.
12. Distinguish between impact and non-impact printers.
13. What is a pointing device? Discuss the functioning of light pen.
14. What is joystick? How is it different from a trackball? Write uses of joystick.
15. When is a bar code reader used for input and how?
16. Differentiate between the characteristics of primary and secondary storage of a computer system.

17. Why are storage devices required? Discuss some common storage devices.
18. List various types of magnetic disks commonly used in today's computer system.
19. What are CD-R, CD-RW and DVD? Write their uses.
20. Why do computers use the binary number systems?
21. Why is binary language often termed as machine language?
22. Discuss the applications of computer technology in pharmaceutical sciences.
23. Convert 243 to binary, octal and hexadecimal forms. (Ans. 111100112, 3638, F316)
24. Convert the numbers-1100112, 111102, 110112 to decimal form. (Ans. 51, 30, 59)
25. Convert the octal numbers-4356028, 526328 to their decimal equivalent. (Ans.146306, 87.6875)
26. Find the binary equivalent of the hexadecimal number-9B.C616 (Ans.10011011.1100011)
27. Draw a flowchart to find the highest mark obtained in the examination given by *n* students.
28. Design algorithm and draw flowchart for exchange of values of two variables.
29. Develop algorithm and draw flowchart to compute the sum of *n* given numbers.
30. Draw a flowchart to find out the lowest common multiple (LCM) of any two given numbers.

Computer Software

1. Differentiate between hardware and software.
2. Hardware and software are like two sides of a coin. Comment.
3. What are various types of operating systems?
4. Classify programming languages with their advantages and disadvantages.

5. Discuss the applications of programming languages with suitable examples.
6. Why are machine and assembly languages often referred to as low-level languages?
7. List the characteristic features of high-level language. Name five high-level languages.
8. Explain how high level language is implemented in a computer?
9. What is the difference between an interpreter and a complier?
10. Distinguish between the functions of compiler and assembler.
11. What do you mean by application software? What are the types of application softwares?
12. Distinguish between application software and system software.
13. What is utility program? List some tasks commonly performed by utility programs.
14. Real-time systems are better than time-sharing systems. Comment on it.
15. Write a short note on the following with their brief history:

    a. COBOL
    b. BASIC
    c. Microsoft Windows
    d. LINUX

Microsoft Windows

1. Describe the salient features of Windows XP.
2. What are the differences between a Notepad and a WordPad in Windows?
3. What are the various options available under Accessories in Windows?
4. What is the use of Recycle bin?
5. What is the role of Windows Explorer in Windows operating system?

6. What is the significance of Task bar?
7. How does Windows Security Center check the status of your computer?
8. What is the role of Firewall and Antivirus software in protecting your computer?

Microsoft Word

1. Enlist the salient features of MS-Word.
2. How many types of toolbars are available in MS-Word? Give brief overview of each toolbar.
3. How can you print a document already saved in MS-Word?
4. What is the advantage of using Print Preview feature in MS-Word?
5. Write a brief account on different types of document views and layouts.
6. What do you mean by formatting of a document?
7. What is word-wrap feature? How is it useful?
8. What are the advantages of find or replace feature of word processor?
9. Give step-wise description of the procedure to check the spelling mistakes in your document.
10. How will you insert Header and Footer in your document?
11. What is a font? List examples of font size and font style.
12. What is the procedure to create WordArt?
13. What is a clipboard? How is it useful?
14. What is data source in context of mail merge?
15. Give advantages of mail merge feature.

Microsoft Excel

1. What is the significance of electronic spreadsheets?
2. Highlight the features of MS-Excel.
3. Write a brief account on basic components of MS-Excel.

4. What are the main uses of Microsoft Excel?
5. What is cell and how it is referred?
6. What do you mean by cell referencing and what are different types of referencing?
7. What is the difference between Save and Save As command?
8. Give the complete process and commands of taking a print graph of graph in Microsoft Excel.
9. Write all steps to prepare a table in Microsoft Excel.
10. Define the term function and reference operators. Write the integral parts of function.
11. Is there any difference between using a formula and using a function for calculation? Explain.
12. Explain different types of functions with examples.
13. How will you perform mathematical calculation using formulae in MS-Excel?
14. Name the various types of graphs which we have in MS-Excel.
15. How will you prepare a chart in MS-Excel?
16. What are different components of charts?
17. Write the steps involved for creating a chart in MS-Excel.

Microsoft PowerPoint

1. What are the various components of a slide? Write their usage.
2. What is the purpose of Autocontent wizard?
3. What is the significance of design template in PowerPoint?
4. What are various views, in which you can open your presentation?
5. How will you insert bullet list in your slide?
6. Which menu and command let you insert animation in your slide?
7. What are action buttons? How can you use them?

8. What is slide layout? Mention some layouts in MS-PowerPoint.
9. You want to insert Clipart in your slide. What is the procedure for doing it?
10. How will you create a custom animation in MS-PowerPoint?
11. Explain various transition effects.
12. What do you mean by Rehearse Timings in presentations? How will you set timings for slides?
13. Write the steps to be followed for adding sound in presentation.
14. Write the steps for inserting and deleting slides.
15. What is the procedure for saving a slide?

Microsoft Access

1. Write the uses of MS-Access. What are Database File, Table, Record, Field and Data-type?
2. Write the steps for creating new and opening existing databases.
3. Enlist database properties. Explain compacting and repairing of a database.
4. Explain different types of action queries.
5. How will you create reports in MS-Access?
6. Write the steps involved to create Mailing Labels for your database.

Introduction to Internet

1. What are different types of networks? Explain.
2. How is LAN different from WAN?
3. What is Internet? Enlist the uses of Internet.
4. Enumerate advantages and disadvantages of Internet.
5. What is protocol? How do protocol affect Internet?
6. What do you mean by e-mail? Write its significance.

7. Internet is a worldwide information network. Comment on it.
8. What is the role of WWW on Internet?
9. HTML is the predominant markup language for web pages. Comment on it.
10. Explain in brief HTML elements, HTML tags and HTML attributes.
11. How will you use Mark-up tags?
12. Enlist commonly used HTML character entities.
13. What are the Form elements? How are forms created for a website?
14. What is a form? What is the function of submit button on a form?
15. How can you set background images in HTML?
16. How will you create and display Table in HTML?
17. What do you mean by framing in HTML? How can you divide a window into frames?
18. Classify website styles. Enlist different types of websites, cite examples.
19. What is a web server? Enlist salient features of web programs.
20. What do you mean by web browser? Explain popular web browsers.
21. What are web search engines? How do they work? Enlist a few important search engines.
22. What is e-commerce? Write an account on advantages of e-commerce.
23. Explain different types of e-commerce with suitable examples.
24. Explain essential Internet tools for e-commerce.
25. Write a brief account on the current scenario and future prospects of e-commerce.
26. What is PubMed? Enlist features and contents of PubMed.

27. Enlist various services provided by PubMed for researchers?
28. What do you mean by the term Patent? Write a brief account on patent databases of different countries and organizations.
29. What are intellectual property rights? Enlist key Internet websites for patent search.

Antivirus Software

1. Define the terms:
   a. Computer virus
   b. Computer worm
   c. Spyware
   d. Trojan horse
   e. Adware
   f. Rootkits
2. What are the signs and symptoms that indicate your computer is infected with viruses?
3. Classify types of viruses with suitable examples.
4. Outline the history of computer viruses and worms.
5. Write in brief characteristics of Trojan horses?
6. How can you protect your computer from malwares?
7. What are antivirus softwares? Give suitable examples. Enlist the important characteristics that antivirus software should possess.
8. **Explain** the principle involved in detection of virus by antivirus program.
9. Explain the concept of firewall. How does it protect computer against intrusions from Internet?

Bioinformatics and eHealth

1. What do you mean by bioinformatics? Enlist major research areas of biotechnology.

2. Bioinformatics is the analysis of biological information using computers and statistical techniques. Comment on it.
3. Classify bioinformatics tools. Write their uses.
4. Enlist examples of bioinformatics software.
5. Write examples of biological databases. Enlist URL of important databases.
6. Write a brief account on applications of bioinformatics.
7. What are electronic health records? State advantages of it.
8. Explain concepts of telemedicine. Enlist its uses.
9. What do you mean by mHealth? Write communication technologies utilized in mHealth.

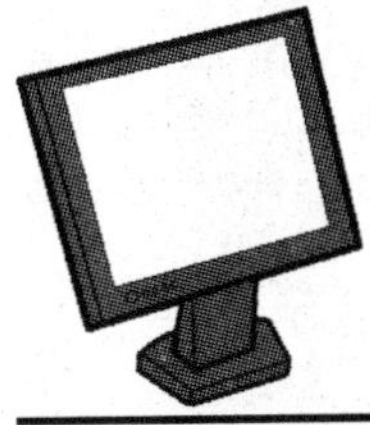

Practical Exercises

1. Write an application to the Principal of your college for grant of permission to attend Indian Pharmaceutical Congress at Ahmedabad. You have to type in MS Word; Font size is 14; font type is Times New Roman.

A Sample Letter

To,
The Principal, Date: 01 Dec., 2009
B.N. College of Pharmacy,
Udaipur.

Sub.: Permission to attend IPC at Ahmedabad.

Respected Sir,
I want to state that this year Indian Pharmaceutical Congress is organized at Ahmedabad and my paper entitled *"Formulation and Evaluation of Colon Targeted Drug Delivery System of Ornidazole"* has been accepted for poster presentation by the scientific committee of IPC.

Therefore, I request you to kindly grant permission to attend IPC, 2009 at Ahmedabad.

Thanking you,
Yours obediently,
Miss. Bindu Goyal
M. Pharm. (Pharmaceutics)-IV Semester

2. Write a letter to the Secretary, Sports Authority of India for getting the information of Sports scholarships to undergraduate students. You have to type the letter in MS Word; font size is 12; font type is Arial.

A Sample Letter

To,

The Secretary, Date: 01 July, 2010

Sports Authority of India,

Delhi.

Sub.: Information regarding Sports Scholarships.

Respected Sir,

I have come to know that Sports Authority of India grants scholarship to those students who show performance in sports activities at national or state level. I have won many inter-state level athletic competitions and I am interested in knowing about the availability of sports scholarships. It will be appreciated if criteria for awarding scholarships to the eligible undergraduate students be sent to our Principal at L.M. College of Pharmacy & Technology, Ahmedabad.

Thanking you,

Yours faithfully,

Vinay Kumar

B. Pharm Part-I,

L.M. College of Pharmacy & Technology, Ahmedabad.

3. Create your Biodata. You have to type in MS Word.

Sample Biodata

Name	: **Mr. Rohit Jain**
Date of Birth	: 16 March, 1984
Father's Name	: Mr. M.P. Jain
Marital Status	: Single
Nationality	: Indian
Permanent Address	: 183, C-Scheme, Jaipur, Rajasthan.
Phone No.	: 2209007
e-mail	: rohit_pharmacy@yahoo.com
Education	: B. Pharm.-IInd year, Sanjeevan College of Pharmacy, Dausa.
Interest	: Reading, Painting and Traveling
Languages Known	: Hindi, English
Extracurricular Activities	: Debate, Basketball, Singing Songs

4. Create a poster inviting staff and students of the college to attend "Farewell Party" of B. Pharm-IV. Type in MS Word, use different tools and insert picture from file or clip art.

Sample Poster

FAREWELL TO B. PHARM.-IV

All the staff members and students are requested to attend 'Farewell Party' of passing out batch of B. Pharm.-IV of our college.

Organized by: B. Pharm.-III Students,
D.K. College of Pharmacy, Jaipur.

Venue: Auditorium, D.K. Campus, Jaipur.

Date: 10 April, 2010 Time: 5:00 pm

5. Create an invitation card for inauguration of Pharmacy Week Celebrations. Type in MS Word.

Sample Card

B.N. COLLEGE OF PHARMACY, UDAIPUR-313 001

Staff and students request your gracious presence on the inauguration of ***PHARMACY WEEK*** on 15 November, 2009 at 11:00 am.

Chief Guest: *Dr. D.S. Rathore,* Ex-Principal, R.N.T. Medical College, Udaipur.

President: *Dr. M.S. Rathore,* Secretary, B.N. Institution.

Guest of Honour: *Dr. T.S. Shaktawat,* M.D., B.N. Institution.

Venue: Kumbha Auditorium, B.N. (PG) College, Udaipur

Dr. M.S. Ranawat	**Dr. Y.S. Tanwar**	**Dr. P.S. Naruka**
Principal	Coordinator	Incharge

6. Your college is organizing an inter-college cricket tournament of pharmacy colleges of Rajasthan. Create a form for registration of the team. Type in MS Word.

Sample Form

M.G. COLLEGE OF PHARMACY, JODHPUR
Inter-College Cricket Tournament
Registration Form

Name of College:

Address of College:

Phone No.:

Name of Coach:

Name of Physiotherapist:

Name of Captain:

Team Members:

1.	2.	3.	4.
5.	6.	7.	8.
9.	10.	11.	12.
13.	14.	15.	16.

Registration Number: .... (leave blank, to be filled by officials).

Signature of coach: **Signature of captain:**

Date:

7. Create a form for admission of candidates to D. Pharm./B. Pharm./M. Pharm. course in your college.

Sample Form

M. A. INSTITUTE OF PHARMACY, JAIPUR
Admission Form
Form No. 25

Name of Student: Paste Photograph

Course: **PPT/GATE Merit List No.:**

Date of Birth: **Sex:** **Nationality:**

Father's/Guardian Name:

Permanent Address:

Phone No.: **e-mail:**

Qualification:

Exam	Board/ university	School/ college	Year of passing	Percentage

Attach attested copies of certificates and mark sheets.

Signature of Candidate *Signature of Parent/Guardian*

Declaration

I hereby declare that I will follow the rules and regulations of Rajasthan University of Health Sciences, Jaipur and the college for the course in which I am admitted.

Signature of Student:

For Office Use

Mr./Miss./Mrs .... s/o or d/o .... is provisionally admitted in the college.

Signature of Principal: *Date:*

8. Prepare a worksheet in MS-Excel based of given data.

List of Students securing First Position Declared by University

Year	*B. Pharm.-I*	*B. Pharm.-II*	*B. Pharm.-III*	*B. Pharm.-IV*
2000	Sandeep Gupta	Deepali Gupta	Sanjay Sharma	Kuldeep Yadav
2001	Ravi Jain	Jagdish Kumar	Motilal Kumawat	Shilpa Sharma
2002	Jagdeep Kumar	Prashant Vyas	Deepa Rathore	Surbhi Singla
2003	Geetangli Bohra	Rakesh Jangid	Manish Mehta	Nitin Tak
2004	Noble Anthony	Prakhil Samar	Jayesh Baghal	Romesh Gaur
2005	Abhishek Jain	Meghna Jain	Ashish Podawar	Gaurav Chaplot
2006	Amit Gosh	Javed Ali	Rakesh Suthar	Anant Nag
2007	Arpan Solanki	Raj Kumar	Piyush Agarwal	Kapil Roy
2008	Rohini Kapoor	Yogesh Jain	Preena Saini	Sunil Negi
2009	Savant Kumar	Kavita Gupta	Mohit Garg	Sumedha Tanwar

9. Prepare a worksheet in MS-Excel based on given data.

Fee Details of Students of M. Pharm.-Ist Semester

Name	*Admission fee (Rs.)*	*Tution fee (Rs.)*	*Library fee*(Rs.)*	*Fine (Rs.)*	*Total fee(Rs.)*
Surbhi Sharma	1,000	10,000		25	
Kapil Sharma	1,000	10,000		-	
Bhavni S. Hada	1,000	10,000		25	
Mohit Jain	1,000	10,000		50	
Sachin Sharma	1,000	10,000		-	
Priyanka Chauhan	1,000	10,000		-	
Piyush Agarwal	1,000	10,000		75	
Nalini Sharma	1,000	10,000		-	

*Library fee= 0.01% of Tuition fee.

Calculate the following using formula in MS-Excel:

1. Calculate library fee as 0.01% of tuition fee for all students.
2. Calculate total fee as a sum of Admission fee + Tuition fee + Library fee + Fine.

10. Prepare a worksheet in MS-Excel based on given data.

Compilation of Result of B. Pharm.-IV Examination, 2009

Roll no.	*Student name*	*P'ceutics (100)*	*Biotech. (100)*	*P'Chem. (100)*	*Total (300)*	*Percentage*	*Rank*
1001	Sandeep Mehta	75	53	73			
1002	Ravi Jain	62	59	67			
1003	Jagdeep Kumar	87	50	71			
1004	Neha Joshi	50	65	52			
1005	Ramesh	71	71	82			
1006	Abhishek Jain	60	62	75			
1007	Amit Gosh	54	52	69			
1008	Arpan Solanki	59	70	73			
1009	Nalini Goyal	77	51	80			
1010	Savant Kumar	67	61	56			

Calculate the following using formulae in MS-Excel:

1. Calculate the total marks as sum of marks P'ceutics + Biotech. + P'chem.
2. Calculate percentage of all students.
3. Calculate rank of students.

11. Calculate the following using functions of MS-Excel:

Number	*Log_{10}*	*Tan*	*SQRT*	*Cos^{-1}*	*Degrees*	*Cos*
9021						
1110.24						
137.81						
1445.9						
15999.01						
16575						
7777						
459.78						
23678						
250.71						

12. Open a new worksheet and type the data given below. Calculate total sales of pharmaceutical products done by different wholesalers in Jaipur region. Prepare a bar chart from the given data.

Apex Pharmaceuticals Ltd., Delhi			
Area- Rajasthan	*Region-Jaipur*		*Year-2008-09*
Month	*Wholesaler A (Rs.)*	*Wholesaler B (Rs.)*	*Wholesaler C (Rs.)*
January	10005559	33225751	17515949
February	11198564	12908654	9990751
March	29876549	12097753	55410076
April	19832400	22245081	21000870
May	2098123	10564308	11111789
June	15611001	9900178	10532987
July	3210087	11118730	32190870
August	45000012	32009841	17531000
September	78099942	9098521	20564321
October	10000458	27051879	11176523
November	58321045	32109843	21009854
December	34577809	21098340	25719530

13. Salbutamol sulphate was dissolved in phosphate buffer pH 7.4 and different diluted solutions were prepared and analyzed by U.V. spectrophotometer at 274 nm. The absorbance of different solutions is given below. In MS-Excel plot a curve between concentration and absorbance; add trend line to display equation of line and R^2 value.

Concentration (mcg/ml)	*Absorbance (274 nm)*
1.00	0.098
2.00	0.182
3.00	0.265
4.00	0.354
5.00	0.443
6.00	0.524
7.00	0.620
8.00	0.705
9.00	0.793
10.00	0.906

14. Dissolution study of marketed tablets of Diclofenac Sodium was performed and the percent drug released at different time intervals is given below. Type the data in a new worksheet in MS-Excel, create formula to calculate percent drug retained (by subtracting the given data from 100) and then perform T-test on drug release data of different brands to determine whether the data is statistically significant or not. Plot the following graphs in XY-scatter type:

i. *Zero-order plots:* Cumulative % Drug Released versus Time
ii. *First-order plots:* Log % Drug Retained versus Time
iii. *Higuchi plots:* Cumulative % Drug Release versus Square Root of Time.

Dissolution Study of Diclofenac Sodium Tablets

Time (min.)	*Cumulative Drug Release (%)*		
	Brand-A	*Brand-B*	*Brand-C*
0	0.004	0.000	0.001
10	11.651	15.095	29.075
20	20.912	31.986	45.071
30	32.8743	45.091	60.230
40	40.159	51.753	72.257
50	55.791	68.210	84.655
60	66.043	70.912	91.240

15. Prepare two slides in PowerPoint based on the following information. Set timings for each slide 5 seconds. Use tools to make your presentation more effective.

Slide 1: Dayanand Hospital, Sector-23, Chandigarh
Slide 2: FACILITIES AVAILABLE

- Ambulance Facility (24 hours)
- Medical and Emergency Facilities
- Pharmacy
- Special Trauma Center
- Alcohol and Drug De-addiction Center
- Health Insurance

16. You are studying in a famous Pharmacy College of Rajasthan. Prepare a presentation in PowerPoint, which shows the salient features of your college.

Slide 1: S.K. College of Pharmacy, Ajmer-305 001 (Rajasthan)

Courses Offered:

- M. Pharm.-Pharmaceutics, Pharmacognosy
- B. Pharm.
- D. Pharm.

Slide 2: *Salient Features:*

- Affiliated to Rajasthan University of Health Sciences, Jaipur.
- One of the oldest college of Rajasthan.
- 20 Faculty Members.
- State-of-the-art Laboratories
- Library with 2000 Books, 05 International Journals Subscribed
- Internet Facility
- Sports and Games Facilities
- Separate Hostel for Boys and Girls

Slide 3:

Result for Academic Session 2008-09

Class	*No. of students*	*No. of merit*	*Ist division*	*IInd division*
M. Pharm.	20	02	20	--
B. Pharm.-I	60	07	41	25
B. Pharm.-II	60	01	52	08
B. Pharm.-III	60	04	45	12
B. Pharm.-IV	59	06	49	10
D. Pharm.-I	60	01	35	20
D. Pharm.-II	59	09	29	28

17. Prepare a PowerPoint presentation on "Applications of Computers in Pharmacy". For preparing these slides you can select any layout of your choice. Set timings and effects to show the slide attractive.

18. Draw the following in Paint.

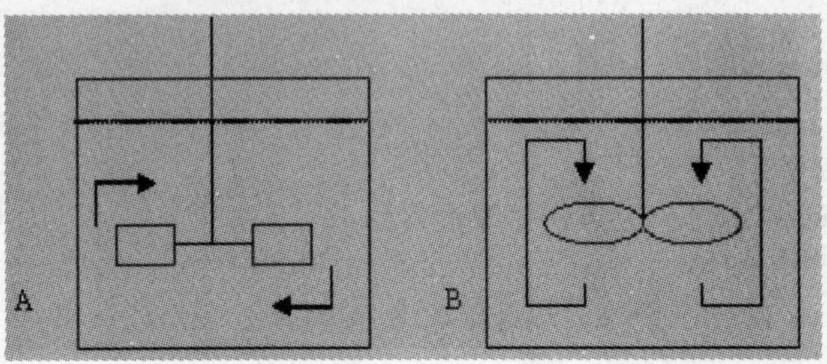

19. Draw the following in Paint.

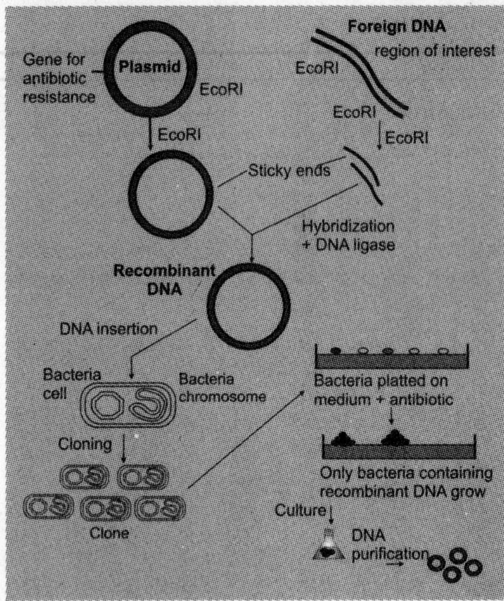

20. Type the names of teaching and non-teaching members of your college in WordPad. Font size is 14; font type is Arial.

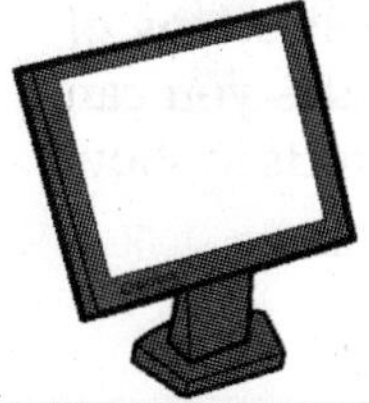

References

1. David William Barron, *Assemblers and Loaders*. Elsevier, 1972.
2. Dean J.M, Booth F.V.M.L. *Microcomputers in Critical Care: A Practical Approach,* Lippincott Williams and Wilkins, 1985
3. Dong, Jennifer Q.; Chen, Bin; Gibbs, Megan A.; Emery, Maurice; Gibbs, John P. *Current Computer-Aided Drug Design.* Volume 4, Bentham Science Publishers, 2008.
4. Ekins S. *Computer Applications in Pharmaceutical Research and Development,* Wiley-Interscience, 2006.
5. Elmasri E., Navathe S.B. *Fundamentals of Database Systems,* Addison Wesley Longman, 2000.
6. Fraade D.J. *Automation of Pharmaceutical Operations,* Aster Pub Corp., 1983.
7. Jain M. *Input Output,* Part-VI, Pragya Prakashan.
8. Jain S. *Introduction to Computer Science,* Vol. I and II, B.P.B. Publications, 1998.
9. Jain S. *O-Level Made Simple (Information Technology),* B.P.B. Publications, 1999.
10. Misener S., Krawetz SA. *Methods in Molecular Biology: Bioinformatics Methods and Protocols,* Humana Press, 2001.
11. Mollah S.A. *Numerical Analysis and Computational Procedures,* Books & Allied (P) Ltd., 2008.
12. Saunders' R. Fleming. *Mathematics and Statistics for Use in Pharmacy, Biology and Chemistry,* Pharmaceutical Press, 1966.
13. Sharma P. *Introduction to Web Technology,* S.K. Kataria & Sons, 2007.
14. Shortliffe E.H., Blois M.S. *Medical Informatics: Computer Applications in Health Care,* Springer, 2001.
15. Sinha P.K., Sinha P. *Computer Fundamentals—Concept, Systems & Applications,* B.P.B. Publications, 2007.

16. Tanenbaum A. *Computer Networks,* Prentice Hall PTR, 1996.

17. Wagner J.G. *Fundamentals of Clinical Pharmacokinetics,* Drug Intelligence Publications, 1975.

18. Wille C. *Presenting C#,* Macmillan Computer Publishing, 2000.

19. www.microsoft.com

20. www.nebi.nlm.nih.gov/**pubmed**/

21. http://en.wikipedia.org/wiki

22. www.**patent**office.nic.in/

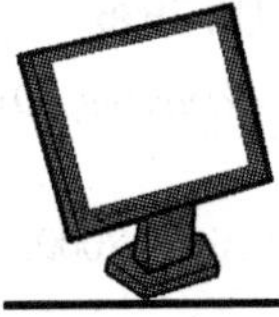

Index

Reader's Notes

Reader's Notes

Reader's Notes

Reader's Notes